The Magnesium Factor

The Magnesium Factor

Mildred S. Seelig, M.D., MPH
Andrea Rosanoff, Ph.D.

Avery
a member of
Penguin Group (USA) Inc.
New York

Every effort has been made to ensure that the information contained in this book is complete and accurate. However, neither the publisher nor the authors are engaged in rendering professional advice or services to the individual reader. The ideas, procedures, and suggestions contained in this book are not intended as a substitute for consulting with your physician. All matters regarding your physical health require medical supervision. Neither the authors nor the publisher shall be liable or responsible for any loss, injury, or damage allegedly arising from any information or suggestion in this book. The opinions expressed in this book represent the personal views of the authors and not of the publisher.

While the authors have made every effort to provide accurate telephone numbers and Internet addresses at the time of publication, neither the publisher nor the authors assume any responsibility for errors, or for changes that occur after publication.

Most Avery books are available at special quantity discounts for bulk purchase for sales promotions, premiums, fund-raising, and educational needs. Special books or book excerpts also can be created to fit specific needs. For details, write Penguin Group (USA) Inc. Special Markets, 375 Hudson Street, New York, NY 10014.

a member of
Penguin Group (USA) Inc.
375 Hudson Street
New York, NY 10014
www.penguin.com

Published simultaneously in Canada

Library of Congress Cataloging-in-Publication Data

Seelig, Mildred S., date.
The magnesium factor / Mildred S. Seelig, Andrea Rosanoff.
p. cm.
Includes bibliographical references and index.
ISBN 1-58333-156-5
1. Magnesium deficiency diseases—Popular works. 2. Magnesium in the body—Popular works. I. Rosanoff, Andrea. II. Title.
RC627.M3S434 2003 2003045337
616.3'96—dc21

Printed in the United States of America
10 9 8 7 6 5 4 3 2 1

Acknowledgments

There are so many people who helped make this book possible. Family, friends, agents, and editors all came together to encourage, suggest, and help from the earliest to the final stages of this project. We especially want to thank two people who read (and re-read) the manuscript for us: Dr. Charles Boris Seelig carefully surveyed most of the manuscript for medical accuracy, and Mr. Steve Sparks helped us make sure that in achieving medical accuracy we still had a readable book for readers not trained in medicine. Amy Tecklenburg, our publisher's editor, was most helpful in suggesting changes that improved the book as well as calling to our attention expressions that needed clarification.

Dennis Hibbert was kind and professional, a combination always well received, in surveying cities' water companies for us, and Kellie Chang found even the most elusive journal articles with a competence rarely seen. To these, and all the others who contributed to the production of this book, we offer our gratitude.

But most of all we wish to thank all those researchers and their many helpers who have studied magnesium over the years. In this book, we have described *some* of their results, for to present it all would take volumes. It is to these researchers that this book is dedicated.

M. S. Seelig, M.D., MPH
A. Rosanoff, Ph.D.

Dr. Rosanoff would also like to thank Nancy Rosanoff, Andy Washburn, and Karl Slinkard for their generous acts that significantly facilitated the writing of this book.

Contents

1

Magnesium: The Mineral That Combats Heart Disease and Keeps Blood Vessels Healthy

We know the scene—its inherent drama puts it into screenplay after screenplay: The patient is surrounded by hustling figures in masks and gowns. The doctor, holding two defibrillator pads, one in each hand, calls "Clear!" The pads are on the patient's chest and then *thud.* The patient jolts.

We all know what's happening. A human heart has stopped beating. If the treatment works, the heart will start beating. Life! If the monitor shows a straight line, it means death. All other health issues are suddenly put aside. The gowned figures around the patient wait. The anticipation is intense. No beats. They repeat the heroic procedure—"Clear!" and the patient jolts again.

Of the more than half-million Americans who will die this year from heart disease, many don't have to die.

Of the millions taking expensive medications—some of which have potentially serious side effects—to treat conditions that increase the risk of heart disease, many could be just as healthy taking lower doses—or not taking them at all.

Of the millions struggling with no-fat, low-fat, high-fat, low-salt decisions, and feeling guilty when they regularly miss the mark, many could keep their hearts and blood vessels healthy *without* all this dieting stress.

The solution to heart disease has been with us all along, and it is nutritional. Most modern heart disease is caused by magnesium deficiency. A vast and convincing body of research, largely ignored, has convinced us and many of our colleagues of this fact. The diet of the industrial world is short on magnesium, and this is causing an epidemic of heart disease in the modern world.

How can we say this? These are bold claims. Is there real evidence? Evidence from placebo-controlled, double-blind research studies—the highest standard for medical research? The answer is a resounding *yes!* We hope the evidence in this book will help you to decide for yourself whether, and how, taking supplemental magnesium may help you, your family, and your friends.

A Typical Story

Jack's experience is typical of present-day heart treatment. In his forties, he had a pain in his chest strong enough to send him to the emergency room. Suddenly he was surrounded by doctors and medical technology of the most advanced kind, and when he came out, alive and grateful, he was taking a diuretic for high blood pressure, a statin drug for high cholesterol, and a beta-blocker for angina pain. He tried to lower his intake of fat and salt, as prescribed, but it was too difficult; he couldn't stick to it. Jack's goal of exercising three times each week brought guilt as often as joy and exhilaration. His doctor was encouraged by the fact that Jack's cholesterol level and blood pressure went down, and urged Jack to keep up the medications. But Jack felt tired all the time. He had muscle aches and even became impotent. And the pains he felt in his chest area were just getting worse. He often felt depressed, probably because he didn't feel he could function fully in an otherwise happy life.

A trained chemist, Jack went to the research journals for information on his plight. His reading gave him the idea that magnesium supplements could help, so he started taking over-the-counter magnesium tablets with his meals. Within days the aches and pains in his legs lessened, and within five months the chest pains were almost gone. On his own he stopped taking the beta-blocker. On his doctor's advice, he started taking it again, even though the chest pains had begun subsiding without the drug. Because his blood pressure had come down, his doctor allowed him to cut back on the diuretic. He couldn't believe how much better he felt. In fact, Jack found it hard to believe that simply taking magnesium pills could make such a difference. So he stopped taking them. Within two months his lethargy was back, along with rising blood pressure, aches and pains in his legs, and some pain in his chest. Convinced, Jack again started taking the magnesium supplements, and once again his health and feeling of well-being began to return. After a year he felt great and was able to stop all of the prescribed medications—even the statin. Now he fully felt that his life had been saved.

Could such a simple remedy eliminate so many signs and symptoms of heart damage? Signs and symptoms that warn of developing abnormalities in blood vessels and signal a danger of long-term, life-threatening heart disease? And better yet, might magnesium supplements safely prevent heart disease? What is the evidence that the entire complex of risk factors for heart disease can be forestalled by one simple but essential nutrient?

Heart Disease—A Twentieth-Century Epidemic

Before 1900 and into the 1930s, heart disease had no medical specialty. None seemed required. Even as late as 1925 to 1935, there was little interest in cardiology and little of it was taught in medical schools. Few realized that an age of heart disease was about to dawn.

By the late 1940s, doctors were calling for more active programs in heart disease because "it seemed to be greatly increasing in occurrence and severity." And it was true. From 1900 to the 1970s, deaths due to heart disease rose steadily (see figure 1.1). Increased longevity could account for some of the rise, but far from all of it. Heart disease is more common in older adults but, more and more, it is showing up in younger people—even in infants. Deaths from heart disease soared from less than 30,000 in 1900 to more than 700,000 in 1970. Since then, the death rate from heart disease has remained rather steady at this high level, while the medical specialty of cardiology has become a major field of medicine. Surgery can now reopen or replace blocked arteries, repair heart valves, and even replace whole hearts. Medications for arrhythmias (irregular heartbeat) and several other risk factors for heart disease, such as high blood pressure, have been developed and are widely used. These medical innovations have saved countless lives, but some have serious side effects. And despite them, the incidence of heart disease has not lessened. Indeed, it continues to increase—as the processed-food–based diet of the industrialized world spreads.

Diet and Magnesium Deficiency

As the heart disease epidemic of the twentieth century was growing, so was the reliance on modern processed foods. There are many things wrong with such a diet. It is high in fat, especially saturated fat; high in cholesterol; and high in sugar and salt, among other things. But not emphasized in the training of many doctors—nor even in that of many nutritionists and dieticians—is that such a diet is low in magnesium. And hearts and blood vessels need magnesium to stay healthy.

The fact is that magnesium deficiency underlies much of the heart disease epidemic that consumes so many of our health-care dollars. Studies have linked low magnesium with many of the major risk factors for heart disease. Other studies show that the average Western processed-food diet is lower in magnesium than is

A processed food diet is often low in magnesium.

Figure 1.1 Change in the Incidence of Heart Disease and Average Intake of Magnesium Contrasted

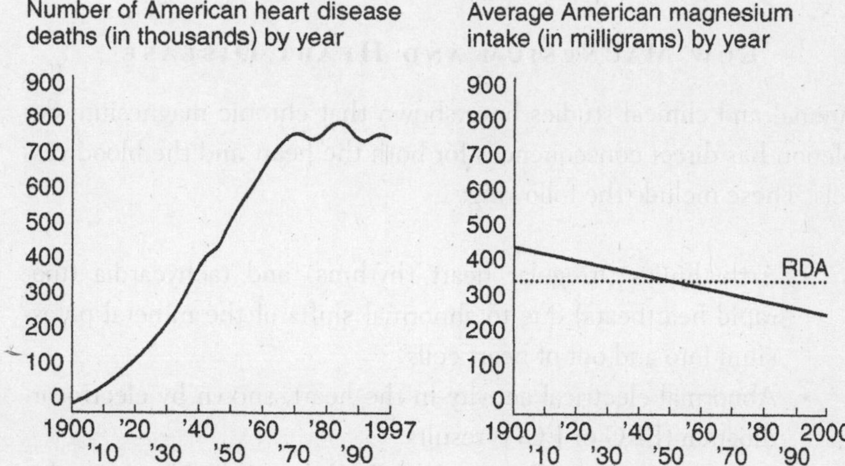

The graph at left illustrates how the frequency of heart disease has gone up since 1900; the graph at right shows the decline in average magnesium consumption during the same period.

Sources: U.S. Centers for Disease Control and Prevention, National Center for Health Statistics, and the American Heart Association, 2000 Heart and Stroke Statistical Update (Dallas, TX: American Heart Association, 1999). © 2003, Copyright American Heart Association. Reproduced with permission; J. R. Marier, "Quantitative Factors Regarding Magnesium Status in the Modern-Day World," *Magnesium 1* (1982): 3–15.

commonly acknowledged. While several essential nutrients are imperative for heart and blood vessel health, the vast research on low magnesium and its impact on heart health has gone unheeded, so much so that much of the heart disease seen today is a direct result of low magnesium consumption. This vitally important nutrient is inadequate in much of our processed foods and water supplies, just when our stressful lifestyle demands that we have more. The effects of a low intake of magnesium can be worsened by the high levels of fat, sugar, sodium, and phosphate in our diets as well as, ironically, by the use of calcium supplements, which has become widespread because of our awareness of calcium's value for bone health.

Let's look at some of the evidence that magnesium deficiency can cause heart disease.

Low Magnesium and Heart Disease

Animal and clinical studies have shown that chronic magnesium depletion has direct consequences for both the heart and the blood vessels. These include the following:

- Arrhythmias (irregular heart rhythms) and tachycardia (too-rapid heartbeats) due to abnormal shifts of the mineral potassium into and out of heart cells.
- Abnormal electrical activity in the heart, shown by electrocardiogram (EKG or ECG) results.
- Arteriosclerosis (stiffening and inflexibility of the blood vessels). This can develop even in children.
- Constriction of the arteries and spasms in blood vessels.
- High blood pressure.
- Angina (chest pain due to heart disease).
- Myocardial infarction (damage to heart cells—better known as a heart attack) due to ischemic heart disease (an insufficient flow of oxygenated blood to the heart) that is associated with too much calcium and not enough magnesium in heart cells.
- Sudden death due to arrhythmia or infarction.
- The formation of blood clots within blood vessels, which can lead to heart attack or stroke.
- Heart valve disorders such as mitral valve prolapse.

The medical profession has responded to this myriad of symptoms by treating each symptom individually, with drugs or surgery or both (see table 1.1). The result is high-tech, expensive chasing after symptoms that may stave off death but does not restore health. How much better it would be to prevent much of the damage from this disease by treating the magnesium deficiency that underlies all of its symptoms, giving the body the simple nutrient it needs for

Hearts and blood vessels need magnesium.

Table 1.1 Symptoms Associated with Heart Disease That Can Be Brought on by Magnesium Deficiency—and Common Medical Treatments for Them

Magnesium deficiency causes:	. . . which is typically treated with
Arrhythmias	Anti-arrhythmic drugs (quindine, procainamide)
Calcium entry into cells	Calcium-channel blockers
Overreactivity to stress hormones (adrenaline)	Beta-blockers, alpha-blockers
Overproduction of cholesterol	Low-fat diets, statin drugs
Blood clotting in blood vessels	Anticoagulation agents
Constriction of arterial muscles	Antihypertensive drugs, vasodilators
High sodium-to-potassium ratio	Low-salt diet, antihypertensive drugs
Insulin resistance	Blood-sugar-lowering drugs
Coronary arteriosclerosis	Angioplasty, bypass surgery
Vulnerability to oxidative stress	Antioxidants (vitamins, drugs)

healthy hearts and blood vessels. Animal studies show that low magnesium levels adversely affect the heart and blood vessels. Clinical studies show that treatment with magnesium, taken at the right time and in the right amount, can lessen heart disease risk factors and even save lives. Might adequate magnesium nutrition lessen the need for heroic surgeries? Might it lessen the need for, or even replace, medications, with their high cost and possible adverse side effects? Drug and surgical therapies could then be reserved for people with heart disease for whom adequate magnesium nutrition is not enough.

Additional Evidence

We know that there are connections between low magnesium consumption and the major risk factors for heart disease. In addition, research has found that there are very low levels of magnesium in the heart muscle of people who have died of heart disease. In one study, the hearts of such individuals had 24 percent less magnesium than did the hearts of people who had died in accidents. Other studies have been performed on cadaver hearts classified by cause of death—death due to heart disease versus death from other causes, usually accidents. The "heart-disease" hearts had anywhere from 12 to 27 percent less magnesium than the "other causes of death" hearts. What's more, damaged areas of hearts from people who had died of heart disease had 40 to 50 percent less magnesium than undamaged areas of the same hearts.

Another interesting finding is that cadaver hearts from people who had lived in areas with hard drinking water (water that contains relatively high levels of dissolved minerals) had higher amounts of magnesium in them—6 or 7 percent higher, on average, than cadaver hearts from soft-water areas. Maybe this is why death rates from heart disease are lower in hard-water communities. Although early nutritional studies in animals proved magnesium to be vital to both hearts and blood vessels, this knowledge was not linked to the rising level of human heart disease seen in the first half of the twentieth century. In the late 1950s, some epidemiological studies (research on populations) pointed to the association.

In 1957, an important Japanese study showed that when hardness of drinking water went up, the rate of death from cardiovascular disease went down. Then more studies from other parts of the world showed the same trend; there was something about hard water that protected people from heart disease death. Whether in South Africa, Greenland, Finland, England, Wales, Canada, Australia, or the United States, cardiovascular and overall death rates were found to be lower in hard-water areas than in soft-water areas. (See figure 1.2.)

Further evidence for this water factor came with a study of British towns observed between 1951 and 1961, a time of rising cardiovascular disease. The towns whose water supply became softer during that decade experienced a 20 percent rise in heart disease death rates, while towns with no change in water hardness showed a rise of only 11 percent in such deaths. Towns whose water supply became harder had only an 8 percent rise in heart-disease deaths.

There was something about soft water that went with higher rates of heart disease death. Coming as it did at the peak of the rise in heart

Figure 1.2 Comparison of Heart Disease Death Rates in Hard-, Average-, and Soft-Water Areas

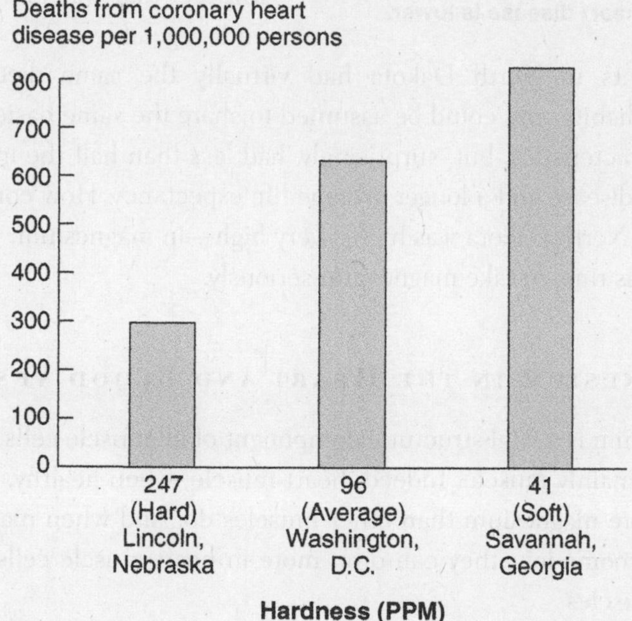

The graph above represents the number of deaths from ischemic heart disease among white men aged forty-five to sixty-four years in American cities with the hardest, average, and softest water.

disease, this information was very intriguing, and medical scientists and doctors naturally wondered what it was in hard water that was protective, or what was it about soft water that was dangerous to hearts. Research soon showed that the protective water factor, in most cases, was magnesium. Calcium, another hard water component, also can be protective because it makes water less corrosive and less likely to leach toxic trace minerals, such as cadmium and lead, out of metal pipes. Calcium shares its direct effect—interfering with the absorption of fat from the intestines—with magnesium.

Hard water's protective effect is illustrated by the case of Finnish immigrants living in North Dakota. Finland, at the time of the study (the early 1960s), had a very high rate of heart disease—one of the highest in the world. The Finns also had high levels of tobacco and alcohol use,

In areas where drinking water is high in magnesium, the death rate due to heart disease is lower.

plus a high-saturated-fat, high-protein, high-calcium, high-salt diet that was low in fruits and vegetables. The Finnish immigrants in North Dakota had virtually the same dietary and lifestyle habits, and could be assumed to share the same basic hereditary characteristics, but, surprisingly, had less than half the incidence of heart disease and a longer average life expectancy. How come? The water in North Dakota was high—very high—in magnesium.

It was time to take magnesium seriously.

Magnesium in the Heart and Blood Vessels

Magnesium is a vital structural component of all muscle cells, and the heart is mainly muscle. Indeed, heart muscle, when healthy, contains even more magnesium than other muscles do. And when magnesium levels become low, they can drop more in heart muscle cells than in other muscles.

Each molecule of myosin (muscle protein) has an atom of magnesium in it. Muscles therefore have to have magnesium to work. About 27 percent of the body's magnesium is in muscle tissue, including the small muscle cells that make blood vessels contract or relax as blood, driven by the heart muscle's pumping, flows through them. If a magnesium deficiency begins to affect the heart's muscle cells and the "nervous conduction system" of the heart, this organ, which must beat regularly and continuously, may run into trouble. The availability of magnesium within the heart affects the rhythm of the heart both directly and indirectly by controlling potassium and calcium levels. This also affects the conduction system. A low level of magnesium in the heart muscle cells can bring on heart arrhythmias ranging from the merely disturbing, such as palpitations, to the severe, including disturbances that can be life-threatening.

Blood vessel muscle cells need healthy amounts of magnesium to relax properly after each contraction. They can become stiff and inflexible if their magnesium gets too low.

Magnesium in Enzymes

Early in 2002, a pharmaceutical ad on television stated that each human being has thousands of enzymes, and that their proper function is needed for health. This is true. Enzymes are what make the body's chemical reactions take place at the proper times, at the proper speed, and in the proper amounts.

Any biochemistry student can tell you that including Mg^{++} (the symbol for magnesium ion—magnesium in its electrically charged form) in a reaction has a good chance of giving you the right answer to test questions. That is because magnesium is a necessary catalyst for all sorts of life reactions. Among the enzymes that have been studied intensively, over 350 need magnesium, directly, to do their jobs properly. For the sake of comparison, the mineral zinc, for example, is required for about 200 enzymes; copper, for less than 20; and selenium, for 10 that have been identified in animal studies so far. To mention just a few, magnesium is directly necessary to the enzymes that break down glucose (blood sugar), control the production of cholesterol, make nucleic acids such as DNA, make proteins (all enzymes are proteins), and break down fats. Importantly, magnesium is necessary to the enzymes that keep potassium inside cells—including those of the cardiovascular system—where it is necessary for cellular activity, and to keep sodium outside the cells, thereby preventing edema or swelling. Without adequate magnesium, these enzymes either will not act or will act at the wrong rate or at the wrong time—or both.

In addition to the more than 350 enzymes for which magnesium is directly necessary, it is indirectly required for thousands of others. One especially important reaction that needs magnesium is the one that controls the molecule adenosine triphosphate, or ATP. ATP is present in all the living world. You can think of it as life's batteries—a substance that can store and release energy back and forth, like a switch. (See figure 1.3). But to do so, it needs magnesium. Literally every energy-consuming reaction in life involves ATP and thus needs magnesium to proceed. This is what puts the number of enzymes that need magnesium into the thousands. (For one illustration, see "HMG-CoA Reductase" on page 13.)

Figure 1.3 ATP and Magnesium: The Batteries of Life

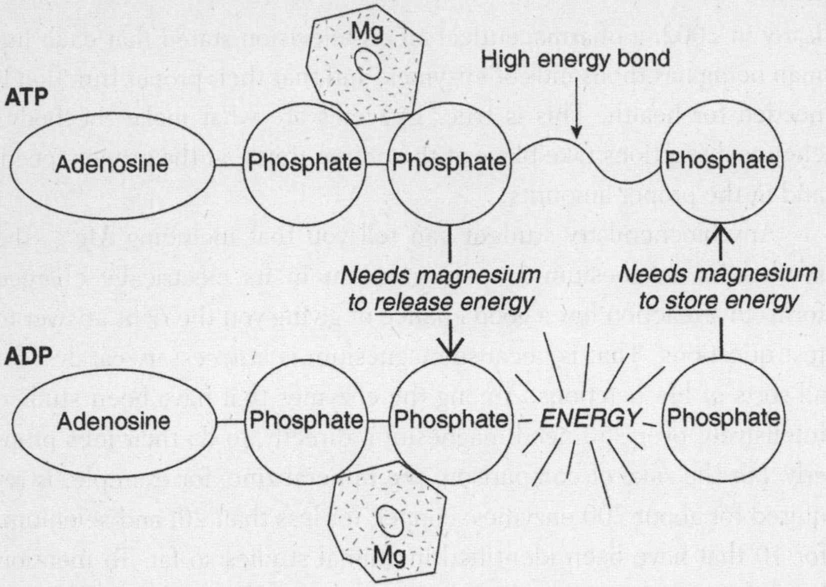

The drawing above represents how magnesium and ATP work together to produce cellular energy. ATP enters into a reaction involving magnesium that releases energy while forming a related compound, adenosine diphosphate (ADP). Another magnesium-related reaction converts ADP back into ATP, storing energy.

It would be hard to overestimate magnesium's importance in enzyme function, both directly, as a cofactor, and indirectly via ATP reactions.

Muscle contraction requires energy, and thus requires ATP and magnesium. The pumping heart is a muscle that alternately contracts and relaxes. The contracting and dilating of blood vessels are due to muscles contracting and relaxing. All of this activity requires magnesium, both directly and indirectly through ATP. No wonder low magnesium can affect the heart and its blood vessels.

Magnesium in the Cells

In addition to all of its enzyme functions, magnesium is an important component of cell membranes. As a result, it is vitally important in reg-

HMG-CoA Reductase

An important example of an enzyme that needs magnesium-activated ATP is the enzyme that controls cholesterol synthesis. There are several enzymes necessary for the body to make cholesterol, but one in particular, known as 3-hydroxy-3-methylglutaryl coenzyme A reductase—or HMG-CoA reductase—seems to regulate how much cholesterol is made by turning the whole sequence leading to cholesterol synthesis on or off. When this enzyme is turned on, cholesterol is produced. When it is turned off, cholesterol production is stopped.

You may think, "Well, cholesterol is bad, so let's just turn this enzyme off." Actually, this is what the class of drugs known as statins do. However, no normally occurring enzyme is all bad. The body needs cholesterol, and this enzyme has the important function of making sure that it is made in the proper amounts for the body's health. Like the enzyme, not all cholesterol is bad. Some cholesterol becomes part of important hormones such as testosterone and estrogen—certainly hormones that are needed. (The beneficial and harmful aspects of cholesterol will be discussed in detail in chapter 5.) No one wants to turn off the production of these hormones in their proper, healthful amounts. So turning off cholesterol production has some consequences. Rather than inhibiting this important enzyme, it is better to regulate its function, allowing it to continue producing needed amounts of cholesterol, but not too much. Magnesium, by activating ATP, has just such an effect on this enzyme. If proper amounts of magnesium are present, HMG-CoA reductase can easily be turned off. If magnesium is in short supply, however, this enzyme can be turned on, and its regulation becomes faulty. So the amount of magnesium present is one determinant of whether or not cholesterol is produced. If not enough magnesium is available for this important function, one result is that HMG-CoA reductase is turned on all the time and too much cholesterol is produced.

ulating what goes into and what comes out of all the body's cells. This makes magnesium crucial to mineral balance.

In simple solutions, such as salt water, all dissolved minerals are evenly dispersed. This is not so in living cells, where they are distributed differently, depending on their functions. This specialized distribution requires energy and is vital to life processes and health. Calcium and sodium ions, for the most part, are kept outside cells, while magnesium and potassium are kept inside cells. These four minerals are the most plentiful in the body, and collectively they are known as electrolytes. Magnesium is crucial to their specialized distribution.

If the level of magnesium within cells falls below normal, calcium and sodium rush inside, while potassium and magnesium leak out. This can cause big problems. If this occurs in heart muscle cells, normal function is impaired, and there is a tendency toward excess contractility. During cardiac surgery, this can cause what doctors call a "stone heart." In the arteries, this phenomenon can lead to stiffness and high blood pressure. Drastic results, indeed. Doctors routinely prescribe calcium-channel–blocking drugs to forestall this abnormal movement of calcium into cells because it is so dangerous for hearts and blood vessels. Magnesium is nature's calcium-channel blocker.

Magnesium and Calcium: A Delicate Balance

Magnesium and calcium are very similar in their chemistry, but biologically, these two elements function and react very differently. In effect, they are two sides of a physiological coin; they have actions that oppose one another, yet they function as a team. For example:

- Calcium exists mainly outside of cells, whereas almost all magnesium is found inside cells.
- Calcium excites nerves, whereas magnesium calms them down.
- Calcium (with potassium) is necessary for muscle contraction, whereas magnesium is necessary for muscles to relax.
- Calcium is necessary for the blood-clotting reaction, which is so necessary for wound healing, whereas magnesium keeps the blood flowing freely and prevents abnormal coagulation within blood vessels, where clotting reactions would be dangerous.

- Calcium is mostly found in bones and gives them much of their hardness, whereas magnesium is found mainly in soft structures. Bone matrix, the soft structure within bone, contains protein and magnesium, and gives the bones some flexibility and resistance to brittleness.

The normal concentration of magnesium ion inside cells is easily 10,000 times that of intracellular calcium ions—under healthy conditions. But if the amount of magnesium in a cell falls, for any reason, calcium ions flow into the cell. With this abnormal situation, a couple of things happen:

1. Higher than normal calcium inside a cell excites a lot of reactions. It puts the cell into a hyperactive state. Heart and blood-vessel cells are especially excitable because they need to react rapidly during sudden stress situations. As such, they are truly vulnerable to deficits in magnesium that allow abnormal rises in calcium, with resulting hyperactivity.

   Sometimes, a hyperactive state is just what you want. It is the essence of the body's fight-or-flight reaction to danger. For example, when in danger, the body needs muscles to contract rapidly and strongly so that one can fight or flee. The cells need to have calcium rush inside, get things excited, and, together with several other substances, make muscles contract. Without calcium, there is no muscle contraction, and without muscle contraction there is no fight or flight.

   But in usual circumstances, you do not want excess muscle contractions. The muscles would soon cramp, bringing on severe muscle pain. To relax, the muscles need magnesium. Magnesium, physiologically the opposite of calcium, relaxes muscles. Under normal, healthy cellular conditions, magnesium levels inside muscle cells are high and calcium levels are low, so that the muscles can relax. This is just one way in which calcium enhances and allows the fight-or-flight reaction while magnesium calms it all down. (For a quick sum-

A body needs a healthy magnesium status to properly utilize calcium.

Table 1.2 Opposing Effects of Magnesium and Calcium in the Fight-or-Flight Response

Function	Magnesium's influence	Calcium's influence
Muscle tension	Promotes relaxation	Promotes contraction
Blood cell clumping	Discourages	Encourages
Blood clotting	Discourages	Encourages
Nerve excitation	Discourages	Enhances
Adrenaline response	Downplays	Enhances

mary of the opposing effects of magnesium and calcium in the so-called fight-or-flight reaction—the physiological response to stress—see table 1.2.)

2. If calcium levels inside a cell get especially high because of low magnesium, the cell physically changes. High calcium tends to make things stiff and hard. But if soft tissue begins to get hard, it is a problem—the problem of *calcification*. In artery and heart cells, the stiffness caused by calcification hampers proper function and can be an important aspect of heart disease.

Figure 1.4 shows the ischemic heart disease rates, plotted against the calcium/magnesium intake ratios, of different countries. If magnesium intake is low, a high calcium intake can make people more vulnerable to heart disease than are people who do not have a high calcium intake. The current promotion of calcium-rich foods and supplements to protect our bones encourages the consumption of calcium. This is fine as long as magnesium nutrition is adequate. But calcium intakes that are unduly high relative to magnesium can intensify the problems caused by the low magnesium content of most modern diets.

Calcium is an important essential nutrient, but it must be guarded and controlled, and balanced by adequate magnesium if it is not to cause damage to the cells and the body as a whole.

Figure 1.4 Ischemic Heart Disease Rates Correlated with Dietary Calcium/Magnesium Ratios

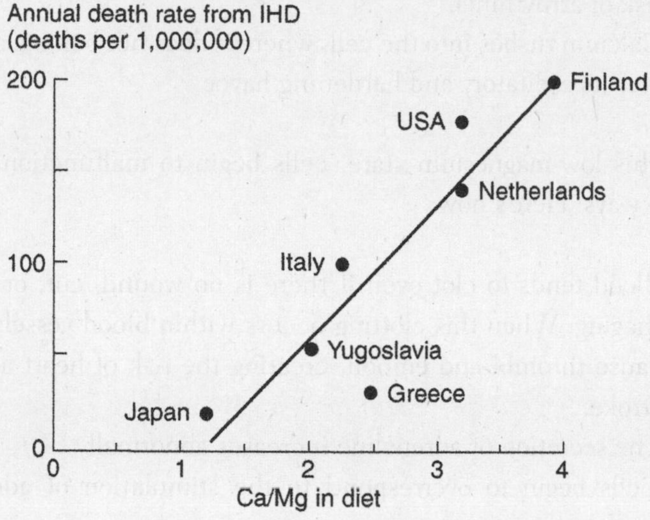

This figure (adapted from Karppanen, H., et al., *Advanced Cardiology* 25 [1978]: 9–24) shows a direct relationship between the incidence of death from ischemic heart disease and the ratio of calcium to magnesium in the average diet. It is interesting to note that Finland, which was the highest of all countries in heart-disease deaths in 1977, is now down to tenth in heart-disease deaths. What did they do? They undertook two important public health measures. First, they worked to educate the population about the importance of reducing dietary salt and fat and eating more vegetables and fruit—foods rich in magnesium and potassium. At the same time, they made available a magnesium-containing salt product that contained less sodium than standard table salt but still had a desirable salty taste, and promoted the use of this product. This high-magnesium salt was also sold to producers of sausage and other processed foods as a replacement for standard salt. Finns in general like salty food, and they accepted foods labeled as containing the new salt in preference to foods labeled low-salt.

Magnesium: The Silent Guardian

If the level of magnesium within a cell becomes too low there are three dire results:

1. There is not enough ATP available for the cell's necessary energy reactions and to maintain the "enzymatic pump" that moves potassium into and sodium out of the cells.

2. Potassium leaves the cell and cannot reenter, and there is a temporary increase in the plasma potassium level, which creates a risk of arrhythmia.
3. Calcium rushes into the cell, where it does not belong, and creates its excitatory and hardening havoc.

In this low-magnesium state, cells begin to malfunction in predictable ways. Here's how:

- Blood tends to clot even if there is no wound, cut, or hemorrhaging. When this clotting occurs within blood vessels, it can cause thrombi and emboli, creating the risk of heart attack or stroke.
- The secretion of adrenaline increases abnormally.
- Cells begin to overrespond to the stimulation of adrenaline stimulation.
- Cholesterol production and metabolism become abnormal.
- All muscle cells, including those in the heart and blood vessels, tend to contract and become unable to relax.
- There is increased production of free radicals and susceptibility to oxidative stress.
- Arteries stiffen and develop a buildup of plaques as a result of too much low-density lipoprotein (LDL, or "bad") cholesterol and too much calcium.
- Glucose is not properly processed as a result of insulin resistance, which can lead to type II diabetes and a whole spectrum of other disorders, all leading to heart disease.

When cells, tissues, organs, organ systems, and bodies have adequate magnesium, these dire consequences do not occur and the heart and blood vessels can be healthy at every level:

- At the molecular level, a healthy magnesium concentration is a natural antioxidant, protecting molecules from free-radical damage.
- At the enzyme level, there is enough ATP for all energy reac-

tions, and enzymes that need magnesium as a cofactor can function well.

- At the cellular level, a normal electrolyte balance is maintained. Calcium, sodium, potassium, and magnesium concentrations shift and adjust as needed. There is no abnormal calcification, hyperexcitability, or tendency to overreact to adrenaline.
- At the tissue level, blood flows freely, without an abnormal tendency to clot, and heart and blood-vessel muscle tissue can relax and contract in proper response to healthy nerve and hormonal signals. When danger comes, the fight-or-flight reaction works—and then subsides.
- At the organ level, proper magnesium levels allow the heart to pump out blood efficiently from the left ventricle; they also forestall high blood pressure by allowing a healthy sodium-potassium balance and preventing arterial spasms and, later, arteriosclerosis.
- At the organ-system level, the heart pumps continuously, without palpitations or arrhythmia, efficiently sending blood into flexible arteries that dilate and constrict in direct response to the body's immediate needs, delivering necessary oxygen and nutrients to all of the body's cells, especially those of the heart.

When the body has adequate magnesium, we don't even know it is there. It is truly the silent guardian of our hearts, blood vessels, cells, and bodies. It is only because many people don't have enough—primarily due to our modern processed-food diets—that we even need to notice.

The value of magnesium in keeping the heart and blood vessels healthy is supported by the fact that people having heart attacks who receive timely treatment with magnesium can have better outcomes than those who do not get this treatment. Several studies from the late 1950s through the early 1990s showed that timely infusion of magnesium during acute myocardial infarction (AMI, the medical term for a heart attack) can

Heart disease rises as the consumption of processed foods spreads.

lower death rates and improve outcome. However, these promising results were not confirmed when tested in large, multicenter trials (termed megatrials) conducted in the 1990s. Such megatrials have become the standard for judging the effectiveness of drugs. The negative results were widely publicized and seemed definitive to much of the medical community. But are they, really? Do they negate the benefit of magnesium therapy during heart attack so promised by the earlier studies? We believe not. Following is a brief history of this work with our short critical analysis.

Early Studies: Timely Magnesium Treatment for Heart Attacks

Several early studies showed magnesium therapy to be highly beneficial during AMI. As early as 1959 in Tasmania (a large island in southern Australia), R. S. Parsons and coworkers gave heart patients magnesium sulfate injections every five days, for a total of twelve injections. One patient out of one hundred died with this regimen. At the same hospital the year before, a similar group of patients did not get any magnesium shots, and thirty out of one hundred died. Timely and consistent magnesium input converted a 70 percent survival rate to 99 percent.

These were remarkable, albeit preliminary, results. Over the years, larger controlled studies confirmed that timely magnesium treatment could drastically reduce death rates for acute heart disease when given either intravenously or as intramuscular shots, or as a combination of the two. A few of these studies are summarized in table 1.3.

In a double-blind Danish study, researchers gave magnesium-chloride infusions to patients with signs of AMI. Patients receiving a forty-eight-hour course of intravenous magnesium chloride soon after the onset of severe chest pains had a 7 percent death rate. In contrast, the death rate among patients who received the same general treatment but were given a placebo instead of the magnesium infusion was 17 percent. When the hospital's ethics committee saw the great difference in mortality between these two groups, the study was stopped because it was deemed unethical to withhold the intravenous magnesium chlo-

Table 1.3 Magnesium's Effect on Mortality in AMI Patients

Year	Author	No. of patients	Timing of magnesium I.V.	Duration of I.V. magnesium	Effect of magnesium on death rate
EARLY STUDIES					
1988	Rasmussen (Denmark)	273	within first 3 hours	48 hours	down 76%
1991	Shechter (Israel)	159	within first 3 hours	48 hours	down 80%
1992	Woods LIMIT-2 (England)	2316	within first 3 hours	24 hours	down 24%
MEGATRIALS					
1995	ISIS-4 partial data (England	10,252	within first 3 hours after fibrinolytic therapy	24 hours	down 3.1%
1995	ISIS-4 partial data (England)	47,794	4–24 hours after fibrinolytic therapy	24 hours	up 6.9%
1995	ISIS-4 whole study (England)	58,046	0–24 hours after fibrinolytic therapy	24 hours	up 5.24%
2002	MAGIC (U.S.)	6,213	initiated a mean of 3.8 hours from onset of symptoms	24 hours	no change

ride from any myocardial infarction patients; the treatment improved the chances of survival so much. Furthermore, the magnesium-treated patients did better during convalescence. Even though only about one-third of the 1,000 subjects originally planned for had been treated with either magnesium or placebo, the magnesium-treated patients did better during convalescence, with only half as many as those on placebo needing anti-arrhythmia therapy during the four weeks after the AMI. At one year, the death rate from ischemic heart disease of the magnesium group was again about half that of the placebo group (15 percent versus 28 percent).

Studies in Israel by Dr. Michael Shechter and his colleagues showed the same encouraging trends, even in older adults and people who could not safely receive "modern" fibrinolytic ("clot-busting") therapy. Such therapy rapidly restores blood flow to an oxygen-deprived heart, lowering the risk of death. Unfortunately, it is given to only about one-third of heart attack patients in Israel (and to somewhat more in the United States), as it can be dangerous. Reestablishing the flow of blood to the heart, paradoxically, can cause further damage to the heart (called reperfusion injury) due to the release of harmful free radicals, which can damage tissues. This danger is especially evident in older adults. The Shechter group showed that starting magnesium-infusion treatment in seventy-eight patients with proven AMI, soon after a heart attack, and sustaining the treatment over a forty-eight-hour period, could lower death rates to 2.5 percent, compared with 12.3 percent for heart-attack patients not given magnesium—an 80 percent reduction. Even in the forty-six AMI patients over seventy years of age (29 percent), the magnesium lowered death rates by 41 percent, to 9 percent from the 16 percent for such patients not given magnesium. But in these elderly individuals, the need for drug treatment for severe arrhythmia fell from 56 percent to 38 percent, and the incidence of lesser disturbances declined from 20 percent to 9.5 percent. These findings—that magnesium treatment could so substantially improve the chance of survival even of people who were not good candidates for clot-busters—was good news. Shechter's long-term follow-up findings of patients over age seventy showed that the favorable effects of intravenous magnesium treatment permitted survival lasting an average of almost five years after the AMI in the magnesium-treated patients.

Magnesium is nature's

- **Calcium channel blocker**
- **Beta-blocker**
- **Blood-thinner**
- **Anticoagulant**

Studies such as these led to a large, controlled double-blind study in England. In this study, known as the second Leicester Intravenous Magnesium

Intervention Trial (LIMIT-2), over 2,300 patients were given intravenous magnesium before clot-busting therapy, which was followed by twenty-four hours' magnesium infusion. At twenty-eight days, the magnesium treatment had reduced mortality among the proven AMI patients—7.8 percent, as compared with 10.3 percent in the placebo. In the cardiac intensive care unit, left ventricular failure—an important cause of severe illness and death after AMI—was reduced by 25 percent in the magnesium-treated group. At one-year follow-up, the death rate was 25 percent lower in patients given the magnesium infusion as compared with the control patients, whose treatment was similar except for the magnesium. These results were less dramatic than the 70 to 80 percent reductions seen in the previous, smaller studies, but among other things, LIMIT-2 gave magnesium for only twenty-four hours, not forty-eight as in the Danish and Israeli studies. Nonetheless, such a large study was very promising.

All these trials showed that intravenous magnesium therapy within the first three hours of heart attack and/or in close association with fibrinolytic therapy could lessen the number of deaths due to AMI.

Drug Developments

While the magnesium studies on heart attack victims were being explored, several new drugs were developed to lower death rates from AMI. During this period, the standard test for such drugs became the large, placebo-controlled, double-blind, multicenter megatrial. New drugs tested in these megatrials gradually have become part of the accepted standard AMI treatment practice. Three examples that are prominent include aspirin plus the classes of drugs known as beta-blockers and angiotensin-converting enzyme (ACE) inhibitors. Interestingly, all of these can result in the body retaining magnesium.

Aspirin

Aspirin has become a mainstay in the treatment of coronary artery disease, whether or not it progresses to heart attack. Aspirin increases the absorption of magnesium in the body and decreases the excretion of magnesium in the urine. These actions raise magnesium levels in the body, which might contribute to aspirin's ability to inhibit blood clotting and to lessen the blood-vessel–constricting effect of adrenaline.

Beta-Blockers

Beta-blockers prevent magnesium and potassium losses in people who take diuretics (water pills), in people undergoing cardiac surgery, and in individuals who have experienced a heart attack. Beta-blockers act by inhibiting the effects of the stress hormone adrenaline. This hormone has a magnesium-lowering effect, so by inhibiting the action of adrenaline, beta-blockers help retain magnesium.

ACE Inhibitors

These drugs are the newest and most effective drugs used to lower mortality after a heart attack. Most of these drugs possess antioxidant activity, which makes them effective at helping to conserve magnesium and protect against heart damage caused by low magnesium levels. ACE inhibitors that lack the antioxidant effect do not cause the body to retain more magnesium.

Additional (Mega) Studies

These drugs having proven valuable in management of AMI, the effects of their administration for the duration of the study were compared with the effects of twenty-four-hour magnesium infusions in two megatrials: ISIS-4 and MAGIC. Summarized results from these two studies appear in the second part of table 1.3. The magnesium infusions showed no advantage over these magnesium-retaining drugs.

The fourth International Study of Infarct Survival (ISIS-4) trial was undertaken, involving 58,050 heart attack patients, at numerous hospital sites. Almost all (94 percent) of both the treatment and the control patients were given daily aspirin tablets (which had been shown in an earlier ISIS trial to improve the survival rates of heart attack patients). Many (about 70 percent) also received thrombolytic (fibrinolytic, or "clot-buster") therapy. The ISIS-4 study also compared the effect of an oral ACE inhibitor or an oral mononitrate drug (comparable to placing nitroglycerin under your tongue), each taken daily in tablet form, with the effect of magnesium infusions over the first twenty-four hours of hospitalization. Patients who received magnesium infusions up to three hours after their heart attacks had 3.1 percent fewer deaths than the control group. Unfortunately, the majority of all the magnesium-treated patients in ISIS-4 (about 82 percent) received their starting dose of intravenous magnesium four to twenty-four hours after their heart attacks and at least one hour after anti-clotting therapy had been provided. Because most of the AMI patients who were given the magnesium received it this late, the lowering of mortality reported in the earlier studies was not confirmed. ISIS-4 reported a 2.0 percent *increase* in mortality from calculations that included all the patients given magnesium, regardless of the treatment's timing. However, if you calculate the difference in death rate based on individuals who received magnesium within three hours after the AMI (18 percent of those who got magnesium for twenty-four hours), there were 3.1 percent *fewer* deaths compared with the control group.

Controversy brewed as criticism of the ISIS-4 mounted. The most important criticism was that magnesium infusions were not given early enough to *all* the patients in whom it was being tested. Because of this controversy, some support was provided by the National Institutes of Health (NIH) for another large multi-institution study of magnesium infusion that was named the *mag*nesium *i*n *c*oronaries (MAGIC) study. The intention was to shed additional light on whether magnesium, given at an appropriate time, is of value for heart attack victims. This test was placebo-controlled and double-blind. Patients received a twenty-four-hour infusion of either magnesium or placebo after an initial loading dose. Treatment began promptly after the infarction. The outcome showed no difference in thirty-day mortality rates between the magnesium and placebo groups.

How can these results be explained in light of the earlier magnesium studies? Funding for the MAGIC study was insufficient to permit researchers to give the magnesium infusions for forty-eight hours or to follow up for more than thirty days as the earlier studies—those that achieved the best results—had done. But perhaps more important, by the time the MAGIC study was performed, drugs proven effective in megatrials were being widely used for heart attack patients. Aspirin, beta-blockers, and ACE inhibitors were given daily to most of the subjects in ISIS-4 and to all of those in MAGIC, including those in the placebo groups. The MAGIC results thus show us that magnesium therapy does not add to the beneficial effect of these drugs on AMI mortality. But the results, unfortunately, do *not* tell us whether magnesium, acting alone, can lower AMI mortality. Such a study, which would require holding back proven medications, would be unethical. All of these drugs, which spare magnesium, would have resulted in a sustained increase in the subject's magnesium levels. Thus we see that, despite assertions to the contrary, the beneficial effect of magnesium on AMI mortality has not been disproved.

How does magnesium help someone who is having a heart attack? The chest pain of a heart attack is a warning that the supply of blood to the heart is insufficient and, as a result, that vital oxygen and nutrients are getting too low for normal heart function or even survival—and that calcium is moving in to replace the magnesium, a serious development. If magnesium is given very early after such onset of pain, it can:

- Protect the oxygen-starved heart tissue from permanent damage
- Protect against increasing cellular calcium at the expense of cellular magnesium
- Protect against rapid and irregular heartbeats
- Dilate smaller arteries that feed the heart
- Help to restore blood flow
- Prevent clotting in arteries that serve the heart
- Protect against free-radical damage

These attributes of magnesium, which protect against heart damage, must surely contribute to the beneficial effects of the magnesium-sparing drugs that are now routinely used to treat heart attacks. The MAGIC study was designed to determine whether intravenous magnesium infusions, given before or at the same time as clot-busting drugs, would achieve better results than were seen with ISIS-4. Unfortunately, neither study considered the complicating influence of the daily administration of magnesium-sparing drugs in both the magnesium-infusion test groups and the placebo groups.

It was disappointing that these studies did not resolve the magnesium controversy. The results from these two studies raise a number of questions:

- Was it reasonable to expect a one-day infusion of magnesium to add to the benefit achieved by drugs that increase magnesium retention and were administered daily for an entire month?
- Can magnesium outperform magnesium-retaining drugs in long-term outcomes such as one-year and five-year mortality rates?
- Might administering daily magnesium supplements after a forty-eight-hour infusion perhaps allow for lower drug dosages, and thus be the best approach?
- Is it reasonable to disregard the remarkable safety record of high-dose oral magnesium (used as a laxative) and intravenous magnesium infusions to manage the high blood pressure and convulsions of severe toxicity of pregnancy when considering its use in the treatment of heart attacks?

Will there be another large study of the effect of magnesium therapy on AMI mortality, testing daily oral administration of magnesium in addition to a timely forty-eight hour magnesium infusion? Could such treatment benefit patients who have had a recent heart attack? Might adequate magnesium therapy also benefit those who have already suffered at least one heart attack?

Dr. Shechter and his coworkers in California and Israel have shown that daily oral magnesium therapy can prevent subsequent heart attacks and improve quality of life in people with stable coronary artery disease. Might adequate magnesium therapy also benefit those who have already suffered at least one heart attack? The high cost of such studies to test the efficacy of a substance that cannot be patented no doubt will prevent substantial industry support. We cannot expect any clinical studies to disregard the benefits of drugs proven to be effective and part of standard practice in cardiology. The low cost of taking oral magnesium tablets daily, and the magnitude of the literature showing its value as a protective agent, may still encourage its use to prevent heart attacks, both in high-risk individuals to prevent a first heart attack, to prevent recurrences in people who have already experienced one or more heart attacks, and to improve the quality of life. But, in the meantime, we are still paying for the publicity given to the failure of the ISIS-4 and MAGIC trials to affirm the very favorable results of earlier controlled studies. ISIS-4 was influential in putting magnesium on the back burner as a treatment for heart disease. Fewer than 10 percent of clinicians now use magnesium for AMI patients, according to the National Registry of Myocardial Infarctions.

Arrhythmias, Sudden Cardiac Death, and Magnesium

When a young or middle-aged person suddenly collapses and dies, and autopsy fails to verify a heart attack, doctors usually suspect a fatal arrhythmia as the cause. Magnesium plays an essential role in maintaining normal heart rhythm, both directly and through its effects on potassium and calcium. The loss of cellular potassium and accumulation of cellular calcium that results from magnesium deficiency gives rise to arrhythmias, including premature beats, tachycardia (too fast a heart rate), and fibrillation (so rapid a rate that the heart quivers chaotically, rather than pushing blood onward with normally spaced, effective beats).

Arrhythmias induced by inadequate magnesium can complicate—or even terminate, through sudden cardiac death—the very conditions for which magnesium-wasting diuretics and other drugs are commonly prescribed, namely heart failure and hypertension. Magnesium deficiency, alone or in combination with potassium deficiency, can cause a change in the electrical activity that governs heart function called a *prolonged QT interval*, or LQT. The QT interval is a portion of the electrocardiogram (ECG) that represents the duration of the electrical impulse that causes contraction of the left ventricle, the heart's main pumping chamber. An abnormally long QT interval is seen in the ECGs of people who develop a potentially lethal arrhythmia called *torsade de pointes*, a condition that responds best to treatment with infusions of magnesium.

Increasing the blood level of magnesium quickly by infusing a magnesium solution has proven effective in treating arrhythmias, both directly and indirectly, by increasing the body's retention of potassium to correct low potassium levels and by blocking the rush of calcium into muscle cells. However, increasing the oral intake of magnesium could make a very significant contribution to cardiac health by helping to prevent arrhythmias in the first place. Magnesium deficiency might provide the answer to the puzzle of sudden death in seemingly healthy individuals, even young people and athletes, who are found on autopsy to have normal, unblocked coronary arteries.

Why Are the Health Benefits of Magnesium Not Commonly Known?

It is a mystery to us why the medical community has not embraced this simple, effective explanation of the heart disease epidemic of the twentieth century. Following are a few of our speculations on the subject.

- Magnesium research information is not made readily available to the busy practicing physician. There has been little organized, sustained effort devoted to informing doctors about magnesium research. When new drugs become available, the pharmaceutical companies that have developed and researched those drugs provide publications and summaries to the physicians most likely to prescribe them. No such organized effort disseminates research information on magnesium. As a result, much of that research remains unpublicized. Thus, many physicians, who lack the time to undertake literature searches, don't know about information on magnesium that holds great promise for improving patient care.
- There is often an undercritical acceptance, by both doctors and the general public, on negative results. This has occurred in two

main areas of magnesium research: the use of magnesium treatment during heart attacks (with the resulting controversy of the ISIS-4 and MAGIC studies, considered earlier) and the water-factor research. During the height of the "water effect" discussion, a few studies reported soft-water areas with no higher incidence of heart disease deaths. This created uncertainty about the promise of magnesium's protective effect, and an editorial in the *Journal of the American Medical Association* (*JAMA*) suggested the whole discussion be dropped. Such negative points of view are often a spur for deeper investigation, so, of course, some researchers continued their studies. Verification of magnesium's benefit was soon available, although it was not discussed on *JAMA*'s editorial page. Water's hardness comes from both magnesium and calcium in the water. At first, results showed that magnesium was indeed often responsible for the lower cardiovascular death rates. But further research showed that not only magnesium, but the ratio of magnesium to calcium in the hard water was the "water factor" for heart disease. A soft-water area could have a beneficial ratio, resulting in less heart disease, and a hard-water area could be so high in calcium that the magnesium's protective effect was obscured. Other issues, such as diet and toxic metals used in water pipes that are leached out of the pipes by soft water, became important details in this vast and complex subject. But, for the most part, the controversy was resolved scientifically, while in the minds of many the negative results still hold sway.

- Magnesium status is hard to assess. If someone has a serum magnesium level that is way below or above normal, he or she is sick and, probably, in the hospital. But within the normal range of serum magnesium, one cannot predict whether any given individual is deficient or adequate in magnesium nutrition. One reason is that less than 1 percent of the body's magnesium is in the serum. This small percentage is not representative of the body's stores of magnesium, which are mostly inside muscle and other cells. Likewise, the magnesium content of red blood cells (RBCs)

Calcium and magnesium need to be in balance to protect against heart disease.

is more indicative of gender, race, and age than of nutritional status. Additionally, magnesium intake at the time RBCs are formed influences the level of magnesium in the cells. Young RBCs contain more magnesium than do old RBCs. Given these facts, a doctor who suspects that magnesium deficiency may be causing early symptoms and orders a test for serum or RBC level will likely not get test results confirming a low magnesium status. Such negative results will likely cause the doctor to disregard (mistakenly) low magnesium as a possible cause of the problem. (The subject of testing magnesium status will be discussed in detail in chapter 10.)

- Conventional medical wisdom teaches that magnesium deficiency is very rare and occurs only in people with severe malnutrition, chronic alcoholism, or other specific disease states. This is taught in most medical and nutrition schools, so relatively few doctors, nutritionists, and dietitians expect or believe that our diets are low in magnesium. Conventional wisdom also teaches that the average American diet is essentially adequate in vitamins and minerals, and that it is the mix of macronutrients—fats, proteins, and carbohydrates—that needs adjustment. What's more, people often think of *malnutrition* (which literally means "bad nutrition") as starvation or undernutrition. But a more common form of bad nutrition in this country is *over*nutrition. Heart disease is caused by overnutrition of some nutrients and undernutrition of others, especially magnesium.
- There is often resistance to the concept that nutritional deficiency can cause disease. The discovery that vitamin C prevents scurvy took years to be accepted, and medical professionals disregarded niacin as the cure for pellagra in spite of overwhelming scientific evidence. On the other hand, the use of fluoride for tooth decay was rapidly accepted. And taking calcium supplements to prevent osteoporosis is recommended by many medical professionals today. Why is some research rapidly accepted—perhaps too rapidly—while other research, such as that on the damage to health caused by inadequate magnesium, is stubbornly rejected?

- Patent laws discourage research into and marketing of nutrients. If a company were to set up a marketing team to tell doctors all about magnesium nutrition research, there is no guarantee that patients would use their brand of magnesium or that doctors would recommend their formulation. They would be essentially marketing any and all brands of magnesium supplements. A company could not guarantee or expect a reasonable return on their investment. Thus, instead, we have pharmaceutical companies concentrating on patented medications to address single aspects of magnesium deficit—antihypertensives for high blood pressure; statins for high cholesterol; calcium-channel blockers and beta-blockers, which combat aspects of magnesium deficit at the cellular level; blood thinners to combat the increased clotting tendency brought on by magnesium deficit; and various medications for insulin resistance. Pharmaceutical companies can market these drugs knowing that they are the only source of that particular drug for a given number of years. They can feel free telling doctors all about the positive research on their patented medicine. The job of corporate executives is to maximize their stockholders' return on their investments, so they cannot be expected to research magnesium—a nonpatentable substance—and then promote that research among doctors.
- Scientists need to be ready to believe something new. This has been shown over and over in the history of medical science and in science in general. Oswald Avery, Colin MacLeod, and Maclyn McCarty proved DNA to be the genetic material back in the 1940s, but it was Alfred Hershey and Martha Chase who got the Nobel Prize for proving it in the 1950s—when molecular biologists were ready to believe it. It has long been generally accepted that heart disease is a problem not generally caused by a specific infectious agent, even though there is some evidence that low-grade infection, perhaps viral in origin, can play a part in the formation of some cardiovascular lesions. Faulty diet has long been implicated in heart disease, but the amount or type of fat (including cholesterol) and the amount of salt in the diet

have been the focus of blame. Much research has been done in these areas, but little attention has been paid to the research, ongoing and growing, that has associated magnesium deficiency with heart disease.

- Magnesium is low-tech. It was an era in love with technology when the epidemic of heart disease peaked. It was a time of Sputnik, nuclear power, and hi-fi recordings; an age for cracking the genetic code, going to the moon, and wiping out smallpox all over the planet. The epidemic of heart disease cried for heroic measures—heart transplants, artificial hearts, bypass surgery, balloon angioplasty, defibrillators and pacemakers, designer foods with no cholesterol and the right kind of fats, and designer drugs to treat risk factors and save lives. A simple nutritional deficiency, quite frankly, didn't capture anyone's imagination. And by the time real results with magnesium came in consistently, we were already highly invested in high-tech heart treatment and training.

The treatment of heart disease today is entwined with big business that provides expensive treatments and entails huge costs. A low-fat diet is not a realistic working solution for most people, and drugs, which are highly researched, thoroughly tested, and extensively marketed—all at great cost—look more and more like the light at the end of this high-tech tunnel. It would be easier to turn around a speeding train than high-tech modern cardiology. We do not expect or even desire that this happen. We don't expect doctors to start telling people who are having heart attacks to go take a magnesium pill. We do expect cardiology to continue to save lives as it refines heart treatment with procedures and medications. But we would like to see these treatments given *in addition to*, rather than in place of, adequate magnesium nutrition.

2

Metabolic Syndrome X, Diabetes, and Magnesium

Michael and his family had always been happy, even though as children and young adults they had been ribbed about being fat, and most of them had put on more weight since immigrating to the United States from Eastern Europe. Since they moved to America, they had eaten lots of sweets and ice cream, which had not been as available to them in the old country since they were a large family and money for extras such as treats was not easy to come by.

But Michael lost his good spirits at his last visit to his doctor. The doctor seemed very serious when he talked to him after reviewing papers on his desk. He said, "Mike, I have the lab results here from the blood samples I took at your last visit.

Your blood sugar and your blood cholesterol levels are too high, and the special tests I ordered show something else. Your blood insulin levels are unusually high and your blood magnesium is a little low. These are troubling, since the last time you were here you told me that your father and some of your cousins have diabetes, and other members of your family also have high blood pressure or heart disease. And your grandfather died of a heart attack at the age of fifty. It seems likely that your relatives, and you, have a metabolic condition that has recently been identified, and that can be dangerous for your heart. I gave you a sheet of exercises for you to try, to get rid of some of that fat on your belly, and told you to cut out some of that cake and candy you've been eating. Have you followed that advice?" Michael looked sheepish and said that he was just too busy to do that bending and stretching, and besides, at his time of life and after working so hard, wasn't he entitled to enjoy the extra treats he could now afford?

The doctor smiled and said, "Well, the results of these tests make me a little more hopeful that, with a few more tests to see if what I suspect is right, we can help you without taking away all of the pleasures of eating. You are resistant to the insulin your body is producing, so there is no point in starting you on insulin injections to control your diabetes. Yes, that is part of your problem. But it is likely that taking magnesium tablets may be an easy way to restore some of your body's insulin's ability to lower your blood sugar. The extra magnesium might even correct some of your abnormal blood cholesterol. I am going to take a little more of your blood to send to a special lab to get a better understanding of why your blood magnesium is only a little low, because I suspect that your body is quite deficient in magnesium. My advice to you, again, is that you at least cut back on sugar-sweetened breakfast cereals, desserts, snacks, and sodas. Substitute fruits, unsweetened fruit drinks, and just plain water or seltzer. If you must sweeten your coffee or tea, use a sugar substitute. Eat more dark-green vegetables, beans, and fish; eat less fatty meat; and use olive oil or canola oil instead of chicken

> fat or margarine for your fried foods. Here is a sheet of advice to give to your wife to help her plan and cook meals. Also, take a magnesium tablet with meals. Start by taking one at breakfast and one with your evening meal. After a week or two, start taking one with lunch also. And come back in a couple of weeks for the results of this special test and to see if you are improving."

Michael was lucky. His doctor was a fairly recent graduate of one of the few medical schools that emphasize nutrition, and he had taken an extra course in diseases that develop because of a combination of hereditary flaws and dietary imbalances. He had also continued to read up on the latest news on how best to test for magnesium deficiency, which plays a role in a newly identified disease, called metabolic syndrome X, which is characterized by abnormalities such as those Michael had told him were present in his family members.

Taking a few magnesium tablets each day was easy for Michael. They did soften his stool somewhat, but this was welcome because he tended to suffer from constipation. Because he felt better, and at subsequent visits to his doctor he found out they were on the right track, he had his four children tested. Three of them showed early signs of metabolic syndrome X, but to a lesser degree than their father had had. They have all now modified their diet (but with occasional allowances for the special desires of kids for at least a little candy and ice cream) and are taking magnesium supplements. Michael also called members of his brothers' and sisters' families together to alert them to this exciting new information that had made him and his children—and even his wife, who was a little overweight and had high blood pressure—feel healthier. They have all lost a little weight, and the blood pressures of those with higher than normal pressures were falling. Michael's high blood sugar level had fallen.

Metabolic Syndrome X

Many people have a condition called "metabolic syndrome X," or the "metabolic syndrome"—a somewhat newly identified disorder. It has been identified in patients with adult-onset diabetes (type II), with or without high blood pressure, as well as in patients with hypertension and no diabetes. Insulin resistance and high blood sugar levels are common in both these conditions. Abnormal fat metabolism also appears, expressed by high levels of the "bad" blood cholesterol—low-density lipoprotein (LDL)—and by midbody fat accumulation. All of these conditions predispose to cardiovascular disease, and are associated with low cellular magnesium levels, which, as discussed in chapter 1, are contributory to abnormalities of heart and arteries.

Beginning in the 1980s, two separate lines of medical research started to be woven together. Investigators in cardiology and diabetes research began to find remarkable similarities in the abnormalities they saw in their subjects. These included the following: high blood pressure, high blood cholesterol, midbody obesity, abdominal obesity (excess weight in the middle of the body), abnormal sugar metabolism (diabetes with a resistance to the action of insulin), and a tendency to increased blood clotting within blood vessels, which were not necessarily narrowed or blocked.

These conditions can occur alone or in any combination, but the current medical understanding is that there is a clear association among them that goes along with a high risk of heart disease. A third line of research has now emerged that links all of these conditions with magnesium. It is this discovery that justifies adding magnesium deficiency to the list of symptoms above and considering cardiovascular disease, diabetes, and magnesium deficiency as part of a single entity that is now known as *metabolic syndrome X.*

A Look at the Research That Discovered Metabolic Syndrome X

Diabetes Line of Research

Diabetes has long been known to be a disease that is characterized by high blood sugar levels and that is associated with a high risk of cardiovascular complications. How has the study of the abnormal glucose metabolism in people with diabetes led to an understanding of metabolic syndrome X, which also is associated with high cardiovascular risks? Glucose is the basic fuel burned by all of the body's cells, but to be used, it must first get into the cells. It is the hormone insulin, secreted by specialized cells in the pancreas, that enables glucose to move from the blood into the cells. In people with diabetes, this system has broken down, either because they do not produce adequate insulin or the insulin is ineffective. Thus, the body's cells are deprived of the fuel they need to function and the blood sugar level becomes abnormally high.

Diabetes researchers, long accustomed to studying people with type I diabetes, who need insulin injections to control their high blood sugar levels, had been increasingly encountering people with a different form of the disorder, type II diabetes. The muscle and fat cells of people with type II diabetes cannot take in normal amounts of glucose from the blood. Their glucose uptake is blocked, sometimes to a great degree, even though they secrete ample amounts of insulin. This condition is called *insulin resistance,* or IR. When given a glucose tolerance test, which measures the body's ability to process glucose, these people have normal or high-normal glucose values, but their insulin values are far above normal. The cells of the pancreas that make and secrete insulin were overdoing both, yet even these high levels of insulin failed to regulate blood sugar. So along with IR, these people have a condition known as *hyperinsulinemia,* or too much insulin in the blood. But that was not all. Many also have certain changes that pose real problems for the heart, including:

- Hypertension (high blood pressure).
- Unhealthy blood-lipid (fat) profiles, with too-low levels of high-density lipoproteins (HDL, also known as "good" cholesterol) and too-high levels of low-density lipoproteins (LDL, or "bad" cholesterol) and triglycerides.
- Obesity, especially with abdominal fat.
- Many also have an abnormal, increased blood-clotting tendency, which poses a risk of thrombosis (the formation of clots in blood vessels).

In looking for the causes of diabetes, researchers found the exact profile of a person at high risk for heart disease. Announced in 1988 by researcher Gerald M. Reaven, M.D., of the Department of Medicine at Stanford University Medical Center, this condition was called *in-*

sulin resistance syndrome, and by 1993 it was termed *syndrome X.* It has long been known that people with diabetes have high rates of heart disease, and now diabetes researchers had some clues as to why those with type II diabetes—those with insulin resistance plus hyperinsulinemia—are at special risk. The excess insulin seems to be at the core of both diabetes and risk factors for heart disease. Clearly, if such a state persists for a long time, heart disease would be the result.

Cardiovascular Line of Research

During the past twenty years, cardiovascular experts have struggled to understand why a substantial number of their patients with angina (cardiac chest pain) seemed to have perfectly healthy coronary arteries (the arteries that supply blood to the heart). This was a mystery because plaques in the arteries, leading to occlusion (narrowing or even blockages) of the coronary arteries, were considered to be the underlying cause of angina due to impaired blood supply to the heart. Coronary angiography tests for these cardiac "syndrome X" cases showed no occlusions that could be corrected with bypass surgery or angioplasty. Nonetheless, these patients had angina, experienced pain with and without exercise, and also had abnormal electrocardiograms (ECG) taken while exercising. This condition was termed *cardiac syndrome X.*

Recent studies have shown many of these people with cardiac syndrome X also have insulin resistance and other abnormalities like those found with insulin-resistance syndrome. To keep this class of individuals distinct, the condition has been termed cardiac syndrome X, but it may actually be a subdivision of the syndrome X that G. M. Reaven associated with insulin resistance. Through the 1990s, the concept of

Metabolic syndrome X can include:

- **Abdominal obesity**
- **High blood pressure**
- **High LDL (bad cholesterol)**
- **High triglycerides**
- **Low HDL (good cholesterol)**
- **High blood glucose**
- **Insulin resistance**
- **Hyperinsulinemia**
- **Increased blood clotting**
- **High cellular calcium-to-magnesium ratio**

syndrome X gradually continued to take hold and, increasingly, cardiac syndrome X is being associated with it.

But these two fields have yet to fully integrate the third line of research initiated by Lawrence M. Resnick, M.D., a practicing physician, researcher, and professor of medicine at Cornell University Medical College. His work gives new insight into risk factors for heart disease by tying them to a cellular imbalance between magnesium and calcium—that is, metabolic syndrome X.

Hypertension Line of Research

Missing in the two lines of thinking that developed the concepts of syndrome X and cardiac syndrome X is the work from the third line of research—the one that links syndrome X with low cellular magnesium levels.

Dr. Resnick's research into factors that affect blood pressure shows how the cellular ratio of magnesium to calcium in hypertensive patients relates both to their development of heart disease and metabolic syndrome X. He and his colleagues observed that the kidneys of some patients with essential hypertension (high blood pressure not caused by a known disease) secreted different amounts of a hormone known as renin, which affects blood pressure. Depending on their renin level, people responded differently to medications and to high salt intakes. The blood pressure of many, but not all, rose if they ate a high-salt diet. Some had their blood pressure lowered by taking calcium supplements, and others by taking magnesium supplements. To find an explanation for these paradoxes, Dr. Resnick and his coworkers explored the mineral balance in the cells of their patients with high blood pressure. In 1984, they published their finding that the level of magnesium inside the cells was low in *all* of their patients with hypertension. By 1988, they found that cellular magnesium was also low in people with insulin resistance. This link between hypertension and insulin resistance pointed these researchers to the role of cellular magnesium in syndrome X. They at first suggested terming the syndrome *generalized cardiovascular metabolic disease.* This has since been shortened to *metabolic syndrome X,* or, simply, *the metabolic syndrome.*

Low Cellular Magnesium and Metabolic Syndrome X

Dr. Resnick and his coworkers have published what they call their ionic theory of syndrome X, according to which a low magnesium ion level inside cells is the key component of metabolic syndrome X. As a cell's magnesium ion level falls, the calcium ion level rises. The result is a low magnesium/high calcium cell ratio. This affects the functioning of various kinds of cells in ways that bring on metabolic syndrome X, as follows:

Type of cells	Respond to low magnesium and high calcium by:	To produce clinically:
Beta (insulin-producing) cells in pancreas	making and releasing too much insulin	Hyperinsulinemia
Fat tissue cells	becoming unable to respond to insulin	Insulin resistance
Muscle cells	becoming unable to respond to insulin	Insulin resistance
Blood-vessel cells	constricting and stiffening	Hypertension
Blood platelets	becoming more likely to stick together and developing a tendency toward thrombosis	Clotting, plaques in blood vessels
Heart muscle cells	enlarging and becoming excessively contractile	Heart disease
Adrenal gland cells	making and releasing too much of so-called stress hormones	Hypertension
Nerve cells	overreacting to stimuli	Nerve irritability
Liver cells	producing too much glucose	Poor glucose tolerance, diabetes
Kidney cells	increasing sodium retention	Hypertension and sodium imbalance

It appears that it is the low-magnesium, high-calcium imbalance that is the fundamental cause of metabolic syndrome X. In blood vessel cells, this causes constriction of the arteries, making them stiff and leading to high blood pressure. The same imbalance causes blood platelets to aggregate (stick together) and leads to an increased tendency toward coagulation within the blood vessels, a condition sometimes referred to as *blood thickening* or *sticky blood*. Muscle and fat cells become unable to utilize glucose normally—they have insulin resistance. At the same time, pancreatic cells overproduce and secrete insulin, causing hyperinsulinemia.

This hyperinsulinemia has been strongly implicated as a cause of many of the abnormalities characteristic of metabolic syndrome X. But it also directly contributes to losses of magnesium, resulting in low cellular magnesium levels, which in turn further exacerbates the condition.

Low cellular magnesium with high cellular calcium is the key to metabolic syndrome X.

The cellular work of Dr. Resnick and his coworkers throughout the 1980s and 1990s more and more defined the underlying problem causing metabolic syndrome X as a cellular imbalance between magnesium and calcium—specifically, a low magnesium/high calcium state inside the cell. This is manifested as impaired glucose tolerance, too much insulin production, hypertension, a tendency for blood to clot, dyslipidemia (an unhealthy balance of blood fats, see chapter 5), diabetes, and cardiovascular disease. This research is also beginning to explain how certain medications, chemicals, and supplements can hurt or help heart disease by affecting magnesium ion levels inside cells. For example:

- Salt lowers cellular magnesium.
- Glucose lowers cellular magnesium.
- Pregnancy lowers cellular magnesium (especially if pregnancy is complicated by diabetes).
- Aging lowers cellular magnesium.
- Insulin temporarily raises blood magnesium, but it causes increased magnesium loss through the urine, ultimately leading to

a lowering of cellular magnesium and increase in cellular calcium. (An exception to this occurs if cellular magnesium is too low to begin with.)

- Captopril (Capoten), a type of drug classified as an angiotensin-converting enzyme (ACE) inhibitor, raises cellular magnesium.
- Glutathione, an amino-acid compound that acts as an antioxidant, raises it. Vitamin E raises glutathione, which then raises cellular magnesium.
- Insulinlike growth factor (IGF), a growth hormone, raises cellular magnesium.
- Estrogen, a sex hormone, raises cellular magnesium, but lowers its blood level.

This third line of research, which first described syndrome X as a metabolic disorder, eliminates the confusion behind heart disease by showing that low cellular magnesium ion levels are the missing link between heart disease in people who have angina despite clear coronary arteries (cardiac syndrome X) and those who have heart disease risk factors in combination with insulin resistance (syndrome X). Unfortunately, along with heart disease, diabetes is either present or on the horizon for these people.

Diabetes, Heart Disease, and Magnesium

Because two-thirds of people with diabetes ultimately die of some form of heart disease, and because low magnesium levels are associated with both diabetes and cardiovascular disease, it is worth examining the evidence that inadequate magnesium is causally linked with both of these major chronic illnesses and death.

Type I diabetes, also referred to as early-onset and insulin-dependent diabetes, is a hereditary condition in which there is inadequate insulin production. In this disease, blood glucose rises to dangerous, even lethal, levels if insulin is not administered. The kidneys must excrete the excess glucose, which causes the kidneys to eliminate magnesium also. Magnesium is needed for insulin to bring glucose into the cells, and to utilize the glucose. The urinary losses of magnesium experienced by people with diabetes can intensify their metabolic abnormalities and increases their risk of cardiovascular disease.

People with type I diabetes need, and respond to, insulin injections. The incidence of type I diabetes is growing because it can now be controlled over the long term with proper medical treatment, allowing many people who have it to live relatively normal lives and have children of their own, passing on the genes that result in this condition. Before insulin was discovered, diabetes usually caused death early in life, so the numbers of those affected did not grow much.

Type II diabetes is different. People with type II diabetes produce plenty of insulin, but their cells do not properly respond to it; they are insulin-resistant. Also known as non-insulin-dependent diabetes, this condition is more commonly called late- or adult-onset diabetes, although it is now increasingly being detected in children. The incidence of type II diabetes is growing as the consumption of modern processed foods increases throughout the world. While this disease has a genetic component, it mostly becomes manifest after years of living on a processed-food diet that is high in refined foods, including sugar, and low in magnesium. When such a lifestyle results in a low magnesium content within the cells, there are metabolic changes in the cells that make them resistant to the action of insulin so that glucose cannot enter the cells. A sustained high blood glucose, or hyperglycemia, results, which—as in people with type I diabetes—increases the excretion of magnesium, as well as glucose, by the kidneys. Since the insulin-secreting cells of people with type II diabetes are functional, their bodies respond to this sustained hyperglycemia (despite adequate secretion of insulin) by making even more insulin. As a consequence, hyperinsulinemia develops in conjunction with high blood sugar, and the abnormalities of syndrome X develop. Thus, type II diabetes is really a magnesium deficiency that manifests as metabolic syndrome X.

In people with either type of diabetes, the tendency toward low magnesium levels increases the risk for heart disease. People with type I diabetes often have a poor magnesium status because constantly high blood glucose levels result in increased excretion of magnesium through the urine. In addition, the utilization of glucose by the cells depends on magnesium, so if there is a large amount of glucose that needs processing, there is an increased need for magnesium. For people with type I diabetes, magnesium supplements can help to prevent heart disease, but they can never make insulin secretion normal. However, they can often improve the response to any insulin that *is* secreted or to the insulin administered by injection.

The sustained high blood sugar in type II diabetes also results in high urinary loss of magnesium. This intensifies the magnesium deficiency that caused the resistance of cells to insulin-induced glucose uptake in the first place, making type II diabetes a progressive disease if not treated. For people with type II diabetes, supplementation with magnesium can improve the response to insulin and can arrest the disease process, especially if combined with exercise and weight loss.

Current Medical Thought on Metabolic Syndrome X

The medical community accepts the clustering of four major risk factors for heart disease, sometimes referred to as the "deadly quartet." These are:

1. High blood pressure
2. Obesity
3. High blood cholesterol
4. High blood sugar/insulin resistance

Despite seeing them as a cluster, doctors customarily treat hypertension with one set of drugs, high blood sugar with another, and high cholesterol with yet another. Insulin resistance may be attacked with one of the new drugs that are becoming available. A low-fat diet and exercise are commonly advised for weight loss. The concept of syndrome X brings all of these abnormalities under one umbrella. Now doctors are increasingly detecting, in people with high blood pressure, some degree of insulin resistance, poor glucose tolerance, high LDL (bad cholesterol) levels, low HDL (good cholesterol) levels, high triglycerides, and a tendency for blood to clot within arteries and veins, in addition to abdominal obesity.

However, for the most part the idea of syndrome X is gaining acceptance without any consideration of magnesium nutrition, which links them all. Since they come as a cluster, it would seem preferable to treat them as a whole rather than as separate diseases. It is therefore worth asking, without magnesium, how do current treatments for the manifestations of metabolic syndrome X fare?

Weight-Loss Diets for Metabolic Syndrome X

Obesity, a result of eating too much food and getting too little exercise, coupled with a genetic component, has been considered a main culprit in many of the manifestations of metabolic syndrome X. Obesity is often associated with insulin resistance and high blood insulin, and this high blood insulin appears to be an important cause of the rest of the problems. Therefore, it has been presumed, if you eat less and exercise more to lose weight, the syndrome will go away, or at least improve. This belief has led to recommendations for weight loss and exercise, long a staple of heart disease treatment and prevention. Unfortunately, it is almost always a losing battle for both patient and doctor. There is also another problem with this approach: Because low magnesium is the underlying cause of metabolic syndrome X, lean people as well as overweight people can have it. Low magnesium/high calcium cellular ratios can happen in lean as well as obese people, causing all the abnormal cell responses discussed earlier in this chapter. Diabetes is found in lean as well as obese people. So is heart disease. Nonetheless, diet and exercise remain a major treatment recommended for metabolic syndrome X.

Specific diets were recommended for people with cardiovascular risk factors before the clustering of syndrome X was recognized. If hypertension was the focus of the diet, low sodium and weight loss were stressed. If cholesterol and lipid profile were unhealthy, a diet low in total fat, saturated fat, and cholesterol was prescribed. If obesity in general was seen as the problem, a low-calorie and, usually, low-fat diet was recommended. More recently, another diet has been recommended—a diet with moderate fat and carbohydrate levels, because low-fat diets are essentially high in carbohydrates, which, in some people, make high insulin levels worse.

How can all these different diets be right for different expressions of the same syndrome? The answer is that diet is vitally important as the cause of metabolic syndrome X and all its associated ills. But the culprit is not to be found in the percentage of fat, protein, or carbohydrate, or even in obesity *per se,* but in the total amount of magnesium available from the diet. Also, as with the example of hard water we saw in chapter 1, the ratio of magnesium to calcium is vitally important. Doctors who have no knowledge of Dr. Resnick's work establishing that low magnesium is the cause of syndrome X now tend to recommend switching from one type of dietary fat to another rather than lowering total fat intake, as well as changing the types of carbohydrates eaten as a way to deal with metabolic syndrome X. What this approach misses is that more magnesium will help, while a diet lower in magnesium, even if it results in weight loss, can worsen it. A more direct approach is to recommend a diet high in magnesium-rich foods, such as vegetables, whole grains, nuts, and fruits. This is a better means of correcting the disease than are weight-loss diets that may inadvertently also cause losses of magnesium. For those who resist such a healthy diet, magnesium supplements can serve well.

Drugs for Metabolic Syndrome X

Doctors are painfully aware of how difficult real lifestyle changes can be. And what are they to recommend for people with metabolic syndrome X who are lean, or who are obese but who cannot or will not lose weight—or for either type of individual, when dieting is ineffective? Current medical practice relies on drug therapy. However, treating just hypertension with a drug that may further impair glucose tolerance is counterproductive in a disease that also involves insulin resistance. Treating high blood glucose separately may have a negative impact on hypertension or cholesterol. The emphasis now is on mixing drug therapies that enhance each other, or at least that do not interfere with one another. Some of the types of drugs recommended are oral hypoglycemics, nitrates, calcium-antagonists, beta-blockers, ACE inhibitors, statins, estrogens, and alpha-blockers—even antidepressants, even tranquilizers, since so many people with metabolic syndrome X also suffer from anxiety and tension. This multidrug approach, however, is filled with risks, frustration, and costs.

The acceptance of the idea that syndrome X is driven by insulin resistance has given rise to the development of new drugs that restore insulin sensitivity as the means to treat the whole syndrome. The best candidates so far are a class of drugs known as thiazolidinediones, three of which have undergone large-scale clinical trials. One of these, troglitizone (Rezulin), had been approved by the U.S. Food and Drug Administration (FDA) but has since been taken off the market because it was found to cause liver damage. The other two, rosiglitazone (Avandia) and pioglitazone (Actos) may be less damaging to the liver, but have not been used long enough for their full safety to be assessed. Time will tell.

These drugs do several things beneficial for people with syndrome X, not the least of which is raising the intracellular magnesium level. But they do not correct poor magnesium nutrition. If the drug is stopped and the magnesium deficiency is still there, the consequences come back. The drug producers are not thinking about bringing magnesium status and nutrition up to par. Rather, they are trying to fix a consequence of magnesium deficiency, insulin resistance, with a drug that will repair that one specific metabolic abnormality.

Comprehensive Treatment for Metabolic Syndrome X

It is estimated that up to 10 to 15 percent of the adult population in industrialized societies have metabolic syndrome X. It is hard to treat because, up to now, treatments have been designed to address only one risk factor for heart disease or diabetes at a time. Thus, we see many medications specific for the management of hypertension, high blood glucose, high cholesterol (especially high LDL cholesterol), and obesity. Physicians have observed that treating one symptom, without considering that treatment's impact on the others, is not a cure and may even be dangerous. As so well stated by S. S. Ready:

> It is possible that treating blood pressure levels alone while ignoring or worsening other strongly associated risk factors has resulted in minimal effects on the incidence of coronary heart disease.

Doctors must treat the whole of metabolic syndrome X, and it doesn't seem easy. If there is no discernable blockage of the coronary arteries, bypass surgery and angioplasty are not appropriate treatments. Diet, especially calorie restriction, is assumed to help those with syndrome X who are overweight, because obesity is commonly considered the cause of syndrome X. Exercise seems to help such individuals as well. But the traditional low-fat, high-carbohydrate diet that has been promoted as heart-healthy for so long can make syndrome X worse.

Magnesium is the real key to treating metabolic syndrome X and heart disease risk factors.

The discovery that low cellular magnesium and the resulting rise in cellular calcium underlies metabolic syndrome X, with its several risk factors for heart disease, is a major advance in medicine. It gives new insight into the malfunctions that can occur in the heart and blood vessels when nutritional magnesium is inadequate. The chapters that follow take this concept to the other major risk factors for heart disease and discuss how they relate to magnesium.

3

High Blood Pressure, Salt, and Magnesium

In 1896, Scipione Riva-Rocci, an Italian internist and pediatrician, invented the inflatable cuff still used to measure blood pressure, but it was fifty years before practicing physicians began to use it routinely. Life-insurance physicians made the earliest practical use of this measuring tool, and they were the ones who found that people with high blood pressure had an increased risk of premature death. Their job was to provide reliable calculation of the life expectancy of insurance policy applicants, and during the first four decades of the twentieth century, their efforts led to the concept that hypertension (high blood pressure) is a risk factor for an early death. At the time, the few physicians who thought about blood pressure at all believed that a moderate elevation in blood pressure was beneficial. Even into the 1920s, any association of high blood pressure with stroke or heart failure was nebulous at best. Hypertension's status as a major public health problem began to emerge just after World War II. Easy to measure and shown to be statistically linked to heart disease by the vast amount of data gathered by life-insurance companies, this first risk factor for heart disease became important to treat as the heart disease epidemic was reaching its peak.

The life insurance statistics were right about high blood pressure. Associated with stroke and heart disease, it continually strains the heart, blood vessels, and kidneys, often for years and often unnoticed. Almost a third of individuals who have high blood pressure are unaware of their precarious condition. Often, there are no overt symptoms until development of kidney problems, a stroke, or heart disease. Its stealth has earned it the title the "silent killer," and it is on the rise. About 50 million Americans have hypertension, and from 1987 to 1997, the number of deaths attributed to this hidden disease rose by over 35 percent. People with untreated high blood pressure can expect, at worst, a permanently disabling stroke or chronic illness or death from heart disease. At best they face rejection by life and/or medical insurance companies and even by some employers. To walk around with high blood pressure is to constantly roll the dice against living a healthy life. *No wonder the American Heart Association has made it a top priority to warn people about this underlying yet quiet cause of heart disease and to help find ways to treat it.*

Much knowledge has been gained from the well-supported, ongoing research into causes of essential hypertension (high blood pressure of unknown cause). We know a lot about hormones that control or contribute to elevated blood pressure, especially those that control blood volume by regulating kidney function. We have learned that even the endothelium (lining) of the blood vessels produces substances that affect blood pressure, some by dilating them and others by constricting them. We know that a high salt intake adversely affects these hormones, at least in some people. It has been shown that a too-low potassium intake can bring on high blood pressure in some, an effect

Low magnesium and high calcium levels contribute to high blood pressure.

that is intensified by a diet high in salt. For some people, excessive calcium intake can also increase blood pressure. For the most part, research findings about causes of essential hypertension have been complicated, conflicting and confusing. Recently, Dr. Lawrence M. Resnick of Cornell University Medical College and his coworkers discovered a unifying factor: low cellular magnesium, in association with high cellular calcium, is found in all people with essential hypertension as a part of metabolic syndrome X. (See chapter 2.) In today's world, many people are short on magnesium and/or potassium. Either or both can cause high blood pressure. This chapter will present direct evidence and evaluate current treatments for this silent killer from this often-neglected nutritional point of view.

The Effect of Magnesium on High Blood Pressure

Magnesium has direct and indirect effects on blood pressure—both of which are substantial.

Directly, magnesium makes blood vessels relax and dilate, a necessary condition for normal blood pressure.

Indirectly, normal magnesium status is necessary for keeping in balance the electrolytes, or ions (the form in which minerals circulate in the body), that are important for normal blood pressure. These are sodium, potassium, magnesium, and calcium. Low potassium, by itself, can bring on high blood pressure. But even adequate potassium intake cannot normalize high blood pressure if magnesium is too low. Without enough magnesium (and potassium) in our bodies, we cannot expect normal blood pressure.

Normal magnesium is also necessary for another indirect effect on the blood pressure. It is needed by the endothelium (the cells that form the lining) of the blood vessels to maintain its normal structure and function. The endothelial cells produce substances, called prostacycline, thromboxane, and endothelin, that affect the blood pressure. Prostacycline, the production of which is increased by magnesium, acts to dilate arteries. The synthesis of thromboxane and endothelin, which constrict arteries, is inhibited by magnesium.

The path to the discovery of low cellular magnesium as an important link to hypertension has been full of seeming dead ends. In the past, some researchers had tried using magnesium supplements to treat hypertension, with conflicting results. As a result, many physicians became convinced that low magnesium had no role in high blood pressure. Let's look at the evidence and try to see why.

Magnesium and Hypertension Research

Most studies of the effect of the recommended dietary allowance (RDA) of magnesium on hypertension have shown that low doses of magnesium such as the recommended dietary allowance (RDA)—the amount officially considered adequate to maintain health—do not lower a high blood pressure. This has fostered resistance to the premise that magnesium might be useful in treating hypertension. However, in higher doses, magnesium has been found to reduce high blood pressure. Table 3.1 demonstrates the importance of dosage. It summarizes sixteen clinical trials of magnesium on subjects with high blood pressure.

In general, a daily magnesium intake of 480 milligrams or more lowered high blood pressure, while taking only the RDA (360 milligrams per day) did not. These results were widely interpreted to indicate that magnesium does not help high blood pressure. On the other hand, since hypertension is an unhealthy state, it makes sense for studies to try magnesium doses higher than an amount believed adequate merely to maintain good health. The studies that employed the larger supplements of magnesium did in fact show it has ability to lower high blood pressure.

Taking more than 400 milligrams of supplemental magnesium has normalized high blood pressure.

Doctors are accustomed to blood-pressure studies that evaluate the effects of medications by trying several doses of the drug being tested. This is called *titrating*. It means that subjects are given a low dose first, and the dosage is then raised, stepwise, to the level that achieves the desired effect. Titrating is a logical technique to use in hypertension studies because it mimics the way in which doctors are instructed to prescribe medications for high blood pressure: Start low,

Table 3.1 The Effect of Magnesium on Blood Pressure

The following table represents the findings of sixteen research studies on the effect of magnesium on people with high blood pressure. These studies are listed in order of increasing magnesium dose. Note that 360 milligrams represents the RDA for magnesium. See References for study citations.

Study No.	Daily magnesium dose	Effect on blood pressure
1	240 mg	No change
2	360 mg	Drop
3	360 mg	No change
4	360 mg	No change
5	360 mg	No change
6	360 mg	No change
7	360 mg	No change
8	360 mg	Drop only when magnesium was taken after placebo
9	360 mg	No change
10	360 mg	No change
11	360 mg	No change
12	480 mg	Drop
13	480 mg	Drop
14	600 mg	Drop
15	360 mg 720 mg 960 mg	No change Drop Drop
16	960 mg	No change

and if it doesn't work, increase the dose. This is recommended because antihypertensive (blood-pressure-lowering) drugs have side effects, some potentially severe, and doctors want their patients to be on the lowest effective dose possible. Most nutrients do not have side effects anything like those of drugs. Starting at the lowest nutrient dose but not then titrating up to higher doses limits the information a study can provide. Study 15 in table 3.1 did take the titrating approach and tried three different levels of magnesium. The investigators found that magnesium did reduce high blood pressure, but only at a daily dose of 720 milligrams or higher.

But what about studies 2 and 8, which provided 360 milligrams per day and did show an effect on blood pressure? Do they support the magnesium hypothesis? Study 2 was conducted with subjects already on long-term diuretic therapy. Since such therapy causes the body to lose magnesium, these subjects were probably magnesium-deficient, and apparently even the low dose of 360 milligrams of magnesium per day might have been enough to at least partially repair the magnesium deficiency and help to normalize the patients' high blood pressure. Study 8 was done in what is known as a crossover design. This is entirely appropriate for studies on medications, but not for studies of nutrients (see "Problems with Crossover Design Studies When Testing Nutrients," page 56).

There is another basic difference between medications and nutrients: Blood-pressure medications *lower* blood pressure even in people who do not have hypertension. Proper nutrient therapy *normalizes* it. People who have normal blood pressure probably have adequate body levels of magnesium. We would neither expect nor desire magnesium supplements to cause low blood pressure in normal, healthy people. But some of the studies cited above made a point of reporting that magnesium does not lower normal blood pressure. Study 11, which was done on a large population, is an example. Large studies are influential in the medical research community, and this one could be seen by many doctors as proof that magnesium does not affect blood pressure. In reality, however, they are expecting magnesium to act like blood pressure medications, which lower blood pressure whether it is normal or not. A dose of antihypertensive medication can cause temporarily low blood pressure in a healthy individual. An oral dose of magnesium, in contrast, will not lower a normal, healthy blood pressure. If you consume more magnesium than necessary on any given day, your body will absorb and use what it needs and let any excess be excreted. Study 11 used 360 milligrams of magnesium, which, as we have seen, is not enough to lower high blood pressure. In addition, the subjects in this study had *normal* blood pressure to begin with. There-

Problems with Crossover-Design Studies When Testing Nutrients

A crossover-design study works in the following way. Let's say we are going to test a substance for its effect on high blood pressure. We need two groups, a treatment group that will receive the treatment and a control group that will receive a placebo, a dummy or inert pill. This way we can really know it's the substance, not the experiment, that makes any difference. So far, so good. Further, no one—neither the researchers nor the subjects—knows who is getting what. This makes the study double-blind, and eliminates the possibility that the results observed will be colored by people's expectations. Good again. Then, at the halfway point comes the crossover part: The subjects switch. Those who had been getting the test substance now get the placebo, and vice versa. Sometimes at this crossover point, there is also a washout period, a time when the subjects receive neither the treatment substance nor a placebo so that their bodies presumably wash out all of the test substance before the second test period begins. At the end of the entire study, you average all the blood pressures taken while the subjects took the test substance and compare that with the average of all the blood pressures taken while on the placebo. The difference, if any, is deemed to be the effect of the test substance.

When testing medications, the crossover design makes total sense. Medications act on specific, pinpointed functions, and then wash out of the body, some slowly, some rapidly. One has to keep taking the medication to keep the action working. A drug can be fully washed out of the body, and sometimes the patient must increase the dose of a particular drug to maintain the desired effect. This is not true of nutrients, however. And magnesium is not a medication, it is an essential nutrient. Giving someone with a nutritional deficiency a nutritional supplement first corrects the deficiency and then builds up a body store of that nutrient. Less is then needed to maintain the sufficiency. If the supply of that nutrient is then cut off, the body will conserve that store by minimizing its loss. Hope-

(continued on page 57)

(continued from page 56)

fully, no one ever completely washes out any essential nutrient, for this would mean sickness or even death.

These basic differences between medications and nutrients could present problems with the crossover design in tests of nutrients. For example, study 8 in table 3.1 was conducted on adult subjects who had moderate hypertension who were already being treated with beta-blockers. It showed a drop in blood pressure only when magnesium was given after the placebo period. Those who were on magnesium first and then switched to the placebo may have gotten enough magnesium during the first half of the study to correct a borderline deficiency and even build up a small store. When these people went on the placebo, such stores may have seen them through the zero magnesium supplement period, keeping their placebo blood pressure value lower than it would have been if they had never taken the magnesium—a falsely low result. The results of the tests on such people would be skewed, minimizing the effect of magnesium on blood pressure. This is what could be at work in study 8, in which only those subjects given magnesium *after* the placebo period showed a significant drop in blood pressure. Giving subjects magnesium after a placebo period, without a crossover, may be a better test of supplemental magnesium's effect on hypertension in studies of this duration (weeks to months).

fore, this study does not prove that magnesium has no effect on hypertension. It demonstrates that the design of the study should be appropriate to the objective, and that results must be carefully studied before valid conclusions can be made. (See References for study citations.)

What are we to do with study 16, in which subjects were given a whopping 960 milligrams of magnesium per day and showed no normalization of high blood pressure? This was a study of thirteen subjects who had been repleted with magnesium at the beginning of the trial. This means that they all had enough magnesium for their bodily needs, and yet still had mild hypertension. This suggests that their magnesium status was not the problem, so even the relatively high dose of 960 milligrams per day could not alleviate their high blood pressure. It is quite possible that these subjects, with diets that provided adequate magnesium, had a potassium intake that was too low to balance their sodium. True, magnesium must be adequate for potassium to do its work, but if the magnesium status is good and the potassium intake is too low, one can still have hypertension. What these subjects probably needed was potassium supplements, not magnesium.

The Role of Potassium

Chad rushed into the deli restaurant, ordered a Reuben sandwich, and waited impatiently for his noon meal. He was so stressed about it all that his usually calm Hawaiian manner was unrecognizable. He looked like a man condemned, waiting for his executioner rather than his lunch. When asked what was troubling him, he said that his blood pressure was too high and that his doctor had told him to "lose weight and cut out the salt!" The sandwich he had just ordered was exactly what he had been warned against. Chad had lost forty pounds and was doing pretty well, but today he just couldn't handle it. He had to have a Reuben, and he felt terribly guilty and troubled about it. His good job, wonderful family, and life in Hawaii had given him an almost stress-free life. But now, high blood pressure was threatening—both him and the family who loved and needed him. His worry and stress were palpable.

"Try this," I [AR] said to Chad, holding up a small container of a salt substitute. "It's got half the sodium of regular salt, the rest is potassium," and I began to explain how he probably just needed some more potassium to balance the sodium as long as he had enough magnesium to help the potassium. He really didn't need to cut out salt, and losing weight wouldn't really change things. I pointed to my 260-pound husband, making one of the best Reuben sandwiches ever, and proudly claimed that he had been on the salt substitute and magnesium supplements for over ten years and had completely normal, even low, blood pressure. Chad's stress level didn't allow him to listen very carefully to this nutrition lecture in the middle of lunch hour, but a week or so later he returned. "What was the name of that salt?" he asked, and my husband threw him a small container saying, "Take it home. Try it. They're cheap!"

The next time I saw Chad, he was a different man. Calm, happy, and content again with his good life in paradise; his blood pressure was normal and he had bought all the salt substitute in the grocery store because he didn't ever want to run out of it. He was cured! And such a simple cure! His doctor thought it was because he had lost forty pounds. However, the last time I saw Chad, his weight was back up (to almost 400 pounds!), and although he was struggling unsuccessfully to lose weight, his blood pressure was still normal. This was more than three years after that first encounter, and the simple cure was still working. "I have told some friends about it," Chad told me, "and they all seem to have the same luck I have had with it." Being overweight is cumbersome for Chad, and he is starting to walk on weekends because his age is making the weight harder to bear without pains. But blood pressure? No problem!

How could something as small as a common half-potassium/half-sodium salt substitute, costing less than one dollar per container, make such a difference? It really sounds too simple. Could it actually accomplish more than sophisticated prescription medications derived from comprehensive research? And what does it have to do with magnesium anyway? Perhaps, since he is Hawaiian, Chad's dietary intake of magnesium might have been adequate, because Hawaii has some of the highest water magnesium levels and one of the lowest rates of heart disease in the United States. In Chad's case, merely cutting down the sodium and increasing the potassium worked. But, in any case, isn't this what scientists call anecdotal evidence, and therefore worthless?

Before 1900, humans lived in a low-sodium, high-potassium, relatively high-magnesium world—a world where plant foods, such as whole grains, fruits, and vegetables, appeared at every meal and processed foods were not available. We evolved in a world of plant foods that are naturally low in sodium and high in potassium and magnesium. In fact, in the natural world, sodium is difficult to get. Have you seen dairy cows come to lick the salt bars the farmers leave out for them? They get so much potassium eating grass and foliage that they need to supplement their diet with sodium to maintain a proper sodium/potassium balance. If we were living as our forebears did, as hunter-gatherers, we might need more sodium too. It surely wouldn't be available at the local grocery shops. In such cultures, sodium salt is a rare and precious commodity. Our kidneys bear the evidence of our environmental history in that they actually retain sodium while letting potassium pass out in the urine. The average kidney can slow the loss of sodium to a tiny 10 milligrams per day if it is in short supply. But the daily minimum potassium loss can be as high as 240 milligrams, twenty-four times that of sodium. The kidneys' ability to retain magnesium falls between the two. Even if there is a deficiency of magnesium, there is an obligatory loss through the urine of a little more magnesium than that of sodium, but if the blood level of magnesium rises above the normal upper limit, the kidneys excrete it at a great rate.

Our bodies invest an enormous amount of energy in balancing sodium with potassium. Keeping potassium inside cells and sodium out of them is an energy-consuming process that supports normal life functions. If there is not enough potassium relative to sodium, the ability to keep potassium inside the cells is overwhelmed, and sodium begins to replace the cellular potassium. The body now has to continue to expend energy trying to achieve the higher level of potassium within cells, which requires a constant supply of enzymes to pump sodium out and potassium in. The enzyme needed for this work is adenosine triphosphatase (ATPase), which is one of the many enzymes that are dependent on magnesium (see page 11)—and many of us do not obtain enough magnesium or potassium from our salt-heavy diets to maintain a normal sodium-potassium-magnesium relationship. To rid potassium- and magnesium-low bodies of excess sodium, doctors prescribe diuretics,

Most of us have a low-potassium, low-magnesium, high-sodium diet.

medications designed to cause sodium excretion by increasing the production of urine.

Today more and more of us are in a low-potassium state compared with our sodium intake, and our magnesium status is also precarious, as can be seen in table 3.2.

As you can see, since 1900 the average sodium:potassium ratio has increased seventy-five-fold and the sodium:magnesium ratio has increased fifty-fold. Instead of taking in thirty times more potassium than sodium each day, we are getting more than twice as much sodium as potassium. We eat few fresh fruits and vegetables and a lot of pure sodium chloride (table salt), plus processed foods that are liberally

Table 3.2 Changes in Average Mineral Intake, Mineral Ratios in the Diet, and Hypertension

This table shows the change in the average mineral intake and balances that has occurred among the American population between 1900 and 2000. Note the great rise in sodium and the decline in both magnesium and potassium—and the rise in the incidence of high blood pressure that accompanied these changes.

Indicator	1900	2000
Average daily sodium intake	200 mg	5,000 mg (25 times higher than in 1900)
Average daily potassium intake	6,000 mg	2,000 mg (⅔ lower than in 1900)
Average daily magnesium intake	400 mg	250–300 mg (¼–⅜ lower than in 1900)
Average sodium:potassium ratio	1:30	2.5:1 (75 times higher)
Average sodium:magnesium ratio	1:2	25:1 (50 times higher)
Incidence of hypertension	Low	High

salted. Our cells valiantly try to keep all this sodium out, but are handicapped by not having enough potassium inside them to do the job. And the amount of magnesium needed to keep enzymes functioning at optimum levels, so as to maintain the appropriate sodium:potassium ratio, is not supplied by the diet many of us consume.

High blood pressure is the body's way of trying to help with this situation. When the sodium:potassium ratio is too high, the body tries to get rid of the excess sodium via the kidneys, even though they are better at conserving sodium than eliminating it. With higher blood pressure, more blood flows through the kidneys, and their limited ability to excrete sodium is fully utilized. Unfortunately, this process spills out the precious potassium, too, since the kidneys do not naturally conserve potassium as they do sodium. The result is chronic high blood pressure. When Chad hit age forty after living on a high-salt, low-potassium diet all his life, the natural result was high blood pressure. Restricting his sodium intake would help somewhat, in that it would lower the sodium:potassium ratio. But this dictated such a drastic lifestyle change that Chad couldn't keep it up day after day. When he started using the half-sodium/half-potassium salt, he was essentially supplementing his potassium without having to take a pill. With enough potassium in his system, he was able to balance the sodium in his diet properly, and his high blood pressure normalized.

In 1928, decades before the advent of any medications for high blood pressure, Dr. W.L.T. Addison, a practicing physician in Toronto, published a now-classic study showing that potassium lowers blood pressure and sodium raises it. He worked with individuals, carefully measuring their blood pressure while giving them large amounts of either sodium chloride or potassium chloride, alternately. Whenever he administered the sodium salt, the blood pressure went up. Whenever he administered the potassium salt, it went down. To make sure the chloride part of the salts was not in play, he repeated the experiment, with the same results, using potassium and sodium bromide. With such clear results, why didn't potassium salts become an accepted treatment for high blood pressure? Admittedly, Dr. Addison studied only a few subjects—too few to qualify as a significant standard ac-

Low potassium, coupled with too much sodium, can cause high blood pressure.

cording to modern statistical standards. And it was not a double-blind investigation. But this was acceptable in his day. In most cases, the subject and the doctor both knew when sodium or potassium was being administered. So it could be argued that their knowledge and expectation might have had an effect on resulting blood pressure. Not such a far-fetched idea, and reason enough, in this day of modern statistical studies, to be unconvinced by Addison's work. But it is not reason enough to totally disregard his findings.

In the early 1930s, another Canadian researcher, W. W. Priddle, lowered the high blood pressure of 100 percent of his forty-five subjects with a therapy that combined a low-sodium diet with potassium citrate supplements. Why didn't this approach take hold? Richard Moore and George Webb, in their excellent book *The K Factor,* postulate that medical students of this period—and up to the present—have been taught that potassium is very dangerous. Any doctor so taught and wishing first to do no harm would be reluctant to give patients potassium, regardless of what Drs. Addison and Priddle found. Additionally, the work of neither investigator is well known in medical circles and it is not widely taught in medical schools. So we have to accept that past history and go on to modern studies testing potassium's effect on high blood pressure. If you ask most doctors today, they will tell you that studies show potassium supplements cannot lower blood pressure. This is true for people with normal blood pressure. Like magnesium, potassium supplements will not lower *normal* blood pressure. But potassium supplements *do* lower high blood pressure.

Magnesium and Potassium in the Regulation of Blood Pressure

Okay, you say. I need more potassium, not just less salt or sodium. But what does all this have to do with magnesium? A good question. Early nutrition studies in humans found that magnesium deficiency lowered potassium levels in the blood even if potassium intake was high. At the same time, the amount of sodium in the blood remained normal. These two trends yielded a higher sodium/potassium ratio even though potassium and sodium intakes were acceptable. Only the magnesium intake was low. If the magnesium was replenished, potassium status became normal—and *all* of this took place while potassium intake was adequate. Thus, it is safe to assume that if Chad's diet had been deficient in magnesium, the potassium-containing salt substitute would not have lowered his high blood pressure.

Much of the essential hypertension in today's society is due to low-potassium diets that provide too much salt. But low-magnesium states, which are becoming more and more common, make adequate amounts of potassium unavailable to the body, even if potassium consumption itself *is* adequate, and this also causes high blood pressure. It also causes more heart disease—not because of the high blood pressure, but because of the low magnesium state.

Low magnesium causes a low-potassium state, even if potassium intake is adequate. If magnesium is adequate, extra potassium can normalize high blood pressure.

With this new knowledge, let's evaluate current medical treatment for high blood pressure.

Current Treatments for Hypertension

The current medical approaches try to lower blood pressure with drugs in order to lower the risk of heart disease. A population survey analysis suggests that lowering blood pressure by as little as 2.0 millimeters of mercury (2 points) could reduce the risk of coronary artery disease by 6 percent and that of strokes and ischemic attacks by 15 percent. Yet does this approach really lessen heart disease? If one lowers a high blood pressure without bringing the magnesium and/or potassium status up to normal, will risk of heart disease go down? The answer to this question is no! Instead of feeling better, people who take antihypertensive medications often suffer from numerous side effects that make them feel far from well. Worse, some people who are treated with medications for hypertension are actually at greater risk for heart disease if their magnesium loss is ignored than those with the same blood pressure who remain untreated. In fact, lowering blood pressure while ignoring magnesium can be dangerous. The following is some evidence from scientific studies:

- The Multiple Risk Factor Intervention Trial (MR FIT) of 1982, when published, was a bombshell. It showed that, among people with moderate hypertension, there was no reduction in the death rate among those who were treated "successfully" (in that their blood pressure was lowered) with medications. But people with mild hypertension who were treated with medications had *increased* death rates. These two groups make up about half of all people with hypertension. So this study was a jolting wake-up call indicating that medications do not help and could even hurt half of those who are taking them, even if they lower blood pressure.
- L. H. Lindholm of Lund University Health Sciences Center in Dalby, Sweden, writing in 1991, reported "a high remaining risk of cardiovascular disease, even though the hypertensive patients have been well cared for and their blood pressure controlled."
- An article in the prestigious medical journal *Lancet* in 1999 stated: "Most cases of myocardial infarction and stroke attributable to blood pressure occur at levels of blood pressure below those defined as clinical hypertension," and heart attacks and stroke "among the small proportion of the population at high risk of cardiovascular disease—those with essential hypertension—are outnumbered by those cases that arise among the large number of people at moderate risk." In other words, most cases of heart attack and stroke occurred in people whose blood pressure was in the normal range.

These findings indicate that even successful treatment of hypertension does not reduce the risk of cardiovascular disease. Nevertheless, current medical treatment tries to lower high blood pressure by recommending the use of one or both of two basic approaches:

1. Antihypertensive medications
2. Diet and/or lifestyle changes

What do these treatments do? Are they safe? Given what we now know about the magnesium and potassium factors, do they actually achieve their therapeutic objectives?

Medications for Hypertension

In one way or another, antihypertensive medications replace only one of magnesium's natural functions. In contrast, magnesium has many antihypertensive actions. It is a beta-blocker (it blocks the action of the stress hormone adrenaline, which raises blood pressure), a vasodilator (relaxes blood vessels), and a calcium-channel blocker (inhibits the flow of calcium into cells)—all properties possessed, individually, by different categories of antihypertensive drugs—all in one. Magnesium also has a calming effect on people with anxiety, a desirable effect because emotional stress increases the production of adrenaline. And whereas each antihypertensive drug acts selectively, usually at one site, magnesium acts at all sites in vascular smooth muscle. Furthermore, magnesium is central to the regulation and control of blood vessels' contraction and relaxation. The physiologic magnesium/calcium balance allows blood vessel muscles to relax. A normal ratio between these two minerals also keeps the heart from overresponding to nerve or hormonal stimulation. Maintaining adequate magnesium levels is the best way to achieve these effects. Antihypertensive medications may mask the symptoms of deficiency of magnesium without replenishing it. Some even make the deficiency worse by increasing loss of magnesium in the urine.

In 1957, a class of medications known as thiazide diuretics became available to treat hypertension, reflecting the beginning of a multibillion-dollar-a-year business, with drugs such as chlorothiazide (Diuril), hydrochlorothiazide (HydroDIURIL), and indapamide (Lozol), among others. More antihypertensive medications were designed, and the pharmacological treatment of hypertension became standard. By 1999, over half of Americans and Europeans with diagnosed hypertension were receiving antihypertensive medications. In about half of those treated with these drugs, the high blood pressure was controlled. But it seems that:

1. Patients presumably must take these medications for life, yet
2. The medications don't always work

The growing awareness that hypertension is often a part of metabolic syndrome X further challenges doctors to lower high blood pressure without making other aspects of the syndrome (such as high triglycerides, low HDL ["good"] cholesterol and/or high blood sugar) worse. In addition, with medication side effects such as weakness, diarrhea, nausea, and loss of sex drive, their patients just do not feel good. Besides, the risk of malpractice suits if a doctor does not use the conventional treatments and a lack of better alternatives keep doctors prescribing the growing arsenal of antihypertension medications. Might taking advantage of evidence from the magnesium and potassium research allow for improved patient care?

Diuretics

Diuretics, or water pills, are usually the first prescription medication patients are given to manage high blood pressure. These drugs increase the excretion of water and salt in the urine, lowering the total blood volume and thus the blood pressure. They work especially well in salt-sensitive hypertensive individuals, but since it is difficult to determine who is truly salt sensitive (special tests are needed to detect salt sensitivity), doctors prescribe them for almost all people with high blood pressure. There are side effects, the most important for the sake of our discussion being the loss of potassium and magnesium along with the sodium. The long-term use of diuretics increases the chance of heart arrhythmia (irregular heartbeat) due to low serum potassium and magnesium, which occurs in 10 to 50 percent of those who take them. Because serum potassium is a good determinant of the body's status, replenishing potassium that is low as a result of taking diuretics is common practice. Serum magnesium, however, is not a reliable index of its deficiency, so its replenishment is less common, even though magnesium deficiency also can be intensified by diuretic therapy. Diuretics were studied in the MR FIT trials on 12,800 hypertensive men. This study found that thiazide diuretics lower blood pressure but do not decrease the death rate among people with moderate hypertension. For those with mild hypertension, the death rate actually increased. In response to this knowledge, so-called *potassium-sparing diuretics* were developed, and most diuretics prescribed today are given with potassium-sparing drugs such as amiloride and triamterene. These allow sodium loss but retain potassium. Some potassium-sparing diuretics also spare magnesium, but others cause it to be lost. Perhaps this is why the long-term use of these drugs has been shown to increase the incidence of heart failure.

The medical value of diuretics cannot be negated. The MR FIT study showed that people with hypertension who had diastolic blood pressures (the second number in the standard blood-pressure reading) above 100 benefited from their use, and the strong loop diuretics ethacrynic acid (Ectecrin) and furosemide (Lasix, Myrosemide), which actually cause even more magnesium loss, are essential for people with very severe hypertension and/or severe fluid retention. It is people with mild and moderate hypertension who either are not helped or who are made worse by the long-term use of these drugs. We suggest that nutritional adequacy be the first priority for such individuals, before or with drug therapy, because long-term benefit is not achievable if a nutritional magnesium deficiency exists.

A 1986 review from Australia by M. J. Field and J. R. Lawrence showed that this was especially true for older adults treated for high blood pressure with diuretics. These people experienced a number of complications, half of them associated with further loss of potassium. The most serious resulting problems of the treated elderly patients were cardiac—which the investigators blamed on several metabolic changes, but especially on magnesium loss. They made reference to work from Sweden by T. Dyckner and P. O. Wester that showed that cellular magnesium was lowered by diuretic treatment and that adding magnesium to the treatment improved the lowering of blood pressure and also protected against cardiac arrhythmias caused by diuretic-induced low levels of both potassium and magnesium.

Diuretics can make glucose tolerance and dyslipidemia worse, so they are not appropriate for the treatment of hypertension that is part of metabolic syndrome X. (See chapter 2.)

Beta-Blockers

If diuretics are not enough to lower a person's blood pressure, inhibiters of the hormone adrenaline, such as beta-blockers, are used. Beta-blockers slow the heart rate and keep blood volume low, thus decreasing blood pressure. These antihypertensive drugs decrease the demands on the heart by reducing its workload and are useful after a heart attack. But their slowing of heart rate and cardiac output can lead to fatigue and a less efficient heart. Additionally, their long-term use can lead to higher blood levels of triglycerides and lower levels of HDL ("good cholesterol") in the blood, both of which are seen in metabolic syndrome X. (See chapter 2).

Magnesium is a natural beta-blocker—one without the side effects caused by drugs with this activity. It is worth determining whether adequate magnesium might reduce the need for artificial beta-blockers. Beta-blocker medications can have side effects, including impaired circulation, palpitations, dizziness, nausea, and slight constriction of airways, but most important, they cannot supply the magnesium-deficient body with the nutrient so necessary for healthy cardiovascular function. There is some evidence that the side effects of some beta-blockers can be reduced by taking magnesium, but clinical studies of whether magnesium supplements might make it possible to decrease the dosage of beta-blockers needed remain to be done.

Lowering blood pressure with drug treatment does not improve an inadequate magnesium or potassium status.

A word of warning: You should

not stop taking beta-blocker medication suddenly. Discontinuation of these drugs must be done gradually and under the care of a physician. Suddenly stopping could bring on a heart attack.

Alpha-Blockers

Alpha-blockers act similarly to beta-blockers, by interfering with signals from the nervous system that speed up and intensify heart contractions. They block the type of receptors known as alpha receptors, which respond to adrenaline. Since alpha receptors are found in both the heart and blood vessels, these drugs cause the heart to beat with less force as well as causing blood vessels to relax rather than to contract.

Angiotensin-Converting Enzyme (ACE) Inhibitors and Angiotensin Blockers

Angiotensin II is another hormone that increases constriction of the arteries, causing retention of sodium and loss of magnesium and potassium. If the action of angiotensin is blocked, the result is both relaxation of arteries and sparing of magnesium and potassium, as well as a loss of sodium—both desirable effects in people with high blood pressure.

A very interesting study of ninety-six subjects with high blood pressure, reported by A. Haenni and colleagues at the Department of Geriatrics of Uppsala University in Sweden showed that ACE-inhibitor treatment not only raised serum magnesium but also lowered serum calcium levels, lowered triglyceride levels, and decreased insulin resistance. These make this class of medications uniquely useful in treating cases of metabolic syndrome X with hypertension.

ACE inhibitors act by inhibiting the enzyme that converts a relatively inert form of angiotensin to angiotensin II, a potent arterial constrictor. Angiotensin-blocking agents act by blocking the cell receptors for angiotensin II. Since magnesium also relaxes arteries, using it together with these inhibitors of angiotensin might well enhance their beneficial effects, perhaps making it possible to use lower doses of these expensive drugs. However, as tempting as it is to recommend combining magnesium with angiotensin inhibitors on the basis of logic, we have not found published articles on such combined usage. *Note:* You should always consult with your physician if you are considering modifying your use of any prescribed medication.

Vasodilators and Central Adrenergic Inhibitors

Vasodilators act directly on arterial muscle cells to relax them, causing the vessels to dilate. Central adrenergic inhibitors, which block signals from the brain that instruct arteries to narrow and the heart to speed up, are occasionally prescribed for hypertension.

Each of these types of drugs functions to relax blood vessel muscles in order to lower high blood pressure. Replacing deficient magnesium achieves vasodilation as one of magnesium's activities.

Calcium-Channel Blockers

Calcium channel blockers prevent the influx of calcium into tiny channels in artery cells. When these channels are filled with calcium, blood-vessel muscles contract and increase blood pressure. Keeping excess calcium out of these channels allows artery walls to relax and expand, reducing blood pressure. The influx of calcium into cells is an important aspect of metabolic syndrome X, for when cellular magnesium gets too low, calcium rises to abnormally high levels inside the cells. Magnesium is a natural calcium-channel blocker; as long as there is adequate magnesium inside cells, damaging calcium influx does not occur. The need for calcium-channel blockers arises from the breakdown of cell-membrane integrity, which is in turn caused by a magnesium deficiency.

The long-term use of calcium-channel–blocking drugs can be risky. One study found that people who took these drugs had 60 percent more heart attacks than people on beta-blockers or diuretics. To put this in context, of 1,000 people treated for hypertension, ten might be expected to have a heart attack in any given year. For those treated with calcium-channel blockers, the risk goes up to 16 out of 1,000.

The Effectiveness of Antihypertensive Medications

Before 1985, prescribing medications for people with high blood pressure was standard. However, such treatment has rarely been simple, and is effective for only half of those who try it. A doctor never knows how any individual is going to respond to a given drug for high blood pressure. The standard practice is often to start with diuretics and, if those don't work, to increase the dose or switch to another type of medication or to a combination of types. All the while, the physician needs to monitor the patient closely for the drug's effectiveness in lowering blood pressure and for the severity of side effects. And, alas, all the antihypertensive medications can have side effects—some of them severe. Since high blood pressure itself usually causes no symptoms, the fact that medications prescribed to treat it can suddenly cause adverse side effects can pose real problems for both patient and physician. If the inconvenience is bad enough, a person may stop taking the medications altogether, leaving the blood pressure to rise again (if, indeed, it was lowered in the first place). And we haven't even started to consider the cost of medication.

Lowering blood pressure with drug treatment does not always lower the risk of heart disease.

As a result of such complexities, some of which may be dangerous, and which must be weighed against the risk of a future event that may or may not happen, the medical community has been trying since 1985 to try nondrug approaches to essential hypertension. This means they want to control the blood pressure, and hopefully normalize it, without using drugs, and to do this they turn to diet and lifestyle changes that have been proven to lower blood pressure and are assumed to have no dangerous side effects. Can such an approach be effective?

Diet and Lifestyle Changes for Hypertension

The most common diet and lifestyle changes recommended for high blood pressure, in descending order, are admonitions to:

- Lose weight.
- Lower salt intake—"cut out the salt!"

- Lower fat intake—"cut out the fat!"
- Exercise.

Needless to say, successfully making such changes, especially on a consistent, long-term basis, is much harder than taking a pill. Books abound on how to make these changes. They can improve health and have been proven effective in studies. But they are not easy. They go against the current of what's around us and put us on a seemingly upstream swim that we are supposed to maintain for a lifetime. Some who can make these changes and adhere to them do lower their high blood pressure and otherwise improve their health. But many fail in the attempt and become frightened, discouraged, and depressed, and feel guilty and stressed. Might taking magnesium help to achieve the desired objectives?

Does Weight Loss Improve Hypertension?

We shall see in the next chapter how weight relates to magnesium status. People who go on weight-loss diets usually increase their consumption of fruits, vegetables, and whole grains while lowering their fat intake. This results in their increasing both potassium and magnesium consumption. For people on such weight-reduction diets, it is not so much their weight loss as enough improvement in magnesium (and potassium) status that normalizes their high blood pressure.

Is Salt Restriction Safer than Antihypertensive Medications?

Before 1980, doctors knew there was some relationship between sodium intake and blood pressure, but they were very cautious about recommending salt-restricted diets, and then only under a very watchful medical eye. This is because salt is a recognized nutrient, one we all need in order to live healthfully, and sometimes a low-salt diet can do more harm than good. One study found that moderate salt restriction caused a *rise* in blood pressure for 15 percent of subjects. This same study showed a rise in LDL ("bad" cholesterol), as well as disturbed sleep patterns, with sodium restriction. There is sodium, even in a salt-restricted diet, that comes from grains, dairy products, and meats, including poultry and fish. But restricting foods in these three groups also reduces the amounts of calcium, iron, magnesium and vitamin B_6 in the diet, since these same foods are primary sources of these nutrients. And we have to mention the disclosure of a small but significant association of low-salt diets and all causes of death, as well as an increased risk of heart attack in men on salt-restricted diets.

Salt is a wonderful preservative and has been used by humans for millennia. In any culture, salt is an important, even precious, commodity. In many traditional processes, salt is made from sea water. If the process includes total evaporation, this does not yield pure sodium chloride (table salt), but rather a salt rich in all the minerals of the sea—including magnesium and potassium, as well as trace minerals (see Appendix D: Magnesium in Salt Substitutes).

Sodium appears to be the only essential nutrient that, when low, actually causes craving. Sodium deprivation alters the taste response. Ever read in a recipe the phrase "Salt to taste"? We all have. Sodium is the only necessary nutrient for which this instruction makes any sense. We need at least 500 milligrams of sodium daily for life. Too little sodium is perhaps more of a problem than too much in most healthy people.

So the story on salt and hypertension is complicated, but when we consider our low intakes of both magnesium and potassium, the puzzle nears solution. Sodium and potassium must be in balance, or at least in a ratio that is not too high on the sodium side, and magnesium must be adequate for blood pressure to be normal. All three minerals are thus important for maintaining acceptable blood pressure. For a person with adequate amounts of tissue magnesium and potassium, almost no amount of salt is too much. It would take injections of sodium salt solution into the bloodstream to induce high blood pressure in such individuals. But even if dietary sodium and potassium are in balance, a low magnesium level can lay the groundwork for development of metabolic syndrome X—and, with it, hypertension. If magnesium status is normal and cellular magnesium balances well with cellular calcium, low potassium intake coupled with high salt intake can cause essential hypertension that is not associated with metabolic syndrome X.

Magnesium and Special Cases of Hypertension

So far, we have been considering essential hypertension and elevated blood pressure associated with metabolic syndrome X. There are also other forms of high blood pressure that create serious medical problems and that have also been associated with low levels of magnesium. The most common are preeclampsia and eclampsia, which are severe complications of abnormal pregnancy that cause not only severe illness and, sometimes, death in the mothers, but also premature births and increased risk of stillbirth. Magnesium deficiency and the efficacy of magnesium treatment have been proved in this form of hypertension. The prevalence of hypertension among African-Americans is responsible for their higher rates of heart disease and strokes than is seen in whites. Hypertension in blacks has not been as clearly associated with inadequacy of magnesium or response to magnesium, as it has in pregnancy, but there are hints that this might be so that call for further study. Let us look at each of these in turn.

Pregnancy-Induced Hypertension

The first use of magnesium for hypertension was in the first third of the twentieth century, in women with the very severe toxemia of pregnancy known as eclampsia. It became a standard of treatment in the United States and continental Europe for pregnancy-induced high blood pressure, and even for convulsions of eclampsia, ever since F. P. Zuspan of the Ohio State University College of Medicine, in the mid-1950s, showed magnesium injections to achieve better maternal and fetal outcomes than did antihypertensive and anticonvulsant drugs. Most American and a majority of continental European obstetricians use magnesium for these conditions, but in the United Kingdom, a 1992 paper reported that only 2 percent used magnesium for women with eclampsia. By 1995, a collaborative eclampsia trial confirmed the studies that had demonstrated the advantage of magnesium treatment in the United States forty years earlier. The delay in accepting the earlier work in England was termed a scandal in 1996.

A large international trial, run from Oxford University in England, compared intravenous infusions of magnesium with placebo infusions in over 10,000 women with preeclampsia to find out if magensium could prevent the development of the severe hypertension and convulsions of eclampsia. This was called the *Mag*nesium for *P*revention of *E*clampsia (MAGPIE) trial. Half were given magnesium and half were given placebo. The women who were given the magnesium had a 58 percent lower incidence of eclampsia than those who were not. Also recorded was the comparative condition of the infants born to the two groups of women. It is important to note that the incidence of preterm deliveries, low birth weight, and infant death was higher among the women who did not receive magnesium than it was among those who did. In view of these two studies, we assume that the use of magnesium in treating pregnant women with hypertension is increasing in England.

Hypertension in African-Americans

African-Americans have a higher incidence of hypertension than white Americans. Indeed, persons of African descent living in the Western hemisphere have the highest prevalence of hypertension in the world, and it causes at least twice the mortality as in American whites. Dietary salt (sodium chloride) is an important factor in this; an inability to prevent blood pressure from increasing to hypertensive levels in response to the comparatively high salt content of Western diets characterizes the majority of hypertensive African Americans. In addition, the chosen diet of this segment of the population tends to be very low in magnesium.

Both genetic and environmental factors have been hypothesized to explain the higher prevalence of hypertension in African-Americans than in both black people residing in western Africa and in white Americans. It has been speculated that the extreme conditions endured by enslaved people who were transported from Africa to the Americas favored the survival of salt-sensitive individuals. Continually subject to salt-depleting diseases such as diarrhea, fevers, and vomiting during their crowding in slave ships, individuals with a genetically based ability to conserve salt might have had a survival advantage and were, therefore, more likely to survive and bequeath their genotype to their descendants in the colonies. However, pointing to the role of magnesium and metabolic syndrome X in this population is the fact that obesity, glucose intolerance, insulin resistance, and hyperlipidemia, in addition to salt sensitivity, are associated with hypertension in African-Americans. Further, the chosen diet of this segment of the population tends to be very low in magnesium. It is possible that promoting the use of magnesium supplements by this segment of the American population might reduce their high rate of essential hypertension.

Nine Steps to Healthier Blood Pressure

For many people, high blood pressure can be corrected with enough magnesium and/or enough potassium. Also, healthy people with ample levels of magnesium and potassium have been shown to handle high-salt diets without developing high blood pressure. In fact, a high sodium chloride intake in these adults has been associated with the lowest blood pressure in the society. Given our current environment, how do we achieve this?

Putting Magnesium to Work for You

Programs for people with normal blood pressure who want to prevent heart disease will be outlined in chapter 11. If you have hypertension, however, the following program of action is for you:

1. Find out whether you have primary or secondary hypertension. Most people with high blood pressure have primary, or essential, hypertension (see pg. 40). However, some have hypertension not because of a lack of magnesium or potassium, but because of an underlying illness such as a tumor, kidney disease, or other condition. This is known as *secondary hypertension.* To lower the blood pressure to normal, such people must be treated for the predisposing factor. If your doctor has not already done so, see him or her to rule out secondary hypertension as a first step.

2. Determine if you have mild, moderate, severe, or refractory hypertension. The severity of your hypertension must dictate your program and determine how rapidly or slowly you can safely make changes. Work with your doctor and decide together to take the safe road to health. Take it one step at a time and regularly reassess your status with your doctor. If your blood pressure is dangerously high, do not refuse immediate drug therapy while you make long-term dietary changes. Trust your doctor while, together, you make a long-term commitment to change your magnesium and potassium status.
3. Determine whether your hypertension may be part of metabolic syndrome X by evaluating any risk factors you may have. Use other risk factors to decide how likely it is that your hypertension is part of metabolic syndrome X. Do you have low HDL cholesterol? A tendency to high blood glucose? Abdominal obesity? These other symptoms may or may not be present if your hypertension is caused by the low magnesium/calcium ratio seen in metabolic syndrome X. If some or all of the findings of metabolic syndrome X are present, you can be pretty sure that your magnesium status is low and that magnesium therapy will be helpful. If aspects of that syndrome (other than hypertension) are not present, you may have adequate magnesium status but a low potassium intake. If that is the case, switching to a potassium-containing salt, which will simultaneously lower your sodium intake, can make a big difference. But remember that magnesium is necessary to utilize potassium properly, and that hypertension and low magnesium can be present without any other symptoms of metabolic syndrome X.
4. Assess your medications. If your treatment for hypertension includes a potassium-sparing diuretic such as triamterene (Dyrenium) or spironolactone (Aldactone), you may want to consult your doctor about switching to another medication before supplementing your potassium. If you do not switch, be sure you and your physician monitor

Salt substitutes containing magnesium and/or potassium can help to prevent high blood pressure.

your plasma potassium closely so that it does not become dangerously high. If you are on a beta-blocker, consult your doctor before adding potassium because this type of drug can raise potassium levels. (See Appendix H: Common Medications that Affect Magnesium Status for a list of beta-blockers.) Beta-blockers reduce control of plasma potassium during potassium loading. The two are not a good mix. If you are on a thiazide or one of the stronger loop diuretics, you may want to switch to another type of medication since they cause the loss of both potassium and magnesium (see appendix H for a list of diuretics).

5. If possible, have your magnesium and potassium levels determined before starting treatment. The serum (blood) potassium level tends to reflect total body potassium and can serve you and your doctor as a benchmark with which to assess your program. If your potassium is low (below 4 milliequivalents per liter [mEq/L]), have it rechecked every two to three weeks until it is in the range of 4 to 5 mEq/L. Then you can have it checked monthly until all of your program changes are made and your potassium status is stable. Be aware, though, that there are other causes of low serum potassium besides inadequate intake. Go over these possibilities with your doctor. Determining magnesium status is more difficult, since the serum values do not reflect total body magnesium. As a result, other tests are necessary to get a true picture. These may include measuring cellular free magnesium (Mgi) by means of nuclear magnetic resonance (NMR), a magnesium load test, ion selective electrode (ISE) testing, and two proprietary tests—called the IMg2+ test and the Exatest. The latter two are particularly recommended. (These techniques will be discussed in detail in chapter 10.)
6. Fill out our Magnesium Status Questionnaire. Decide how important magnesium replacement is for you.
7. Replenish your potassium and magnesium—gradually! There are three ways to do this.
   - Diet
   - Magnesium-containing salts.
   - Magnesium supplements.

Table 3.3 Studies Showing the Effect of Vegetarian Diet and Magnesium-Containing Salts on High Blood Pressure

PanSalt is a compound of sodium, magnesium, and potassium. A lacto-ovo vegetarian diet excludes meat and poultry but permits eggs and dairy products in addition to all fruits, vegetables, grains, beans, and nuts.

Study No.	Magnesium Source	Effect on Blood Pressure
1	PanSalt	Drop
2	PanSalt	Drop in systolic blood pressure (the first measurement).
3	Lacto-ovo vegetarian diet	Drop

We recommend trying diet and, if necessary, magnesium-containing salts before resorting to magnesium supplements. Table 3.3 summarizes the results of studies showing that both a vegetarian diet and magnesium-containing salts can normalize high blood pressure.

Make dietary changes that work for you. You can raise your intake of both magnesium and potassium by including more fruits and vegetables in your diet. You can maximize the level of magnesium already in your diet by reducing the amounts of fat, sugar, and refined carbohydrates you eat and by making sure you don't take excessive amounts of vitamin D and calcium. You can also decrease your need for potassium by lowering the amount of sodium in your diet. (A program for making these changes is detailed in chapter 11.)

If dietary changes are unrealistic for you or do not give the desired result, you can change your potassium and magnesium status by using a salt substitute. If your magnesium questionnaire result shows you to be at risk for magnesium deficiency, try a salt substitute containing magnesium first. (See appendix D for a list of these salts and how to obtain them.) If results of your magnesium questionnaire show that your risk level for magnesium deficiency is very low and you still have hypertension, you may benefit from a potassium-containing salt substitute. Your goal should be to get 2,600 to 3,500 milligrams of potassium per day.

8. After a few weeks of dietary changes and/or salt substitute supplements, gradually start to lower the dosage of hypertension medication(s) you take. Do this in a series of steps, with a physician's supervision, monitoring your blood pressure as you go. Taper off the medications by decreasing your dose every one to four weeks, depending on your blood pressure. Again, work closely with a physician as you do this. Do not just do it on your own, and do not make sudden changes in blood pressure medications.
9. If necessary, add traditional nutritional supplements to your regimen. If using a salt substitute does not normalize your blood pressure or allow you to discontinue medications, you will need to add magnesium and/or potassium supplements. Keeping the changes you have already made, you can try adding 700 milligrams of magnesium per day, taken in divided doses with meals, and titrate (see page 53) up to 1,200 milligrams per day. Do this gradually, giving each dose several weeks to work, and be ready to back off a bit on the dosage if diarrhea results. With potassium, begin with 2,600 milligrams per day and titrate up to 3,600, again giving each dose at least three to six weeks to make a difference. Work with your doctor on this. Remember that if you have had hypertension for a very long time, you may not lower your blood pressure even as you bring your magnesium and potassium status into balance—but it is not the high blood pressure *per se* that causes heart disease, but the underlying magnesium deficiency. The risk of stroke and heart disease may be reduced by correcting your magnesium and/or potassium status, even if you continue to have some degree of high blood pressure. It is important to have your doctor's supervision if you reduce any medications you now take for hypertension. And again, the watchword here is *gradual change.* Do not add large doses of supplements or stop medications abruptly. Gradually improve your nutritional status and let your body normalize its

blood pressure as it is gradually weaned from the antihypertensive medications. If your blood pressure is too high to allow for complete cessation of medications, make sure the ones you are taking are not making your magnesium and/or potassium status worse. A word of caution here: If you have severe kidney disease (renal failure), *you must not take any magnesium and or potassium supplements.* In any case, you should not attempt to change your program and/or lifestyle drastically, suddenly, or without the supervision of a physician.

10. If you are completely off potassium- and magnesium-wasting medications, and if high blood pressure persists even after months of using appropriate salt substitutes and/or taking further supplements, and if your serum potassium is still below 4 mEq/L, you may need to try intramuscular injections to improve your magnesium status. You need to work with your doctor on this. (Guidelines for this treatment approach are discussed in appendix F.)

Can taking magnesium be dangerous? No. Even administering magnesium intravenously, which provides much more magnesium than you would take as a dietary supplement, is generally quite safe, although intravenous infusion can sometimes inadvertently cause serum magnesium to go above normal ranges. But this method is increasingly being used in hospitals without causing harm. Milk of magnesia (magnesium hydroxide) has been sold over the counter and used safely by millions of people for 125 years. The dose recommended as a laxative—1,000 to 2,000 milligrams of magnesium for adults—is higher than any oral supplement levels recommended in this book. Used as an antacid, the recommended dose of milk of magnesia provides 165 to 500 milligrams of magnesium. These are the levels generally recommended in this book. High doses of oral magnesium supplements have a laxative effect, and if you absorb more magnesium than your body needs, healthy kidneys rapidly pass any excess into the urine, and it is excreted. Although it is best to get all our nutrients, including magnesium, from foods, this often is not feasible, and oral magnesium supplements are very safe (unless you have kidney failure). Too-low intakes of magnesium, in contrast, *are* dangerous. Without enough magnesium, many serious disorders can develop in the heart, arteries, and other tissues.

What about taking potassium? When potassium is given intravenously in a hospital, infusing too much too fast can cause the heart's rhythm to become abnormal. This is, obviously, very dangerous. Oral potassium supplements also can be dangerous for people with kidney disease, and ordinary potassium-containing pills can cause stomach and intesinal ulcers. These pose no danger for people with normal kidney function. Even over the long term, a high intake of potassium from foods is not associated with any chronic problems. An intake of 3,500 milligrams per day is beneficial to health. A twelve-year study on women over the age of fifty showed that those who got less than 1,900 milligrams of potassium per day had a stroke rate of over 5 per 100. Those who consumed between 1,900 and 2,600 milligrams of potassium per day had an incidence of stroke of only 2 per 100. Those with potassium intakes of more than 2,600 milligrams per day had *no strokes at all.* Similar results have been seen in men. A person who eats a chronically low-potassium diet or suffers from low-potassium status due to medications he or she is taking is at increased risk for stroke and heart disease. Being potassium-deficient is clearly more dangerous than taking potassium supplements.

All in all, the program outlined above is generally quite safe. However, it is important to always remember that everyone is different. Even though research findings tell us that 90 to 95 percent of people with mild to moderate primary, essential hypertension can normalize their blood pressure if they get the right amounts of magnesium and potassium for a long enough time, research does not tell us how much of each nutrient any given individual needs. Nor does it tell us how long it will take any one person to replenish his or her stores of potassium and/or magnesium. An additional complication is that, obviously, for 5 to 10 percent of people with primary hypertension, this will not work. In one early study in which individual subjects' blood pressure were provided (rather than just the average of all subjects, as is often the case), one person's reacton was just the opposite of everyone else's. So there are what researchers call "unusual responders," and if you are one of them, it is best that you and your physician know that exceptions exist. Studies may not include unusual responders in their results. But if you are one of the few whose responses differ from those of most people, more careful evaluation may prove necessary as you take measures to restore your magnesium status. Also, you should *not* attempt to change your lifestyle and nutritional or medical programs drastically, suddenly, or without your physician's advice.

Our knowledge of the role of insufficient magnesium in cardiovascular disease tells us that hypertension, a known risk factor for heart disease, might well result from low intakes of magnesium and potassium, coupled with a high intake of sodium. Further, the findings of many studies indicate that it is not high blood pressure *per se,* but rather the underlying magnesium deficiency associated with it that makes people with hypertension so vulnerable to cardiovascular disease. Correcting high blood pressure without correcting an existing magnesium deficiency cannot and will not prevent cardiovascular disease. It may even make things worse if side effects of medications or the high stress due to an individual's inability to make prescribed dietary and lifestyle changes end up increasing the severity of the underlying nutritional deficiency.

4

Obesity, Physical Activity, and Magnesium

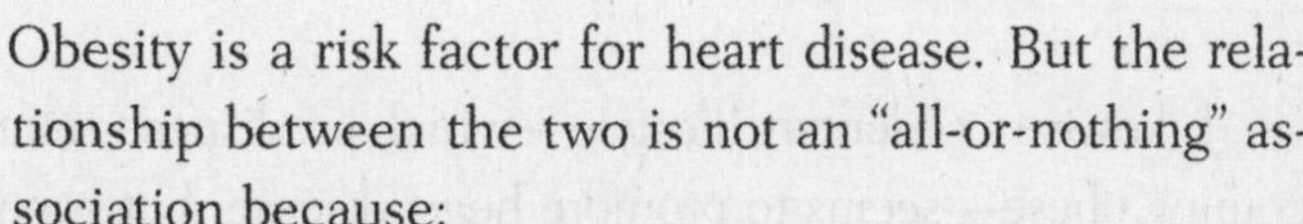

Obesity is a risk factor for heart disease. But the relationship between the two is not an "all-or-nothing" association because:

- Not all fat people have heart disease
- Not all people with heart disease are fat

As one example, Dave Alexander has successfully finished 276 triathlons since 1983, even though he is considered obese at five feet eight inches and 260 pounds. Even people with body weights in the recommended range have a 25 to 35 percent chance of getting heart disease. And, for those in the obese category, that risk climbs—but to 37 to 46 percent, not 100 percent.

Figure 4.1 Obesity as a Risk Factor for Heart Disease

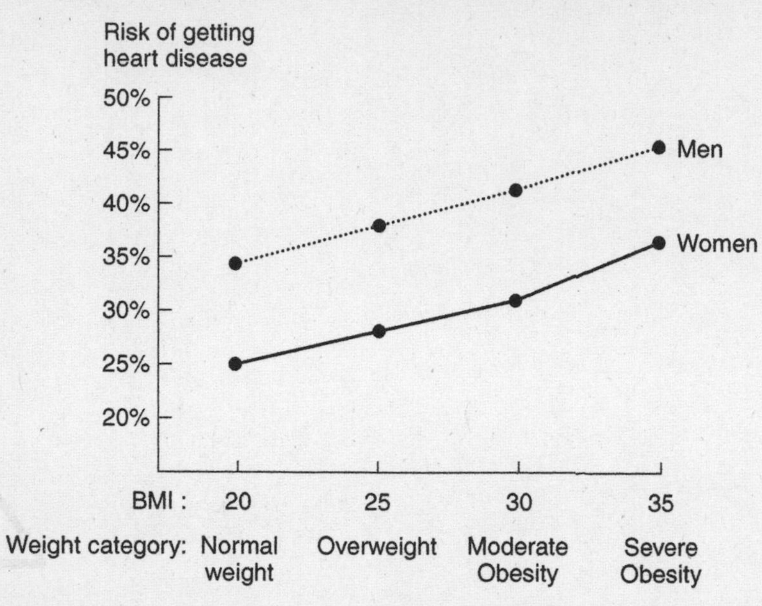

This graph represents the way in which the incidence of heart disease increases as the degree of overweight (as defined by body mass index, or BMI, which takes account of height and weight) increases.

Adapted from American Heart Association, "Lifetime Risks and Costs of Heart Disease Much Higher for Obese," American Heart Disease Abstract 2519, 10 October 1998.

Likewise a sedentary lifestyle—which predisposes many people to becoming obese—seems to promote heart disease, but even active athletes sometimes die of heart failure. Consider these seeming anomalies:

- Ex–National Football League quarterback Joe Gilliam, Jr., died of a heart attack when his fitness level was at near the highest of his life.
- It is rare, but 1 out of 100,000 young athletes die of heart disease each year.

These less than bold associations belie the prevailing view in our modern industrialized culture that being too fat and inactive makes a

Fit or unfit, fat or thin, you can still have a magnesium deficit. Or not.

person a "heart attack waiting to happen." For many, weight loss and exercise seem as imperative as they are elusive. The reality is that our modern diet, so high in processed foods, promotes *both* magnesium deficiency and obesity. Obesity often occurs with a magnesium deficit, but not always. Lean people who eat the typical modern diet can have magnesium deficits, too. Low magnesium is the link with heart disease. Let's see how obesity and magnesium deficit are interrelated, and how physical exercise influences both.

How Processed Foods Take Out Magnesium and Increase Calories

Food processing separates plant food sources into components, then remixes these components into tasty, processed food. Often, magnesium is removed during the separation process, and rarely if ever is it replaced during remixing. In the case of oils from seeds, olives, corn, peanuts, and other sources, the loss of magnesium is complete. These refined oils appear in our foods as unsaturated oils (olive, canola, corn, and other oils) and as hydrogenated or partially hydrogenated oils (in margarine and vegetable shortening). All of these refined fats and oils have almost or absolutely no magnesium. Butter, which is essentially refined milkfat, also is very low in magnesium. White wheat flour, a major staple of our processed-food diets, is made by refining out wheat bran and germ, which not only lowers the magnesium content by 80 percent, it also increases calories by just under 7 percent. This may not seem like much, but over a lifetime, 7 percent more calories can make a big difference. A similar trend can be seen in the refining of granulated sugar.

These and other refined food staples are mixed and remixed to make a vast array of tasty, processed foods. Such remixing allows for addition of oil or other fats and/or sugar to enhance taste. This adds more calories, but not more magnesium.

Processed foods have magnesium separated out but not put back in.

The hardening of oils to make margarines or lardlike or butterlike fats—making them useful as spreads or for use in baking, and increasing their shelf life—requires hydrogenation, a chemical step that adds hydrogen to the oils. This alters the molecular structure of the oils and may improve taste, but it also increases the risks to the heart and arteries, even more than do the extra calories provided by the oils.

The Consequence of Overeating Refined Foods

With the delicious concoctions of processed flour, sugar, and oil, and other fatty ingredients always around us, designed to please our taste buds, few people can say no for long. As we consume more sugar, more calories, and less magnesium, those of us with a genetic susceptibility respond by becoming overweight, or even obese, while at the same time developing magnesium deficiencies. What's more, the more refined flour, sugar, and fat we eat, the more magnesium we need and the less likely we are to get it in adequate amounts. If restaurant, homemade, or store-bought food contains fat, refined flour, and/or sugar as one or more of the major ingredients, it is a low-magnesium, and quite possibly a high-calorie, food. A steady diet of such foods, year after year, can produce magnesium deficit and, with it, metabolic syndrome X—a major factor in heart disease (see chapter 2). No wonder that, as processed food becomes available to more and more peoples of the world, obesity and cardiovascular disease have become a general, worldwide problem.

Eating a diet rich in refined sugar, fat, and refined white flour predisposes us to obesity and, in some people, even to metabolic syndrome X. In chapter 2, we presented evidence that magnesium deficiency, leading to low cellular magnesium, is the intrinsic characteristic—and probably the underlying cause—of metabolic syndrome X, which is also characterized by insulin resistance. Let us consider how the food culprits we are implicating relate to the magnesium deficit that underlies the syndrome.

Refined sugar and fat provide no magnesium, and refined white flour provides precious little. The body reacts to high blood sugar (glucose, stemming mostly from the sugar we eat, but also from other

A diet rich in refined sugar, fat, and refined white flour predisposes us to obesity.

carbohydrates, such as flour) by secreting insulin. As the insulin helps the circulating glucose enter the cells, the blood glucose level falls. This process can create cravings for more sugar—which, if eaten, sets the cycle going again. The cells, being fed with more and more glucose, store it as a complex sugar called *glycogen,* and then convert it into fat, if you take in more calories than you need to meet your immediate needs.

While this is going on, the kidneys do their best to rid the body of the excess glucose. The trouble is that the excretion of magnesium increases along with the increased urinary glucose. This can compound the risk of magnesium deficiency created by eating magnesium-poor foods. Now the body's cells develop the low cellular magnesium level that characterizes metabolic syndrome X. Further, magnesium normally helps the cells to respond to insulin, but if there isn't enough magnesium, the insulin is unable to assist in the cellular uptake of glucose. The result is that we now have the beginnings of insulin resistance, another prime characteristic of metabolic syndrome X.

It probably takes a genetic vulnerability to react to dietary indiscretions in these ways. But because of their cravings, people with such an innate susceptibility tend to eat too much of precisely those foods that are causing their problems. For such people, living in a society faced with an abundance of readily available foods that are high in these and other refined staples, overweight and obesity *is almost inevitable.* Since low magnesium is the key to metabolic syndrome X, with its risks of heart disease, we can see how a diet rich in refined foods can promote magnesium deficiency and, with it, obesity and metabolic syndrome X. Obesity *per se* does not cause this syndrome, but it often goes along with it and can worsen its complications (see figure 4.2).

A diet of highly processed foods promotes both obesity *and* magnesium deficit.

When people diet to lose weight, they often consume less fat and less sugar while adding foods that are fiber-rich, such as whole grains, beans (legumes), fruits, and vegetables, all of which are rich in magnesium. Such a diet provides not only more magnesium but also fewer calories. Many researchers and much of the medical community assume that the resulting weight loss is what lessens the clinical signs of metabolic syndrome X or heart disease. This contributes to

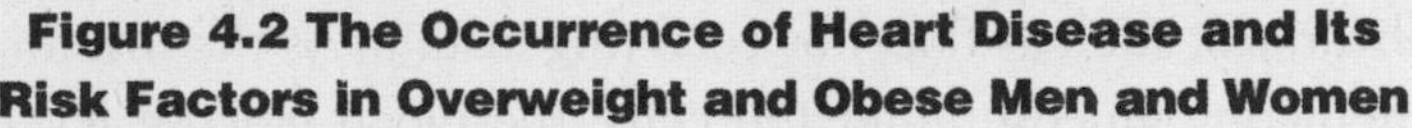

Figure 4.2 The Occurrence of Heart Disease and Its Risk Factors in Overweight and Obese Men and Women

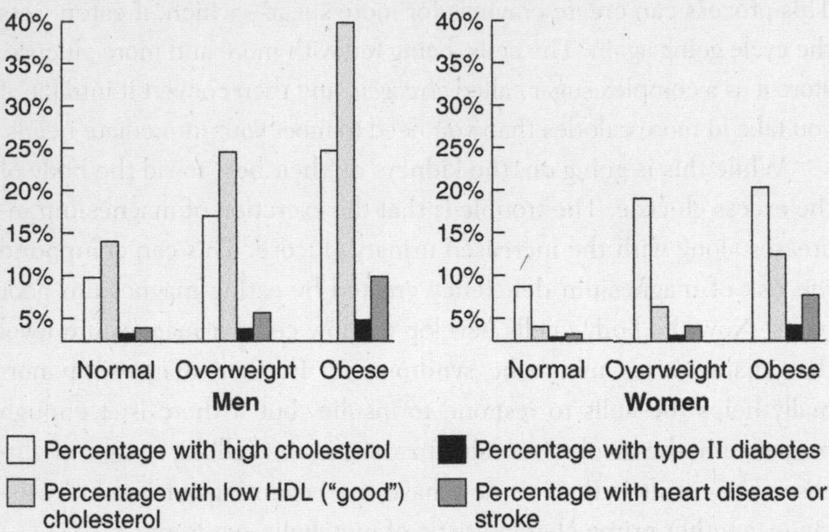

The graphs above show the percentages of men and women, respectively, who are of normal weight, overweight, and obese and who also have high total blood cholesterol, low HDL ("good") cholesterol, type II diabetes, and heart disease or stroke. Across the board, the occurrence of heart disease and its risk factors are clearly higher in the overweight and obese than in those of normal weight.

Adapted from M.E. Lean, "Pathophysiology of Obesity," *Proceedings of the Nutrition Society* 59(3) (August 2000): 331–336.

the improvement, but replenishing his or her cellular magnesium content is the major factor that results in improvement.

Abdominal Obesity, Heart Disease, and Magnesium

It is the laying down of *abdominal* fat that relates most obesity to heart disease and metabolic syndrome X. In the past twelve years, researchers have discovered that obesity of the abdomen is much more closely associated with metabolic syndrome X and cardiovascular disease than is overall obesity. This type of obesity is called *abdominal obesity, central obesity, visceral obesity,* and several other names—including *apple fat,* because people with this type of fat deposition (seen predominantly in men) have a torso profile that resembles the shape of an apple, in contrast to the most common pattern of fat deposition in women, which results in a body profile that is more like the shape of a pear. Of the 10 to 15 percent of the population who have metabolic syndrome X, as many as 70 percent can be identified by their waist measurement alone. Abdominal obesity becomes more prevalent with age and with the degree of overweight. Your waist measurement tells you if you have abdominal obesity (see table 4.1). This is much more a risk factor for heart disease than is overall obesity because it is so much more associated with the insulin resistance and high blood insulin of metabolic syndrome X.

Studies show that abdominal obesity is associated with low levels of magnesium, zinc, and vitamins C and E. There is also a very telling study of men with heart disease or heart disease risk factors who were on low-fat diets. The subjects were divided into two groups. Both

Table 4.1 Waist Measurement and Health Risk

If you know both your waist measurement and your body mass index (BMI), a measure of your weight as related to your height, you can determine whether you have abdominal obesity as a risk factor for heart disease and metabolic syndrome X.

BMI Measurement*	Waist Size (in Inches)		Risk Category
	Men	Women	
20–25	less than 37**	less than 31½**	Healthy
25–30	37–40	31½–34½	Some risk
above 30	above 40	more than 34½	High risk

*Instructions for determining your BMI can be found on page 100.

**Note that this table does not include a *lowest* "safe" waist measurement for either men or women—but you *can* be too thin! (*See* Do You Really Need to Lose Weight? starting on page 98.)

Adapted from: M.E. Lean, "Pathophysiology of Obesity," *Proceedings of the Nutrition Society* 59(3) (August 2000): 331–336.

groups were advised to follow a somewhat lower fat diet. One group was also advised to eat almost a pound of fruits and vegetables each day and to get a little exercise. It is safe to assume that the fruit-and-vegetable group were consuming more magnesium, as well as potassium, zinc, and vitamin C. After three years, those advised to exercise and eat vegetables and fruits had reduced their abdominal obesity 80 percent more than those on the low-fat diet alone. The addition of exercise and fruits and vegetables also resulted in lower blood pressures and weight; lower levels of glucose, insulin, triglycerides, and LDLs ("bad cholesterol"); and fewer symptoms caused by coronary artery constriction (angina) or heart attacks. They also gave rise to higher levels of HDLs ("good cholesterol"). These facts support the idea that the low magnesium, at the core of metabolic syndrome X is a factor in abdominal obesity. When the diet provides adequate magnesium and other micronutrients, abdominal obesity is reduced.

Abdominal Obesity, Insulin Resistance, and Magnesium Deficiency

Researchers have found that the abdominal area of the body extracts over half of the blood's insulin. It is the tissue that is by far most responsible for getting insulin out of the blood. When insulin secretion increases beyond normal, as happens in people with insulin resistance, the abdominal area extracts all the insulin it can. But it has its limits. At very high blood insulin levels, it cannot remove as much insulin as is secreted. Could it be that abdominal obesity is a response to the body's having to deal with more and more glucose and often, subsequently, excess insulin on a regular basis? Contributing to this is what can happen to people eating low-magnesium foods as described earlier in this chapter: Magnesium-deficient cells' response to insulin, and their capacity to metabolize the glucose to produce energy, can become lower than normal. As a result, an alternate path is followed—that of converting excess sugar to fat—especially in those prone to obesity. If the fat is deposited in the abdominal area, it is possible that

Fat or thin, low magnesium can bring on syndrome X and heart disease.

the body may be able to extract more insulin from the blood, allowing the body to stave off the adverse effects of high blood insulin. Is abdominal obesity a physiological adaptation to diets low in magnesium and high in refined carbohydrates? Is abdominal obesity a body's attempt to stave off adverse effects of metabolic syndrome X? We don't know. Further studies are needed.

People who live at high altitudes undergo physiological adaptations to the low oxygen content of high-altitude air, and these adaptations can even change body stature. Is it possible that our modern diet, so high in sugar and refined flour, and so low in magnesium and micronutrients, engenders so much insulin production that, in order to keep going, the body responds by increasing abdominal girth to maximize the ability to extract excess insulin from the blood? There is a hint of evidence for this view in some animal studies, but it has not been put to the test directly in humans. In one human study, removing abdominal fat did not affect the development of metabolic syndrome X. So perhaps we speculate too much. But the fact remains: Abdominal obesity, rather than general obesity, has the strongest link to metabolic syndrome X, diabetes, cardiovascular disease, and magnesium deficit.

The Effect of Exercise on Obesity and Metabolic Syndrome X

Fitness, or aerobic, exercise, done on a regular, ongoing basis, builds an extensive network of blood capillaries in the body's tissues. It also increases the number of mitochondria, the energy-producing structures within the cells. An aerobically fit body can bring more blood and insulin to muscle cells, maximizing glucose uptake. The numerous mitochondria in cells of a fit body that is supplied with optimal amounts of magnesium can burn glucose efficiently, allowing even more glucose uptake. Less glucose in the blood means less of a stimulus for insulin production. This is how regular aerobic exercise militates against metabolic syndrome X. These physical adaptations to regular aerobic exercise occur in all tissues, but especially in those of the muscles, including the heart. No wonder death rates go down with higher fitness levels.

People living in the modern industrial world can easily choose a sedentary lifestyle over one that leads to fitness. This can cause the body to respond by lessening the number of capillaries in our tissues and decreasing the number of mitochondria in our cells. This condition diminishes blood flow to cells and lessens efficient glucose uptake, which, in certain circumstances, can promote high blood insulin levels. If this adaptation to a sedentary lifestyle is coupled with a diet that is low in magnesium and high in refined foods, metabolic syndrome X can easily develop. With the high circulating levels of insulin, which normally lowers blood glucose levels, causing cravings for refined carbohydrates—the food elements the body converts into fat—obesity or overweight becomes likely.

Exercise, on its own, increases blood flow, making it easier for muscle cells to take up glucose from the blood. This increased glucose uptake reduces the likelihood that metabolic syndrome X will develop or progress, especially since exercise enhances the effect of insulin. Exercise and insulin act synergistically; that is, the two together will yield *greater* glucose uptake than the sum of the two acting separately.

Given these facts, exercise seems like a "no-brainer." But caution is necessary. For people in a low-magnesium state, even if they are physically fit, strenuous exercise can be dangerous since exercise increases the body's magnesium requirements. (The reasons for this will be discussed in detail in chapter 6.)

The Effect of Exercise on Magnesium Status

The more intense the exercise, the more magnesium is needed to burn glucose for energy production to meet the needs of the straining muscles. And the sweating caused by vigorous exercise causes magnesium loss. Both of these factors contribute to magnesium deficiency, which in turn increases the risk of arrhthymia or chest pain that can signal coronary artery spasms or occlusion.

When you exercise, whether in short bursts or during intense training, adrenaline is released and magnesium moves—from the blood to the cells and from cells to the blood. Many investigators have tried to determine the effect of exercise on magnesium status by measuring changes in the amount of magnesium in the blood during exercise. But, as we will see in later chapters, serum magnesium (the level of magnesium in a blood sample from which blood cells have been removed) does not reliably reflect the magnesium status of the whole body, so these studies have not yielded consistent results.

In general, blood magnesium levels change during exercise, but not consistently. One study showed that the levels of magnesium in the red blood cells and plasma (the cell-free portion of the blood) stayed the same during the training of eleven athletes, but that there was a loss of whole blood magnesium. The authors did not know if this indicated an actual loss of magnesium from the body or the shifting of magnesium from the blood to elsewhere, perhaps to the muscle cells. Another study showed no change in serum or red blood cell magnesium in patients on a treadmill, whether or not they developed signs of inadequate blood oxygen supply, even though magnesium poured into the whole blood. Where from? The cells? Was this an attempt by the body to keep blood levels of magnesium constant?

In a bout of exercise, such as a forty-minute run, plasma magnesium decreases while adrenaline increases. But such exercise can also cause a rise in serum magnesium because of a shift from the cells and a decrease in plasma volume. With protracted exercise, however, serum magnesium can fall. These dynamics of magnesium, shifting from blood to cells and cells to blood, are complicated and not fully understood. But it is clear that exercise and the release of the adrenaline it stimulates cause shifts of magnesium into the body's exercise-active sites and away from inactive regions. If you do not have enough "backup" magnesium, this can be a problem.

When Exercise Is Bad for You

If the body's cells are low in magnesium, stress—such as exercise—can be dangerous because it causes the release of adrenaline and a sudden shift in magnesium from the cells to the blood, further lowering magnesium in cells to dangerously inadequate levels. The heart is particularly vulnerable to exercise stress–induced magnesium loss because the mag-

Thin or fat, a magnesium deficit makes exercise dangerous.

nesium in heart cells is rapidly exchangeable. This means that the heart can take up magnesium quickly, which is a protective capacity. But it can also rapidly release it, so this capacity is a double-edged sword. When the cells of coronary arteries become deficient in magnesium, a situation that is accompanied by a shifting of calcium into the cells, they constrict, thereby interfering with blood bringing oxygen to heart cells. Even though an exercising, magnesium-low person may be free of ischemic heart disease (see page 6), temporary constriction of the coronary arteries can create the risk of a heart attack or cardiac arrhythmia that can cause cardiac arrest. If the body's cells contain adequate magnesium, a sudden shift of magnesium is not dangerous. The body cells can cope with the "emergency" of exercise and not become too low in magnesium.

If a person's magnesium status is low, excessive strenuous sport or other physical activity can intensify the consequences of a marginal magnesium deficiency. Thus, if magnesium status is low to begin with, exercise or training can use up the available magnesium while increasing the body's need for it. If there are not adequate body stores to back up the initial burst or long-term usage of magnesium, signs of the magnesium deficiency can become manifest. This can happen in the fit as well as the unfit, the thin as well as the obese.

The intense physical exertion of training worsens nutritional deficits, which, if severe, can then become obvious. In someone with a magnesium deficit—even a borderline one, but especially a more severe deficiency—an intense bout of physical exercise or an extended period of intense training can be dangerous regardless of the individual's aerobic fitness or muscle strength. Both athletes and sedentary people who want to begin an exercise program should therefore make sure that their magnesium status is up to par before beginning their program. The rise in adrenaline that comes with a rise in activity level can evoke signs of serious magnesium inadequacy in a person whose magnesium status is borderline, and this can be very dangerous. If the magnesium status is low enough, such a burst of exercise can cause cardiac arrhythmia and even bring on sudden death.

These facts explain why some athletes who are lean and in shape but also low in magnesium can experience sudden, unexpected cardiac arrest and death, while some people who are fat but have adequate magnesium can safely engage in regular exercise.

How Magnesium Status Affects the Response to Exercise

Taking magnesium supplements can enhance exercise performance in people with heart disease as well as in athletes. Adequate magnesium improves both the utilization of glucose and the body's response to the stress of exercise. It also improves strength and endurance and can prevent or reduce muscle cramping during and after exercise.

In a group of the best trained athletes, those who do triathlons, taking 400 milligrams of supplemental magnesium per day for one month before the "big event" has been found to yield better race times as well as better glucose utilization and better stress response during the race.

In people with coronary artery disease, taking 720 milligrams of magnesium per day for six months definitely improved exercise tolerance (as evidenced by better glucose uptake and less of a rise in stress hormones) and made for better blood flow and a lower incidence of ischemic ECG changes during exercise (16 percent vs. 40 percent).

As insurance against inducing magnesium deficiency while trying to lose weight by exercising, it is best to know your magnesium status before starting. The only trouble is that (as will be explained in detail in chapter 11) determining whether you have an adequate supply of magnesium is not easy. Blood serum values for magnesium cannot be relied upon to indicate the body's true magnesium status. Cellular magnesium is a better measure, since over 90 percent of the body's magnesium is inside cells.

In one study of people with coronary artery disease, half of a group of subjects aged forty-two to eighty-two were given 720 milligrams of magnesium a day for six months. Then both groups were tested while they were exercising. Measurement of the magnesium inside their cells (by a procedure

Thin or fat, a solid magnesium status makes exercise beneficial.

that did not require analysis of samples removed from the body) showed that, in both the magnesium and placebo groups, muscle-cell and brain-cell magnesium levels were below normal. But those taking the magnesium supplement had higher cellular magnesium levels—closer to the normal range—than those taking a placebo. The ones with higher intracellular magnesium had better blood flow (almost four times better), better exercise tolerance, and 60 percent fewer ischemic ECG changes during exercise than the placebo group—who, not having taken magnesium, had lower intracellular magnesium levels. The supplemented group still had some abnormal ischemic changes. We believe that these results occurred because this group might not have sufficiently repaired the subnormal intracellular magnesium levels that had contributed to their heart disease, even though they had taken magnesium supplements for six months.

If you are going into physical training or starting an exercise program, magnesium can help, even if you do not know whether you are deficient at the beginning. Supplementation at a level of 2.3 milligrams of magnesium per pound of body weight per day (this comes to about 345 milligrams per day for a 150-pound person) can really help. Higher levels (up to 720 milligrams per day) is recommended for those with coronary artery disease. Magnesium supplements have been shown to improve exercise tolerance in both people with coronary artery disease and trained athletes.

Do You Really Need to Lose Weight?

Obesity has been long associated with shorter life and poor health in Western societies. In other cultures, it has been associated with wealth and status—because the rich, successful, and powerful are the only ones who can afford the foods that make them fat. So they are free of the social stigma that creates stress in the West. However, we are doubtful that it fully protects them from the physical consequences of obesity.

Obesity raises the chance of getting other diseases beyond the obvious cardiovascular problems of metabolic syndrome X, heart disease, and stroke. These include kidney disease, type II diabetes (the insulin-resistant form, which can be part of metabolic syndrome X), gallbladder disorders, sleep apnea, gout, osteoarthritis, accidents, and some types of cancer. Obesity can also make it less safe to undergo surgery. But people who are obese can have lower death rates from other causes, such as tuberculosis, ulcers, and suicide. The obese have more depression and engage in more binge-eating than do the nonobese, and they can suffer from social and economic discrimination. Any or all of these, combined, can adversely affect a person's quality of life and stress level, so it is worth taking a closer look at this condition and defining clearly at what point extra weight presents a health risk.

Overweight and Health Risk

To make the latest research in obesity easier to understand, we must first introduce and define the concept of the body mass index (BMI). This is the modern research measure used for weight risk assessment. BMI is the index of one's weight as related to one's height (see "Calculating Your BMI" on page 100).

As you read about BMI, keep in mind that most of this research has been done on young to middle-aged white people. Also keep in mind that some people who would technically be considered overweight are perfectly healthy that way. In fact, when these genetically larger people lose weight to enter the "normal" range, they may become *less* healthy. Likewise, some theoretically underweight people are perfectly healthy as they are. These genetically thinner people are healthy at a low weight that would have dangerous consequences for most of us. Furthermore, the increased health risk associated with obesity does not hold true for people in all ethnic or racial groups. The level at which a BMI becomes "dangerous" is much higher for African-Americans than for white Americans. For some groups, there is no association at all between mortality (death rate) and obesity. One outstanding example is Pima men, a group of Native Americans indigenous to the southwestern United States. The BMI with the lowest mortality rate for Pima men is 35 to 40, a very dangerous range for white Americans. So let us look more closely at BMI and its association with health risk.

It is when obesity and overweight are coupled with elements of metabolic syndrome X that the risk of heart disease really climbs. For

Calculating Your BMI

Calculating your approximate body mass index (BMI) is simple. All you need to know is your height and your weight. You can use measurements in either inches and pounds or meters and kilograms. Then make the following calculations:

IF USING INCHES AND POUNDS

1. Determine your height in inches (note that 5 feet equals 60 inches; 6 feet equals 72 inches).
2. Multiply your height (the result of step 1) by itself. This is your height squared.
3. Multiply your weight in pounds by 703.
4. Divide the result of step 3 by your height squared (the result of Step 2). This is your BMI.

Example: If you are 5 feet 10 inches tall and weigh 160 pounds, you would do the following calculations:

1. 5 feet 10 inches = 70 inches (your height in inches)
2. 70 x 70 = 4,900 (your height squared).
3. 160 (your weight in pounds) x 703 = 112,480.
4. 112,480 (the result of Step 3) ÷ 4,900 (your height squared) = 22.96 (your BMI).

IF USING METRIC MEASUREMENTS

1. Determine your height in meters. (Note that 1 centimeter is equal to 0.01 meter.)
2. Multiply your height (the result of step 1) by itself. This is your height squared.
3. Divide your weight in kilograms by your height squared (the result of step 2). This is your BMI.

(continued on page 101)

(continued from page 100)

Example: If you are 180 centimeters tall and weigh 75 kilograms, you would do the following calculations:

1. 180 centimeters = 1.8 meters (your height in meters)
2. 1.8 x 1.8 = 3.24 (your height squared)
3. 75 (your weight in kilograms) ÷ 3.24 (your height squared) = 23.15 (your BMI).

Once you have calculated your body mass index (BMI), use the following table to understand what that number means for your weight and your health:

BMI	**Weight Category**
Less than 20	Underweight
20–27	Recommended weight
27–30	Overweight
30–34	Moderately obese
More than 34	Severely or morbidly obese

Be aware, however, that the healthiest BMI for any given height goes up with age (see table 4.3, page 105).

example, obese people with normal blood pressure have almost twice the risk as the nonobese, but for people who are obese and also have high blood pressure, the risk goes up tenfold. The same is true for other elements of metabolic syndrome X when coupled with obesity (see table 4.2). Since low cellular magnesium is identified with metabolic syndrome X, we can see that most health problems of obesity arise when coupled with magnesium deficiency. If we can correct magnesium deficiency with magnesium-rich food and/or supplements, what then do we do about overweight and obesity?

If you graph the rate of death from all causes against the BMI, you get a U-shaped curve (see figure 4.3). This means that those who are

Table 4.2 Relative Heart Disease Risks for People with Symptoms of Metabolic Syndrome X

This table shows the incidence of heart attacks in people of various weight categories, with and without high blood pressure, type II diabetes or high cholesterol. Note that the risk category designated "normal" refers to the overall risk for people of normal weight who have healthy normal blood pressure and do not have diabetes or high blood cholesterol.

Symptom	Weight Category		
	Recommended	**Overweight**	**Obese**
Blood pressure:			
Normal	= normal	1½ times normal	2 times normal
High	4 times normal	5 times normal	10 times normal
Type II Diabetes:			
No	= normal	2 times normal	4 times normal
Yes	2½ times normal	5 times normal	12 times normal
Blood cholesterol:			
Normal	= normal	2 times normal	3 times normal
"High"	3 times normal	4 times normal	7½ times normal

Adapted from: M.E. Lean, "Pathophysiology of Obesity," *Proceedings of the Nutrition Society* 59(3) (August 2000): 331–336.

thinnest and those who are most obese have the highest death rates. Those in the midrange for BMI have much lower death rates. This is termed "the bottom of the U." It is the BMI, or weight range for height, that has the lowest death rate, and it goes up with age (see figure 4.4).

Some older people who are in the categories of overweight traditionally labeled "caution" or even "concern" are actually at the weight that is associated with the lowest death rate *for their age group*. So why are so many of these "overweight" people (those with a BMI of 26 to 29) on weight-loss diets, on orders from their doctors? If your doctor sees that your BMI is in the range of 26 to 27 and concludes that you are in the "caution" or even "concern" weight range, he or she may be

Figure 4.3 The "U" Curve of Body Weight

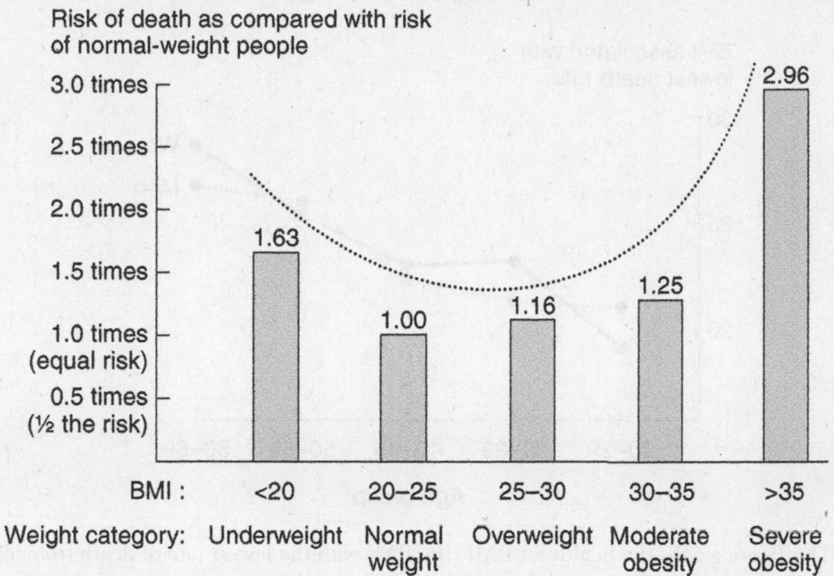

This graph illustrates that the rate of death from all causes is lower among people who are at a recommended weight, overweight, and even moderately obese (with BMIs between 20 and 35) as compared with that for people who are either underweight or severely obese. The number over each bar represents the mortality rate for that group as compared with that of the healthiest weight category (BMI of 20 to 25). Thus, people in the "moderate obesity" category, who have BMIs between 30 and 35, have a mortality hazard ratio of 1.25. This means that there are 25 percent (¼) more deaths than people in the recommended weight category.

Adapted from P. T. Katzmarzyk, C. L. Craig, and C. Bouchard, "Underweight, Overweight and Obesity: Relationships with Mortality in the 13-Year Follow-Up of the Canada Fitness Survey," *Journal of Clinical Epidemiology* 54 (9) (September 2001): 916–920.

missing the fact that, if you are over fifty, that BMI is associated with a very low risk of death.

Weight-conscious people are familiar with the tables of recommended or ideal weights for men and women of different heights. These were created by life-insurance companies to assess risk—not just for heart disease, but for any and all causes of death. But these tables did not take into account age and the fact that "the bottom of the

Figure 4.4 The Healthiest Weight and BMI Get Higher with Age

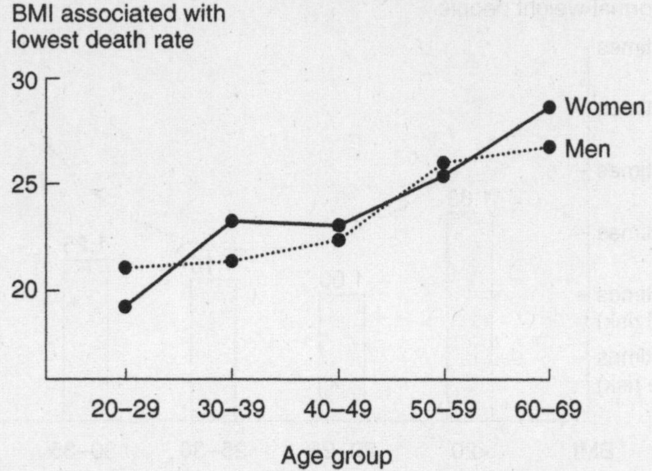

This figure graphs the healthiest BMI (the BMI with the lowest rate of death from all causes) against age. Note that the BMI with the lowest rate of death gets larger with age. Thus, the healthiest body weight for a given height goes up as people age.

Adapted from R. Andres, D. Elahi, J.D. Tobin, et al., "Impact of Age on Weight Goals," *Annals of Internal Medicine* 103 (6, Part 2) 1985: 1030–1033.

U" gets higher with age. Likewise, the expert committee of the National Heart, Blood, and Lung Institute's Obesity Education Initiative, in cooperation with the National Institute of Diabetes and Digestive and Kidney Disorders of the U.S. National Institutes of Health (NIH), that derived *The Clinical Guidelines on the Identification, Evaluation, and Treatment of Overweight and Obesity in Adults: The Evidence Report* defined overweight as above the eighty-fifth percentile of weight in adults aged twenty to twenty-nine years "with no particular relation to a specific increase in disease risk."

Weight tables derived from the work of Dr. Reubin Andres of the National Institute on Aging's Gerontology Research Center and his colleagues are much better assessments of ideal weight for health because they take age and weight of "minimal mortality" into account (see table 4.3). If you are within the weight range for your height and age, you are at the "bottom of the U," and therefore at your ideal weight

Table 4.3 Weight Ranges with the Lowest Mortality

Height	Gerontology Research Center Age-Specific Recommendations* Weight Range for Men and Women by Age (years)				
	25	35	45	55	65
feet-inches			*pounds*		
4-10	84–111	92–119	99–127	107–135	115–142
4-11	87–115	95–123	103–131	111–139	119–147
5-0	90–119	98–127	106–135	114–143	123–152
5-1	93–123	101–131	110–140	118–148	127–157
5-2	96–127	105–136	113–144	122–153	131–163
5-3	99–131	108–140	117–149	126–158	135–168
5-4	102–135	112–145	121–154	130–163	140–173
5-5	106–140	115–149	125–159	134–168	144–179
5-6	109–144	119–154	129–164	138–174	148–184
5-7	112–148	122–159	133–169	143–179	153–190
5-8	116–153	126–163	137–174	147–184	158–196
5-9	119–157	130–168	141–179	151–190	162–201
5-10	122–162	134–173	145–184	156–195	167–207
5-11	126–167	137–178	149–190	160–201	172–213
6-0	129–171	141–183	153–195	165–207	177–219
6-1	133–176	145–188	157–200	169–213	182–225
6-2	137–181	149–194	162–206	174–219	187–232
6-3	141–186	153–199	166–212	179–225	192–238
6-4	144–191	157–205	171–218	184–231	197–244

*Values in this table are for height without shoes and weight without clothes.

Adapted from R. Andres, et al., "Impact of Age on Weight Goals," *Annals of Internal Medicine* 103(6 part 2) (1985): 1030–1033. Used by permission.

for health. Being either above *or* below this range is associated with a higher overall risk of death.

You may be surprised to find you are not "too fat" after all. Being slightly obese or overweight, which many of us are, is not as bad, healthwise, as most of us assume. The overweight (those with a BMI of 28 to 31) have more high blood pressure and diabetes than the nonoverweight, but higher cholesterol values become evident only in those who are obese (those with a BMI greater than 31). And remember: Obesity does not *always* mean low magnesium and heart disease. In one study of people with advanced heart failure, the death rate among those who were obese was not higher than that among those who were not. In fact, the obese patients with advanced heart failure tended to live longer with the condition, than did nonobese individuals. A person with heart disease has a magnesium deficit, whether obese or not, and neither obesity nor leanness defines one's magnesium status.

This is not to say that there are no health problems with obesity. Severe obesity can be quite detrimental to health. A BMI above 35 imposes a health risk for people of any age and also presents a greater risk in a number of other circumstances. These include undergoing surgery and having breathing problems and/or sleep apnea. There is also a tenfold increase in the chance of developing type II diabetes for people above age forty, and a greater chance, in general, of getting breast, endometrial, or prostate cancer. The very obese also have to face severe quality-of-life issues, including mobility, psychological, social, and, often, economic difficulties. These can be very stressful. But ordinary overweight and even slight obesity are much less of a health problem than is either severe obesity *or* being underweight.

There is a psychosocial component to overweight that is immense for some, especially white women, and that can affect the quality of life and even physical health by imposing continual extra stress. These social and psychological aspects of weight are often overlooked by many in a culture obsessed more and more with body image and the belief that fat is *always* bad. It's not. It's only when BMI gets above 35 to 40 that the death rates match and go beyond those of the underweight. In fact, among people over age fifty, the overweight (those with a BMI of 25 to 32) do better than those in any other category as far as longevity is concerned.

So why are so many of us trying to lose weight? As the number of people who are obese has increased over the past fifty years, our belief system has more and more associated obesity with poor health. These trends have set up a social and medical obsession with weight and weight loss. We have demonized the health aspects of moderate overweight. And while we have overemphasized the association of poor health and overweight, we have minimized the health disadvantages of being underweight. Where are the warnings about underweight? The five-foot-eight-inch-tall woman who weighs 120 pounds or less is living in a danger zone, according to research. Where are the magazine articles on how to *gain* weight? Experts are understandably reluctant to relinquish weight-loss goals that they believe to be the solution to the major killer: heart disease

While the numbers of people who are overweight or obese have been rising, magnesium deficiency has also increased. This important factor has been mostly ignored, despite the increasing recognition of magnesium's association with metabolic syndrome X and its risk factors, including abdominal obesity. So the rise in obesity is blamed for the health consequences of our low magnesium. Among those trying to find a solution to the heart disease epidemic, the demonization of the health aspects of moderate overweight has taken precedence, while magnesium deficiency continues to be ignored.

In our culture, we are immersed in a high–processed-food environment, which gives rise to overweight and obesity while subjecting excess weight (and people who carry it) to a social, medical, and psychological beating. The stresses of poor body image, of always trying to diet and feeling inadequate when we "fail," can waste our magnesium, which is already in limited supply from a processed-food diet. It's time for some clarity.

Weight Loss and Cardiovascular Risk

Weight loss can improve cardiovascular risk factors, but it may or may not lessen the overall risk of death. Several studies have shown that losing weight by calorie restriction and physical exercise can lessen some risk factors for heart disease. But not all diets work the same way. Most medically recommended weight-loss diets have focused on the percentage of fat—a macronutrient—in the diet. Only recently has it been recognized that lowering fat means increasing carbohydrate intake. If the added carbohydrate is refined, real problems can arise with triglyceride levels and glucose tolerance. Magnesium and other minerals (mostly micronutrients) are rarely, if ever, measured in weight-loss diets. But diets that are fortified with either supplements or fruits and vegetables give better results in terms of cardiovascular risk factors. Sticking with a diet that provides adequate magnesium and micronutrients improves total and HDL cholesterol, blood pressure, glucose, quality of life, compliance, and weight loss better than a diet with the same of percentage fat but with inadequate magnesium and micronutrients. Adding fruits and vegetables to a low-fat diet lessens abdominal obesity; lowers glucose, insulin, blood pressure, weight, triglycerides, and LDLs; and raises HDLs. The same low-fat diet without fruits and vegetables only lowers LDLs. In one study, subjects on a diet of micronutrient-rich foods had 33 percent fewer cardiac events and a 33 percent lower overall mortality, while reducing central obesity 80 percent more, than those on a nonmicronutrient diet. The macronutrition focus is still being mightily debated, but we need proper mineral nutrition, including adequate amounts of magnesium, to make weight loss healthy.

There is also a genetic component to weight loss. In a study on weight loss that divided groups by a familial (genetic) tendency to become obese, the group from obese families experienced 13 percent less weight loss and had a 75 percent higher incidence of diabetes than the nonobese groups—on the same diet. Studies that do not recognize these differences in micronutrition and genetics report that weight loss helps some risk factors but not all. For example, it can increase the sensitivity of cells to insulin, but does not decrease the oversecretion of insulin. So weight loss, in and of itself, helps some things, but not all; in some people, but not all.

Changing one's diet to induce weight loss can sometimes increase magnesium, sometimes lessen magnesium, and sometimes leave it the same. If only calories, fat, cholesterol, and carbohydrates are emphasized, one cannot really tell if magnesium intake is going up or down. Yet unless the magnesium goes up, cardiovascular risk factors are not as likely to improve with a weight-loss diet.

It has been shown over and over again that medically significant weight loss is hard to achieve and almost impossible to maintain. The total emphasis on fat, cholesterol, and calories has not helped. Is the stress of weight-loss dieting worth it?

Weight Loss and Life Expectancy

There is no doubt that high weight, defined as a BMI above 32, is associated with increased blood lipids, and that abdominal obesity is further associated with even worse dyslipidemia (an unhealthy blood fat and cholesterol profile), as well as hypertension and insulin resistance: metabolic syndrome X. In such cases, losing weight by means of diet and/or exercise certainly can improve all these risk factors. But whether or not weight loss can decrease death rates is a nagging question. Studies have yielded differing results. In some cases, weight loss increases mortality and in others it decreases it. The results are equivocal, to say the least. In general, at this point, it is safe to say that intentional weight loss may often, but not always, lead to a longer life, and unintentional weight loss is hazardous, especially for older adults. The confusion is partly resolved by a study that showed *weight* loss to increase the death rate while *fat* loss lowered it. Weight cycling (the yo-yo syndrome, or weight gain following weight loss, repeatedly) does not improve the prospects for longevity. The people with the best mortality rate are lean women whose weight has been stable throughout their lifetime.

We suggest that if all the diet and mortality studies were reevaluated with magnesium nutrition as a focus, weight loss would be shown to increase the lifespan as long as magnesium nutrition is strong, and to decrease the lifespan if magnesium nutrition is weak.

The Rising Trend of Obesity—A Worldwide Epidemic?

We live in a society that has an ample supply of delicious, fattening food, and our bodies show it. Many of us are overweight, and a rising number of us are obese. Ninety-seven million Americans are either overweight or obese, and in 1997, the prevalence of obesity reported in developed countries ranged from 7 percent in France to almost 33 percent in Brazil. In 2001, Austria's rate of obesity was reported to be 34 to 50 percent and going up with the age of the population. The European mean for obesity is 15 to 22 percent, and this doesn't even count the merely overweight. But the prevalence of obesity in different countries ranges from 7 to 9 percent obese to 22 to 45 percent obese (the lower figures in men, the higher in women). In the United States, more than a third are considered medically obese; the prevalence of obesity rose 40 percent during the 1980s.

At any one time, 25 percent of American men and 40 percent of American women say that they are trying to lose weight. Yet in the last decade, the number of obese people in the United States has increased rapidly, even though 50 million people reportedly tried to lose weight. As this population-wide weight gain occurs, there is an increase in the number of people who are considered morbidly, or grossly, obese—obese to the extent that it prevents normal activity or functioning. Morbid obesity is associated with serious medical complications.

Obesity is a problem not only in the developed world but also in the developing world—anywhere highly processed foods become available. It is first seen in women, followed closely by men, and then starts to show up in children and adolescents.

Worldwide, over one-half billion people have this chronic nutritional disorder. It is becoming a worldwide epidemic. The number of overweight people now equals the number of underweight people in the world. Obesity is starting to replace undernutrition and infectious diseases as the most significant contributor to ill health in the world. Generally believed to be caused by trends toward more urban living, less activity in general, and more food availability, obesity may become the foremost chronic disease of the world as worldwide affluence spreads.

With such widespread growth, the worldwide epidemic of obesity and its consequences for our health, health-care systems, self-image, and self-esteem are substantial. Such an intractable condition, growing as it is with the spread of processed foods, is in large part a threat to global well-being because it is accompanied by magnesium deficiency.

If You Decide You Want to Lose Weight

Dealing with obesity means separating the two goals of weight loss: body health and body size. You may be dealing with both, or you may be dealing with one or the other. But before you jump into a program for weight loss, it is best to sit down for a minute and decide what your real goals are. Do you want to lose weight because you are worried about your health? How much of your goal involves losing weight to change your body size for your psychological and/or social comfort? Both goals are worthy. We shall provide information and recommendations to maximize the health aspects of intentional weight loss—whatever your goals. If you want to lose weight to lower your risk of heart disease, to enhance your confidence and self-esteem, or to do both, the following information can help you make a difficult endeavor a bit more directed and less chancy.

Losing Weight for Health

If your doctor tells you to lose weight, the first thing you should do is to find out if you really need to lose and, if so, how much. Begin with the following:

1. Take your waist measurement.
2. Calculate your BMI and determine your weight category (see "Calculating Your BMI," page 100).
3. With the results of steps 1 and 2, above, consult table 4.1, Waist Measurement and Health Risk, to determine whether you have abdominal obesity and what your risk category is. For men, increased risks begin at waists larger than 35½ inches. For women, they begin at 31½ inches.
4. Refer to table 4.2, Relative Heart Disease Risks for People with Symptoms of Metabolic Syndrome X, to the effect of your weight category on your various health risks.

Note that just being "overweight," or even "obese," is not necessarily dangerous in and of itself. If you are into the overweight or obese category, look up your weight for age and height on table 4.3, Weight Ranges with the Lowest Mortality. Are you outside the optimal range for your age and height? Do you really need to lose weight for health? How much? Do you need to gain? Again, how much? Filling out the form in My Weight Goals, below, can help you to think through this question.

My Weight Goals

1a. My BMI, waist measurement, and weight show me to be (circle one):

underweight | recommended weight | overweight | moderately obese | severely obese

1b. My age, weight, and height show me to be (circle one):

below | within | above

the healthiest weight for my age. (Use table 4.3.)

If you are at the recommended weight and within the healthiest weight for your age, stop here. If you are underweight or at the recommended weight AND below healthiest weight for age, go to step 6. If you are overweight or obese, continue with step 2.

2. To be a healthy weight for my age, I need to lose _____ pounds. (Use table 4.3.)
3. This would take me from __________ (weight category) to the recommended weight category. It would decrease my chance of heart disease from _____% to 25% (for women) or 35% (for men). (Use figure 4.1.)
4. Such a gain in health is worth the weight loss to me (circle one):

   yes | no
5. The gain in social aspects and self-esteem I would experience would make such a weight loss worth it for me (circle one):

   yes | no

(continued on page 113)

(continued from page 112)

If overweight or obese, stop here. If underweight, continue with step 6.

6. My BMI or table 4.3 shows me to be underweight (circle one):

   yes no

7. To be a healthy weight for my age, I need to gain _____ pounds. (Use table 4.3.)

8. The social and self-esteem aspects of such a weight gain are fine with me (circle one):

   yes no

If Your Weight Is in the Recommended Range

If you are in the optimal weight range for your age and height, do not have abdominal obesity, and have no other risk factors for heart disease, you may still want to lose weight for psychological and/or social reasons. This is just fine as long as you do not go below the weight range for your age in table 4.3 and as long as you keep your intake of essential nutrients—including magnesium—at a healthy level. Remember: A considerable number of people with heart disease are not obese and have no other known risk factors. Make sure to keep your magnesium status healthy. (This will be discussed in detail in chapter 11.)

If your weight is in the healthy range but you have cardiovascular symptoms or risk factors, take magnesium supplements as recommended in the chapters of this book that discuss your specific risk factors.

If Your Weight Is above the Recommended Range

If you have abdominal obesity and/or are above the "safe" range of weight for your age and height as given in table 4.3, you can improve your health by changing a few things. If you are under age forty, you are likely to have few symptoms. By taking precautions now, you will be doing the best you can for yourself to forestall the onset of symptoms, starting at about age forty, that generally come in three stages:

Stage 1. Fatigue, breathlessness, back pain, arthritis, sweatiness, poor sleep, depression, and/or menstrual disorders.
Stage 2. Hypertension, dyslipidemia, and/or type II diabetes.
Stage 3. Risk of heart attack, stroke, and some types of cancer.

What should you do if your obesity is a true risk factor? First of all, don't panic! If you have abdominal obesity or a BMI above 32, the best thing you can do is to take supplements of the proper micronutritents: vitamins and minerals. This is pretty easy. The next best things to do are to increase the amount of exercise you get and limit your refined flour and sugar intake. Both of these are difficult. They are difficult to initiate and they are difficult to maintain, but doing either or both, in addition to taking magnesium supplements, can really help. Here's how to go about it.

NUTRITIONAL SUPPLEMENTATION

Start taking magnesium supplements, increasing the amount gradually, as you are able to tolerate it, until you reach 480 milligrams per day. You can also add 15 to 30 milligrams of zinc, 400 international units of vitamin E, and 250 milligrams of vitamin C per day. If the magnesium supplements give you diarrhea, back off the dose to about 150 to 200 milligrams per day or until your stools are comfortably soft.

A BIT OF READING

During your first thirty days on supplements, read *Aerobics,* by Kenneth H. Cooper (Bantam Books, 1988), and a book on refined carbohydrates. We suggest *Sugar Busters! Cut Sugar to Trim Fat,* by H. Leighton Steward, Morrison C. Bethea, Sam S. Andrews, and Luis A. Balart (Ballantine Books, 1998), or *Lick the Sugar Habit,* by Nancy Appleton (Avery/Penguin Putnam, 1996). Hopefully this will motivate you to notice how much refined carbohydrate you eat and to learn about the benefits of exercise. *But don't start changing your diet or exercising yet.* Wait until you have been taking magnesium supplements for at least a month.

If anything will get you motivated about exercise, Cooper's book will. You can use this month to read about aerobics and figure out which, if any, aerobic activities you like best. Dancing? Walking with a friend? Walking alone? Basketball? Ping-Pong? There are many aerobic activities Cooper does not list. As long as an activity involves continuous movement of the arms and/or legs, it is probably aerobic. But remember: Wait for a full month of regular magnesium supplementation and check with your doctor before beginning your aerobic plan.

EXERCISE AND DIETARY CHANGES

After thirty days on magnesium, if you choose, add either an exercise program or your no-refined-carbohydrate program. Do not try to do both at the same time. Both changes are difficult and both are stressful. (If you know positively that exercise is more stressful than beneficial for you, you can skip it, but keep up the supplements and consider changing your refined carbohydrate intake.)

If you have abdominal obesity or generalized obesity, one of the very best things you can do for yourself after magnesium supplementation is to change your carbohydrates. That means to cut out all the sugar and, possibly, refined flour from your diet. This is not easy. Some people go through actual withdrawal from sugar, with headaches, grumpiness, raging and severe cravings for any form of sugar. If this happens and you can "white-knuckle" it for anywhere from three to fourteen days, the cravings will subside along with the withdrawal symptoms. You can also try to cut back on sugar in stages to lessen the withdrawal symptoms, although this will take longer. Either method is not easy. Even after you are off sugar, it can be a challenge not to relapse by eating sugar again and having to start the process all over.

Some people have a similar reaction to ceasing consumption of refined flour, which is broken down into sugar (glucose) in the body. Others will not have to avoid refined flour so much. You need to get to know how your own body reacts to refined carbohydrates. If this is out of the question for you, seriously consider adding an exercise program to your life, while you continue your magnesium supplements.

It may be easier to cut out the refined carbohydrates if your exercise program is in full swing. With exercise, go slowly, gradually. Less is more. Your goal is to gradually increase your exercise to "fitness" level. When cutting down on sugar and white flour, you can go cold turkey or reduce them gradually to achieve your goal—zero.

Keep up this supplement plus either an exercise or a low refined-carbohydrate regimen for six months. Then add the other program—exercise or low refined carbohydrates—and continue for another six months. This is not easy. Many people benefit from a support group that meets regularly as they make these changes.

REEVALUATION

After one month on supplementation, six months with one component (either exercise or low refined carbohydrates), and six months with the other component, reevaluate your obesity as outlined on page 112. If you are making progress, keep up your supplements, exercise, and/or low refined carbohydrate program. You are getting healthier. If you have truly adhered to all aspects of this program and there has been no change in either your BMI or abdominal obesity measurement, you may want to try a weight-loss diet *in addition to* your existing program.

WEIGHT-LOSS DIETS

If you decide you need to add a weight-loss diet to your regimen, you can go on any of the many diet programs that are out there—the American Heart Association diets, the Dean Ornish diet, the Atkins diet, the Heller diet, the Syndrome X diet, among others—*as long as you keep all refined carbohydrates to a minimum (preferably zero) and maintain your magnesium supplements.*

For any or all of this, you will probably need some support. You may benefit from a consultation with a nutritionally minded doctor, nutritionist, or dietitian. You can find a registered dietitian in your area by contacting the American Dietetics Association. (See Resources.)

If you go this route, be sure to get help in adjusting the three basic aspects of your program: more magnesium, more exercise, and less refined carbohydrate. If you need to add a reduced-calorie diet, be sure your intake of magne-

A weight-loss diet can be beneficial if it improves magnesium status.

sium and other essential nutrients is adequate for you and that refined carbohydrates are minimized. The following are summaries of some of the more popular weight-loss regimens you may wish to explore:

- *The Atkins diet,* named for its originator, cardiologist Dr. Robert Atkins, is a low- or zero-carbohydrate way of life that takes away the cravings carbohydrates can bring to those with hyperinsulinemia (high blood levels of insulin). It also results in fat loss rather than just weight loss, and this has been associated with lower mortality. Also, with the cravings gone, it is much easier to stay on the diet and lose weight. But a support system really helps. Dr. Atkins believes in and depends upon nutritional supplementation, including magnesium supplements, with his diet. Many doctors are concerned that the Atkins diet, which allows for a good deal of fat intake, may increase blood cholesterol. However, if magnesium is adequate, the Atkins diet does not raise LDL or total cholesterol, and triglycerides stay low because there is no sugar or simple carbohydrate intake.
- *The Dean Ornish diet* is a very low fat, vegetarian diet that is high in carbohydrates but emphasizes complex-carbohydrate sources that are high in magnesium such as fruits, vegetables, whole grains, and legumes. Dr. Ornish advises against the low-magnesium sugar and refined-flour products, which can "waste" magnesium. This is a severe but wholesome program. You can lose weight and improve your cardiovascular and glucose tolerance health with it. But remember that some people on this diet still do not get enough magnesium for their situation. Check your water supply. Does it contain magnesium? Consider your past eating habits—could you have come into the Ornish diet with a magnesium deficit? If so, it is best to replenish your magnesium stores with supplements. Does your family history indicate a high magnesium need? Again, supplements can ensure heart health on the difficult (for some) but excellent Ornish program.
- *The Heller diet,* touted as the "carbohydrate addict's" program, is advocated by Drs. Richard and Rachael Heller. It is based on the belief that having all of one's daily carbohydrates in one sit-

ting will cause less insulin production than if the carbohydrate intake is spread out over the day. We have not assessed whether this is true. If you want to try Heller, fine, but remember that refined carbohydrates are still not good for you. To forget this is to ask for trouble on the Heller diet, especially if you are very sensitive to refined carbohydrates.

Jane tried Heller. She was a very thin person, but on the Heller diet she felt that she was becoming obsessed with eating as much pizza, cake, ice cream, and the like in the one hour per day when carbohydrates were allowed. It got so all she really thought about the rest of the day was what she was going to eat, and how she was going to travel from here to there to get it all within one hour. When she realized her life was dictated by food or thoughts of food, she decided to cut out the carbohydrates that caused her trouble altogether, and her cravings subsided. She needed a support group, however, to remind herself that even a little sugar could set off her "addiction."

- *The American Heart Association (AHA) step I and II diets* are traditional low-fat, low-cholesterol diets. They can be safe and beneficial if the carbohydrates you eat come from whole grains rather than refined flour foods, whole fruits rather than fruit juices (added sugar or not), and vegetables. You should stay away from fat-free desserts that substitute refined carbohydrates for fats. The DASH diet, which gets its name from a clinical study entitled *D*ietary *A*pproaches to *S*top *H*ypertension, is a modification of the AHA diet that emphasizes fruits, vegetables, and whole grains. It works well because it emphasizes magnesium-rich foods.
- *The Syndrome X Diet* is moderate in fats (35 to 45 percent of total calories from fat, with only 5 to 10 percent as saturated fats) and carbohydrate (45 percent of calories), with the balance of daily calories from protein. Again, this diet can be fine as long as you make sure to get adequate amounts of all essential nutrients, especially magnesium, and avoid refined carbohydrates.

THE ADDICTION MODEL FOR WEIGHT LOSS

Many people trying to change their lifestyles and/or weight are helped with the addiction model for overeating. This model assumes that some people have a genetically determined physical reaction to certain foods, plus an obsession or compulsion with those very foods:

> Sandy was a teenager. She went on a weight-loss diet to lose fifteen pounds and was successful. She cut out all sugar and desserts, even going without sugar on her daily bowl of bran flakes with skim milk. After staying on this diet for several months, she was delighted with her 116-pound figure (down from 136 pounds) and gave herself a big treat: Rice Krispies with whole milk and a teaspóon of sugar. She did not stop eating for ten years. She gained her twenty pounds back, plus more, and even became bulimic for a while, trying to keep from gaining too much weight. At one point, she topped 160 pounds. Finally, she realized that sugar was the culprit and, with the help of a support group, tried to cut sugar out of her life. The constant cravings subsided, and her weight settled at slightly above ideal. But living in a society where sugar is everywhere all the time makes relapse easy. The knowledge that she is "allergic" to refined sugar helps.

If you wish to explore the addiction model, you can find a support group in your area by contacting an organization such as Overeaters Anonymous, Food Addicts Anonymous, or Compulsive Eaters Anonymous (see Resources).

All that said, if you are overweight but do *not* have abdominal obesity, have no other risk factors, and are over age forty, you may not need to lose weight for your cardiovascular health. You may be a genetically large person whose healthy weight seems high to a weight-obsessed culture. Losing weight may actually make you feel worse. Instead, it may be better to focus on keeping your magnesium status healthy, get adequate exercise, and watch your diet as outlined above. If your weight is in the safe range, your magnesium status appears adequate, you are exercising and off refined carbohydrates, and you still have risk factors, you may benefit from selected medications to treat those risk factors. Consult with your doctor.

If you are approaching your fifties and starting to gain weight, you may be noticing that your knees or other joints are beginning to bother you. Perhaps you are exercising less because of it, or even socializing less. You may find yourself avoiding stairs and other physical habits that make you notice your pains. This can lead to a downward spiral in which you become less active and it becomes easier to gain weight, which in turn aggravates the aches and pains. If you gain enough weight, trying on clothes becomes less enjoyable, leading to less socialization and an overall drop in your quality of life. If this sounds like you, magnesium supplements followed by an exercise and/or low refined carbohydrate diet as outlined above can help keep you healthy.

If your BMI is above 35 or 40 and you are severely or morbidly obese, you probably already have joint problems and may also have sleep apnea (a condition in which you repeatedly stop breathing for a matter of seconds to minutes while you are asleep) and other breathing problems. You may have developed gallbladder disease and the other health problems of the morbidly obese. Losing weight can be crucial for your good health. For you, we recommend the following:

- Take magnesium supplements—work with your doctor and be sure your kidneys are all right.
- Try to get some mild, regular exercise.
- Try to connect with Overeaters Anonymous or some other type of support group. If getting to meetings is too hard for you, try communicating with others who share your dilemma via the telephone or on the Internet.

If you are severely obese, we probably cannot tell you anything about diet; most likely you are already an expert, especially in what won't work. We urge you to try a support group based upon the addiction model of overeating. People who have lost over 100 pounds sometimes have special groups. In consultation with your doctor, you may decide to help your weight-loss plan with the newer weight-loss drugs.

Also, surgery can help, but there are some adverse effects. Be careful. Take good care of yourself.

In summary, if your doctor tells you to lose weight, before going on a weight loss diet:

1. Start taking magnesium supplements before you begin an exercise regimen. Both of these together on a continuous basis will help stave off heart disease.
2. Cut out sugar and refined flour. The many different names for sugar can be found in appendix I. Refined-flour products include white bread, pasta, and most pastries. Start reading ingredient lists on food labels, remembering that ingredients are listed in descending order. Sometimes you will find two or three different forms of sugar listed separately, using alternative forms and names. Also remember that the ingredient listed as *enriched flour* is refined wheat flour that has had most of wheat's magnesium removed.

If Your Weight Is Below the Recommended Range

If you are underweight, you may not have the same social, psychological, or economic pressures as people who are overweight, but there is a health issue you need to acknowledge. It's the underweight and very obese that are in the greatest danger of cardiovascular disease, of early death from other causes, and of magnesium deficiency.

If you binge and purge: This is a life-threatening disease. Run, don't walk to Overeaters Anonymous or some appropriate support group where you can start to cut down on your isolation and begin to join others in your situation. You and your life are precious. You deserve to take care of yourself.

5

Fat, Cholesterol, and Magnesium

Julie was a beautiful, slender, healthy woman in her late thirties, happy in her marriage, with two active, growing children. Her healthy home life gave her a strong base, and she was becoming accomplished in her chosen field of translation. She was living in Berkeley, California, and her life was blossoming. At her annual medical checkup, her blood work came back with high cholesterol and high triglycerides. Alarmed, and unused to being called back for a follow-up, she was stunned to learn she had to go on a low-cholesterol, low-fat diet in hopes of reducing her "at-risk" status for heart disease. Not wanting to make these lifestyle changes, she confided to her women's group the fear, resentment, and new stress in her once satisfying life. She felt guilt every time she ate a "treat" not on the diet and feared she was slowly committing suicide. She had barely felt resentment when she took time from her career for the childrens' early childhood. But now, when her children and husband blithely ate the special things that she made for them and that were suddenly off-limits to her, the resentment was so overwhelming that she began to pick fights with her mystified family. When a friend in the women's group told her about magnesium, Julie jumped at it. She started taking supplements of 360 milligrams per day. At her six-month checkup, the doctor was surprised to see how far her cholesterol had dropped and congratulated her on making "some tough dietary changes." Julie went back to her old ways of eating, but kept the magnesium supplements going on a daily basis. A year after the original high-cholesterol, high-fat scare, her values were still in the normal range, even without the low-fat, low-cholesterol diet. Resentments were gone, and Julie felt relieved as well as healthy.

Could we all be so lucky?

During the 1950s, total cholesterol became strongly associated with heart disease. Alarming rates of heart disease at mid-century needed a solution, a treatment, a means to prevent what was fast becoming an epidemic. This need, along with strong evidence that cholesterol and fat in the diet caused atherosclerosis and increased the risk of heart disease, gave rise to the low-cholesterol, low-fat diet recommendations that are now so familiar.

What Is Cholesterol?

Cholesterol is a lipid—a fatty substance—that is absorbed by the body from the food we eat and that is also synthesized by many of the body's cells, particularly those of the liver and intestines, and that also is a component of cell membranes in all tissues. It is necessary for normal cell membranes and normal cell growth and is a precursor to many vital hormones such as testosterone, estrogen, progesterone, and the stress hormones. It is also converted to vitamin D when our skin is exposed to sunlight.

For years, total blood cholesterol was one of the indicators most widely used by physicians to monitor health. If a patient had a high total cholesterol level, changes in diet were strongly recommended to lower it. In the absence of cholesterol-lowering drugs, dietary modification was the only treatment available. Cholesterol was also studied intensively for its link with the deposition of fat on the walls of arteries and, ultimately, with heart disease. Researchers learned that much of the blood cholesterol is attached to other fatty and protein components to form cholesterol-lipoprotein complexes that are categorized according to their density—high, low, and very low. So we now know that total cholesterol is made up of several classes of cholesterol-lipoprotein complexes, not all of which are dangerous if present in high levels. This has led to a shifting in focus from high blood cholesterol to the balance among the different types of cholesterol-lipoprotein complexes in the blood. The term now generally used for abnormalities of the fatty substances in the blood is *dyslipidemia,* rather than high cholesterol. In general, dyslipidemia is characterized by levels of high-density lipoproteins (HDL) that are too low, with levels of total blood cholesterol, low-density lipoproteins (LDL), very low density lipoproteins (VLDL), and triglycerides (TG) that are too high.

High blood levels of LDL and VLDL cholesterol are indeed associated with hardening of the arteries, a common forerunner of heart disease, so they are often called "bad cholesterol." On the other hand, HDL cholesterol is beneficial. Rather than being deposited in cells in the lining of arteries, like LDL and VLDL cholesterol, HDL cholesterol actually transports fat out of the arteries, preventing the formation of arterial plaques, so it is considered "good cholesterol." A blood HDL level that is too low is a risk factor for heart disease. Blood triglycerides are often measured along with cholesterol. They are not really cholesterol at all but rather another class of fats (lipids) in the blood. Like LDL and VLDL cholesterol, high triglycerides increase the risk of heart disease, and so are often considered a part of "bad cholesterol."

"High cholesterol" is a term we hear a lot, but as you can see, it is a misleading simplification.

The Effect of Magnesium Intake on Cholesterol

There is strong evidence that a high-fat diet—in both animals and people—can cause damage to arteries and the heart. But there is also strong evidence that magnesium deficiency intensifies the harmful effects of a high-fat diet because magnesium helps to protect against the arterial damage induced in the cardiovascular system. One way magnesium protects is in its effect on cholesterol. It was reported in 1957 that magnesium supplements could lower high cholesterol levels in laboratory animals. Two years later, it was proposed that both a high intake of fat and a low intake of magnesium might be responsible for the higher cholesterol levels fround in Australians who (or whose ancestors) had immigrated from Europe as compared with the native Austrilian population. Since then, several clinical studies have verified this speculation. The results of eighteen studies on humans shows that taking magnesium supplements can have the following effects in normalizing cholesterol values and/or high triglyceride levels in blood:

- Total cholesterol dropped by 6 to 23 percent
- LDL ("bad") cholesterol dropped by 10 to 18 percent.
- Triglycerides dropped by 10 to 42 percent
- HDL ("good") cholesterol rose by 4 to 11 percent

Unfortunately, these dramatic effects have not been accepted by the medical establishment, in part because of other human studies that failed to show a lowering effect of magnesium supplements on cholesterol and fat levels. On close examination, we can see that these studies had methodologic problems that explain their failure to confirm the positive findings. Three of them used a crossover design appropriate for testing drugs but not nutrients. (See Problems with Crossover-Design Studies When Testing Nutrients on page 56.) Another of these six negative trials was done on subjects who had familial hypercholesterolemia, a genetic condition that causes

Mangesium supplements can lower total cholesterol 6 to 20 percent.

high cholesterol levels and that is not responsive to magnesium. The other two were done on people with type I (insulin-dependent) diabetes. Such people are not directly comparable to people without diabetes because insulin therapy can increase the loss of magnesium through the urine. Thus, these six negative studies do not negate the positive effect magnesium has on abnormal blood cholesterol levels.

Research on the effect of magnesium on cholesterol has not been much publicized either to doctors or to the public. Thus, medical doctors rarely prescribe magnesium for elevated cholesterol levels. Julie, whose story opened this chapter, was lucky to have a friend who suspected that her high cholesterol might be a sign of magnesium trouble, and that magnesium supplements might help her. She was able to replenish early her dwindling magnesium, staving off the more severe aspects of the deficiency.

How Magnesium Controls Components of Blood Cholesterol

Magnesium exerts its effects on cholesterol levels in two primary ways. First, it regulates enzymes that control cholesterol production. Second, it raises the level of HDL ("good") cholesterol while lowering LDL ("bad") cholesterol. Let us look at each in turn.

Magnesium and Enzyme Regulation

The availability of magnesium controls a crucial step in the enzyme-driven process that results in the production of cholesterol. It can either increase or decrease cholesterol production, depending on the body's needs.

Cholesterol is the product of a series of reactions that start with a crucial one, the conversion of HMG-CoA to a compound called mevalonate, a fatty acid derivative. The process proceeds, stepwise, to the synthesis of cholesterol. (See figure 5.1.) Magnesium, in conjunction with ATP, deactivates the rate-limiting enzyme HMG-CoA-reductase, inhibiting this crucial initial step. As long as there is adequate magnesium, the inhibition of this enzyme can take place when necessary,

Figure 5.1 The Synthesis and Uses of Cholesterol

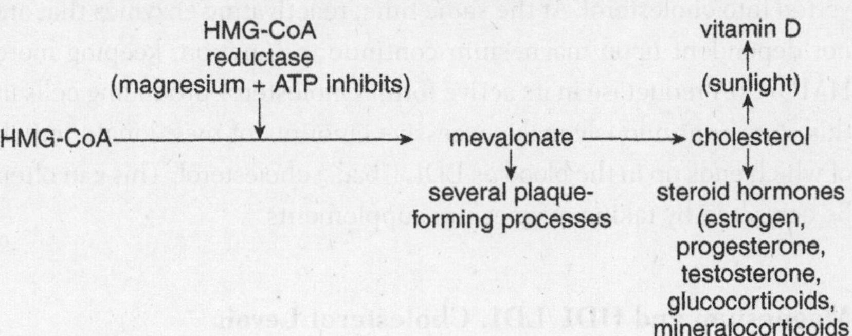

The drawing above illustrates the sequence of events that result in the creation of cholesterol, as well as the things that cholesterol is used for. Cholesterol is necessary but if there is too much, it can be lethal.

stopping or decreasing the production of mevalonate. The end result is that cholesterol production is impeded and less cholesterol is formed. Conversely, if there is a deficiency of magnesium, the conversion of HMG-CoA to mevalonate is enhanced, thereby increasing cholesterol formation. This can give rise to the development of cholesterol-filled atheromas—fatty deposits in the arteries. This is a negative result of having too much cholesterol. However, without adequate cholesterol, important substances cannot be formed. The steroid hormones, such as the sex hormones and the adrenal corticosteroids, derive from cholesterol in a number of enzyme-dependent steps, as does vitamin D, in response to sunlight exposure. It is important to note that the enzymes that are necessary for these processes, are magnesium-activated. In brief, cholesterol is necessary but if there is too much, it can be harmful.

If the body needs more cholesterol for such necessary functions as the production of vitamin D and steroid hormones, inactived HMG-CoA reductase can be reactivated by other enzymes. Some of these reactivating enzymes can use magnesium to function, but they can also rely on other activating minerals.

In brief, if there is a magnesium deficiency, there is an insufficient supply of the magnesium-ATP complex to deactivate HMG-CoA reductase, so there is more production of mevalonate, which is converted into cholesterol. At the same time, reactivating enzymes that are not dependent upon magnesium continue to function, keeping more HMG-CoA reductase in its active form. Cholesterol-producing cells in this state continuously make excessive amounts of mevalonate, much of which ends up in the blood as LDL ("bad") cholesterol. This can often be corrected by taking magnesium supplements.

Magnesium and HDL/LDL Cholesterol Levels

People with high HDL cholesterol—levels above 40 milligrams per deciliters (mg/dL) of blood—have less heart disease than people with HDL cholesterol below this level. Thus, HDL cholesterol is a heart disease risk factor only if the level of it is too *low.* Conversely, LDL cholesterol is a risk factor if levels are too high.

A group of scientists in France discovered that magnesium-deficient animals had reduced activity of an important enzyme that transforms LDL into HDL cholesterol. The enzyme is known as lecithin-cholesterol-acyl-transferase (LCAT). Magnesium is a necessary cofactor for this enzyme, which transfers part of one molecule to another with the result that LDL cholesterol is converted into HDL cholesterol. Thus, magnesium is necessary to convert LDL ("bad") into HDL ("good") cholesterol, the fraction of cholesterol in the blood that transports the LDL cholesterol away from the arteries. This is true for humans as well as for experimental animals, so people with high LDL cholesterol and low HDL cholesterol values can correct and normalize *both* their good and bad cholesterol levels by taking magnesium supplements. Anyone low in magnesium could have higher "bad" and lower "good" cholesterol in addition to higher total cholesterol. Cholesterol measurements can actually be a reflection of magnesium status, not fat intake. Those with poor numbers are more likely to have magnesium deficiencies and, therefore, more likely to have heart disease than are those with levels in the healthy range.

The Plaque Theory of Arteriosclerosis and Magnesium

Doctors and other scientists have observed that the majority of people with heart disease have abnormal blood vessels. Specifically, they have buildups of hard materials along blood vessel walls that, if severe, can narrow the diameter of blood vessels. These buildups of cholesterol, fats, calcium, and clotting factors are termed *atherosclerotic plaques*. Their buildup and the resulting narrowing and hardening of the arteries, especially those that serve the heart, are crucial factors in the progression of heart disease.

What traditional medical science seems to have missed is the fact that magnesium deficiency enhances the production of these fat-provoked atherosclerotic plaques, and that low magnesium can cause additional blood vessel disturbances. A slight, borderline magnesium deficiency can cause damage to blood vessel linings that permits small tears to occur. A slight tear in a blood vessel initiates the healing response of clotting, which leads to scarring inside the vessels and the potential for fat, cholesterol, and calcium to collect and form plaques at these scar sites. Another aspect of a low-magnesium state, "sticky" blood platelets, contributes to the formation of clots, which in turn adds to plaque buildup at these tear sites. Clot formation is also the source of emboli (clots that circulate in the bloodstream) that can block coronary arteries, leading to heart attacks, or obstruct the blood flow in arteries that serve the brain, leading to strokes. If magnesium is low inside these blood vessel cells, calcium tends to rush in where it doesn't belong, which adds a hardening factor to these unhealthy blood vessel cells. Such calcification is the basis of stiff, narrowed arteries—arteriosclerosis. But if magnesium is adequate, a moderately high-fat diet, even in the presence of a high-calcium intake, cannot cause such blood vessel havoc, and the tendency toward plaque buildup is diminished or even eliminated.

The Effect of Fat Intake on Magnesium Absorption

It has long been established that the heavy consumption of fats interferes with magnesium absorption. As long ago as 1918, a small study showed that boys given a high-fat meal absorbed half as much magnesium as they did on their normal diet. This was verified in the 1960s by larger studies on young men and women, who were shown not to retain enough magnesium to remain in balance, despite their consuming recommended amounts, when their fat intake was high. When normal young men were put on a diet similar to the milk-and-cream, protein-enriched diet then prescribed for people with peptic ulcers, they lost magnesium, even though their magnesium intake exceeded what was then thought to be necessary. If a person has a gastrointestinal disease that causes steatorrhea (fatty stools), the fat's interference with magnesium absorption has caused symptoms of magnesium deficiency ranging from muscle weakness or spasms to convulsions, and even thinning of the bones.

Thus, if you have a high-fat diet and inadequate magnesium, you are damaging your blood vessels.

Research has shown magnesium can lower total cholesterol by lowering bad LDL cholesterol and triglycerides, while raising good HDL cholesterol into the normal range. A diet high in saturated fat impairs magnesium absorption. The links between magnesium and the dangers of a high-fat diet are strong. Magnesium deficiency plays a role in atherosclerosis. But we rarely hear about it. Magnesium is rarely prescribed for these conditions. How has the cholesterol/high-fat theory developed so far without this knowledge?

How High Cholesterol Became the Enemy

It started with the eggs. Most of us got the message that eggs are bad for us. After all, they are high in cholesterol and saturated fat, two prominent factors in the type of diet first shown to cause atherosclerosis. Lately, research reports have been telling us that eggs are not so bad. The concept that eggs *are* bad had become so widespread that a television commercial showing eggs getting out of jail actually had meaning for us. Beyond the latest confusion in recommendations—be it three eggs per week rather than two, olive oil rather than margarine or margarine rather than butter—all in all, we know that cholesterol is bad and that whenever faced with a choice between low-fat or high-fat, the healthier choice is always the low-fat one, and unsaturated fat is always better than saturated.

How did this begin? Have our attempts to change our fat and cholesterol intake improved our health? Have all those low-cholesterol, low-fat recipes been worth the time, trouble, and expense? Do they lengthen our lives? And why all the mixed messages? How can we judge all the advice we are getting on diet?

Let's start with cholesterol.

In early studies, laboratory rabbits got atherosclerosis when fed high-cholesterol diets. Few paid attention to the low magnesium content of those early experimental diets. Nor was it seriously questioned that these so-called atherogenic diets produced atherosclerosis or plaques in rabbits, which are herbivorous (vegetarian), while other, carnivorous (meat-eating) animals were more resistant to damage caused by high-cholesterol diets.

Despite these experimental observations, the idea that cholesterol and fat cause heart disease became the popular dogma. It persists to this day, with low-cholesterol, low-fat diets most commonly offered as the solution to the heart-disease dilemma. At least it was something tangible to try. Plus, there was some experimental evidence to support it, especially when results of the Framingham study showed that high levels of cholesterol in the blood were associated with a greater risk of heart disease. The presence of cholesterol in atherosclerotic plaques gave confirming physical evidence. The plaques contain the enemy: cholesterol. However, they also contain calcium and fats other than cholesterol, as well as blood platelets and other elements found in blood clots. But it is still widely taught that these plaques are due to too much circulating cholesterol; that if one could lower the amount of cholesterol in the blood, these plaques would not form or would form more slowly. The conclusion, according to this premise, is that the high rate of heart disease seen in people with high cholesterol levels can be explained by the buildup of these plaques. Thus, physicians, nutritionists, and dietitians have long recommended that—although it is admittedly difficult, even for people at high risk of heart disease—a trustworthy preventive, and maybe even curative, approach is to lower the levels of fat and cholesterol in the blood by lowering the amount of fat and cholesterol in the diet.

By the 1960s, when heart disease deaths hit their peak, cholesterol levels became an obsession. Foregoing butter for margarine and limiting eggs became a life-and-death matter. Population studies were widely publicized showing that people with higher intakes of cholesterol were particularly subject to heart disease (with the blatant exception of Eskimos). Not so widely publicized were the population studies on cardiovascular rates in hard-water versus soft-water regions that began to appear in scientific journals during that time (see chapter 1). Most of these studies attributed the much lower rates of illness and death due to heart disease in hard-water areas as compared with soft-water regions to the rich magnesium content of hard water. Direct studies on magnesium and cholesterol or atherosclerosis appeared mostly in specialized research journals and were not widely circulated nor publicized. High fat and cholesterol remained the generally accepted enemy in heart disease.

The results of low-fat, low-cholesterol diets and the associated efforts to reduce the threat of cardiovascular disease have been, to say the least, confusing. For example, several important studies in the 1970s showed that low-fat diets had little or no effect on serum cholesterol levels, and other studies proved that adding 200 or 300 milligrams of cholesterol per day to the diet could not raise serum cholesterol values. A large clinical trial that successfully lowered serum cholesterol values an average of 6 to 10 percent with drugs showed no advantage of the lower cholesterol values when it came to heart disease and death rates. Many people with heart disease have normal cholesterol levels, and some people with high blood cholesterol have no signs of heart disease. By the 1980s, it was known that magnesium could prevent the atherosclerosis originally produced in those rabbits fed high-cholesterol diets. But again, these results did not receive the publicity that cholesterol and high fat received.

The cholesterol idea persisted.

As refinements in the cholesterol/fat theory of heart disease progressed, cholesterol was subdivided into total cholesterol, "good" cholesterol (HDL), and "bad" cholesterol (LDL). If one's good HDL cholesterol went below 40 mg/dL, there was a definite trend toward more heart disease. LDL cholesterol above 100 to 150 mg/100 cc or triglycerides above 150 mg/100 cc for men

A low-fat diet can lower total cholesterol 3 to 6 percent.

(130 for women) were deemed predictive of heart disease. By 1993, the American Heart Association's National Cholesterol Education Program set the goals of lowering the bad LDL cholesterol to target values with a diet providing no more than 30 percent of calories from fat and, if that failed, with cholesterol-lowering medications. Most people attempting to stay on such diets could not reach such low-fat levels on a consistent basis. And of those who actually achieved this feat for a whole year, only 20 percent lowered their LDL cholesterol values to the target level. But these difficulties have not stopped us from badgering ourselves mercilessly about our diets, and we began to see egg white omelettes, light margarine, dairy-free creamers for our coffee, fat-free pastries, and other such oddities in the marketplace. As if processed foods had not already done enough to us to make us sick, out came super-processed foods with no fat and no cholesterol as a means to make us well. Now we even have available, at a premium price, "rehabilitated" eggs that are low in cholesterol and high in unsaturated fat, developed by feeding hens certain nutrients. The risk factor concept of disease had come of age. Instead of looking for a specific treatment for a specific disease, such as vaccination against polio or antibiotics against pneumonia, treating and preventing heart disease became a matter of reducing as many risk factors as possible. And cholesterol was a most popular risk factor, one to be treated with a low-fat, low-cholesterol diet and/or by drugs.

So it has long been thought that changing our diet can lower our blood cholesterol and fat levels enough to avoid heart disease. This is partially true, but not in the way most of us think.

The True Benefit of a Low-Fat, Low-Cholesterol Diet

A diet that is low in fat and cholesterol can mean that the body has more magnesium. Since too little magnesium contributes to the formation of abnormal cholesterols, and processed foods are low in magnesium, many people in the industrialized world have both abnormally high cholesterol levels and low magnesium levels. Instead of being given magnesium supplements, we are told to lower our cholesterol and fat intake. Not wanting to die of a heart attack, many of us have tried to lower our cholesterol with a low-fat diet. And sometimes low-cholesterol, low-fat diets can indeed reduce cholesterol levels—but *not* because they are so low in fat and cholesterol. They really work because they raise the intake of magnesium.

The typical American diet contains 35 to 41 percent of total calories from fat, with 13 to 16 percent saturated fat. Most of this fat comes from low- or low-to-medium magnesium foods such as meats, dairy products, fried foods, snacks, and butter or margarine. (See Appendix B: Common Foods Classified by Magnesium Content.) The rest of the fat is in baked goods, which come along with refined flour and sugar, both of which are very low in magnesium. Restricting the intake of these foods in an attempt to lower a person's fat intake to 30 percent of calories or below results in nutritional changes beyond the change in fat consumption. In general, people on a low-fat diet get more of some nutrients—vitamin A, beta-carotene, folate, vitamin C, vitamin B_6, iron, vitamin B_1 (thiamin), and vitamin B_2 (riboflavin)—but less of others—vitamin B_3 (niacin), selenium, vitamin E, and zinc. For the purposes of this discussion, magnesium intake is higher with a low-fat diet, and people on such diets, as a group, are less likely to be low in magnesium than people on the typical American diet.

What about lowering the level of saturated fat in our diet? We are told that it is bad for us. How does it relate to magnesium? Saturated fats are mainly animals fats. When the level of saturated fats in the diet is high, several things happen:

1. Magnesium is less well absorbed because excess fat in the intestinal tract—whether from high-fat food or from gastrointestinal disease—interferes with magnesium absorption.
2. Even as less magnesium is absorbed, more magnesium becomes necessary to process the excess saturated fats.
3. Blood vessels, if deficient in magnesium, have fragile linings that are subject to small tears, more so when blood fat is high. These tiny tears can attract cholesterol, clotting elements, and calcium from the circulating blood, as a part of plaque buildup.

When people replace dietary saturated fats with unsaturated fats, they usually stay away from meat and eat more vegetables. This not only lowers their magnesium requirements, but also provides more magnesium and makes it easier to absorb. Such diets have a better chance of providing adequate magnesium nutrition. But if people remain low in magnesium, they are still at risk of heart disease, even if they lower their saturated fat intake.

Problems with Low-Fat, Low-Cholesterol Diets

So it is not surprising that the low-fat, low–saturated fat, and low-cholesterol diets can affect cholesterol values, but not in the way we would suppose and not as reliably as magnesium supplements do. For one thing, what doctors call *noncompliance*—failure to stick with the diet—is a major obstacle. A diet that provides only 30 percent of calories from fat is hard to achieve for most people on an ongoing, regular basis. Pastries are everywhere, as are candy bars, which provide more sugar than is good for someone with dyslipidemia. There is always some sort of celebration with cake or dessert, often at work, or at lunch out with the boss, friends, or coworkers. At the movies, popcorn tastes so much better with the "butter"—just this one time—and there's always the fast-food pizza or burger, fries, and soda bought and eaten on the run. It's just so much easier to eat a high-fat diet when you live in the industrialized world. Indeed, trying to lower your cholesterol level by changing your diet can be very stressful, something a person with borderline or low magnesium especially does not need (more about this in chapter 6).

Despite the difficulties involved, many people try to change their dietary habits and lower their fat intake. Motivated by their fear of the potential consequences of diagnosed high cholesterol, a prior heart attack, or just a desire to remain healthy, they make real efforts to stick to a low-fat diet. But there's a great deal of complexity associated with making a change in one's diet. Lower fat doesn't always mean more magnesium. For example, a person who substitutes fish for red meat will consume less saturated fat, more polyunsaturated fat, and more magnesium. Substituting soymilk for regular whole milk will greatly increase your dietary magnesium intake while reducing both fat and the calcium/magnesium ratio at the same time. This is really different from replacing whole milk with something other than soymilk (such as skim milk), because soymilk is a high-magnesium food and skim milk is not. And we should be aware that soy's high levels of phytate, a dietary fiber derivative, can diminish both magnesium and zinc absorption. In addition, skim milk is high in calcium and phosphorus while soy milk is not. A person who stops eating high-fat pastries and substitutes the remarkable fat-free pastries now on the market will take in a lot less magnesium than the person who substitutes whole-grain bread instead. And fat-free pastries and cholesterol-free candy contain a good deal of magnesium-draining sugar. So any of these changes will lower dietary fat, but only some will increase magnesium intake. If you look at the magnesium rather than the fat, you can see why the results from low-fat diets are so variable and confusing.

If you are attempting to improve your cholesterol and fat levels through diet, a high-magnesium diet is more reliable than a low-fat diet. Five studies on humans have found that all cholesterol and blood fat values improved with high-magnesium diets that did not rigidly lower fat consumption. The results showed that a high-magnesium diet had the following effects on blood cholesterol and triglycerides:

- Total cholesterol dropped by 6 to 13 percent
- LDL ("bad") cholesterol dropped by 7 to 18 percent
- Triglycerides dropped by 10 percent
- HDL ("good") cholesterol rose by up to 10 percent

There are other issues with low-fat diets beyond those of compliance and food selection. If such a diet is actually adhered to for a year—a feat not achieved by many who try it—the current recommended diets, with no more than 30 percent of calories from fat, 10 percent of calories from saturated fat, and 300 milligrams of cholesterol, do change cholesterol values. Such diets can lower LDL ("bad") cholesterol, on average, anywhere from 3 to 13 percent. That's good. What is confusing is that the lowest fat diets, those with only 22 to 25 percent fat, actually *raise* blood triglycerides and lower HDL cholesterol. The effects of such a diet on HDL ("good") cholesterol are the following:

- HDL ("good") cholesterol *drops* by 2.5 to 3.2 percent
- Triglycerides *rise* by 20 to 40 percent

This is going in the wrong direction. These very low-fat diets provide up to 60 or 70 percent of calories taken in as carbohydrates and are, in fact, high-carbohydrate diets. Nutritionists have evidence that, in some people, the excess carbohydrates are stored by the body as fats, and these end up in the blood as triglycerides. There is good evidence that triglyceride values relate more reliably to the amount of refined carbohydrates in a person's diet than to the fat or cholesterol in the diet. Add to this the fact that very low-fat diets, recommended by the American Heart Association's National Cholesterol Education Program in 1993, lower good cholesterol rather than raising it, especially in women. Why? A very low-fat, very high-carbohydrate diet, especially if rich in refined sugars, increases the body's losses of magnesium. Since magnesium intake with these diets can be generally low to begin with, this extra loss in the urine can turn a low or suboptimal magnesium intake into a magnesium deficiency. Since, as we have seen, low magnesium levels increase LDL cholesterol and decrease HDL cholesterol, a diet that intensifies magnesium inadequacy carries with it the risk of making the cholesterol problem worse. One study on women showed that a low-magnesium diet caused low levels of good HDL cholesterol. Such facts raise serious questions about a treatment that is difficult to administer as well as to achieve. This is what we mean by "confusing" results.

These results are not heartening. Recently, the *type* rather than the *amount* of fat in the diet has been emphasized. We see recommendations to eat more monounsaturated fats, such as olive oil, which is widely used in France. The French have a low rate of death due to heart disease despite eating rather high-fat diets. If you must count your cents as well as your calories, you might use the cheaper canola oil, even though it is not as high in monounsaturates as olive oil. The so-called Mediterranean diet is not often described as a high-magnesium diet, but with its emphasis on nuts, seeds, vegetables, whole grains, fruits for dessert, little or no sugar, and very low dairy consumption, we can see (using the information in appendix B) that it is an excellent diet for delivering adequate amounts of magnesium.

At the opposite end of the scale, Dr. Robert Atkins, originator of the Atkins diet, says that we can eat all the fat we want and be perfectly healthy as long as our carbohydrate intake is *very* low. Dr. Atkins gives a very convincing argument that a high-fat diet *combined with* high carbohydrates is the real culprit, because it raises both total cholesterol and triglyceride levels. He claims that his patients do not have high cholesterol values, and that many people with heart disease get well on his diet as long as their high-fat intake is always combined with a low-carbohydrate intake and adequate nutrition, including magnesium nutrition. The evidence from the very low-fat diet studies mentioned above tends to confirm the idea that carbohydrates may be more of a culprit than fats in the triglyceride and cholesterol story. It is certainly possible that Dr. Atkins's patients tend to preserve their magnesium since they completely avoid refined carbohydrates such as sugar and refined flour.

Countering Dr. Atkins and the American Heart Association is Dr. Dean Ornish. Dr. Ornish rightfully claims that plaque formation is stopped in less than one-fifth of people who achieve the 30 percent fat diet, regardless of their cholesterol values, while another 40 percent of people on such a diet develop even more vessel blockages. His solution is an even lower fat diet (10 percent of calories as fat), which makes his diet the one that provides the most carbohydrate of virtually any diet out there. But his dietary recommendations include vegetarianism, which can mean significantly higher than average dietary magnesium, as well as very low intakes of the big magnesium-wasters: refined carbohydrates such as refined flour and sugars. Also, this strict diet comes as part of an overall program for significant stress reduction, which can drastically lower magnesium requirements. (This will be discussed in detail in chapter 6.)

But there is more to consider about the impact of the currently recommended low-fat diets. There are substantial individual variations in people's responses to very low-fat diets. For example, changes in LDL cholesterol ranged from an increase of 3 percent

Switching to a high-magnesium diet can lower total cholesterol 6 to 13 percent.

to a decrease of 55 percent for men, and an increase of 13 percent to a decrease of 39 percent in women. That means that while some people lowered their bad cholesterol by more than half, other people raised their levels of bad cholesterol after a year on these diets. Despite such complexities and confusions, the belief persists that lowering blood cholesterol, especially LDL cholesterol, is somehow the key to fighting heart disease. With this frame of mind, dietary intervention studies show the low-cholesterol, low-fat diets to be "successful" if they reduce the numbers of people who need to go on cholesterol-lowering drugs. And if LDL cholesterol is lowered enough, this goal is achieved. Up to 20 percent of people who go on these diets will not have to take cholesterol-lowering drugs. The other 80 percent presumably will. What are these drugs and how do they work? *What are they getting into?*

Cholesterol-Lowering Drugs Compared with Magnesium

Very high doses of the B vitamin niacin have been used to lower cholesterol levels quite successfully, as have drugs classified as fibrates, such as gemfibrozil (Lopid). But as with low-fat diet therapy, there are side effects, and no great drops in the incidence of heart disease or death from heart disease have been noted. But medical science, persisting in its quest to lower cholesterol, now specifically targeting LDL cholesterol, has achieved a breakthrough: statin drugs.

The Effects of Statin Drugs

Responding to the perceived need to lower LDL cholesterol levels in order to prevent or at least retard heart disease, the pharmaceutical companies looked for a way to cut cholesterol off at its source. And they came up with an ingenious idea. Why not inhibit the enzyme responsible for cholesterol synthesis? After devoting much research to the enzyme HMG-CoA reductase, the rate-controlling enzyme in the cholesterol synthesis pathway, they developed a series of drugs called *statins.* Examples of statins include atorvastatin (Lipitor), cerivastatin (Baycol), fluvastatin (Lescol), lovastatin (Mevacor), pravastatin (Pravachol), rosuvastatin, and simvastatin (Zocor).

These drugs act by inhibiting HMG-CoA reductase, an enzyme that needs magnesium for proper regulatory control. By inhibiting this enzyme, these drugs can lower LDL cholesterol levels by very large amounts, in the 35 to 65 percent range. They are especially effective in people with the highest LDL cholesterol levels. But there's more. Much more. When these drugs were studied, they were found to do more than lower LDL cholesterol. They also reduced total mortality (the number of overall deaths), cardiac mortality (the number of deaths due to heart disease), and the total incidence of heart attacks, angina, and other nonfatal cardiac events. Not only that, they lowered the number of deaths due to stroke. These drugs appear to be, literally, lifesavers. After repeated good news from trials on patients with high cholesterol levels, the effects of these drugs on people with heart disease who had normal cholesterol values were studied, and again researchers encountered the clinical benefits of lower mortality and fewer cardiac events. The excitement has been profound, and has been expressed in articles in medical journals about the benefits of taking statins.

Intuitively, doctors and researchers knew that the greater than expected benefits of statins could not be due only to their ability to lower LDL cholesterol. So they began looking closer. What they found was that statins were achieving several other things as well:

- They made blood platelet cells less "sticky." Because the platelets did not aggregate so much, there was less risk of clotting in the blood vessels and less chance of emboli (see page 129) or thrombosis (the lodging of an embolus in a blood vessel), as well as of plaque formation—so important in the atherosclerosis process.
- They slowed the progression of plaques and stabilized them. There was some evidence that taking statins could even reverse the process of plaque formation, which had long been thought to be a one-way process only.
- They reduced inflammation in blood vessel tissue.

All of these processes and more were found to be a result of less mevalonate, the direct result of the activity of HMG-CoA reductase, the enzyme the statin drugs inhibit (see figure 5.1). In studies on animal cells, all of these beneficial effects could be undone by adding mevalonate. The inhibition of HMG-CoA reductase and, with it, the amount of mevalonate in the system turned out to be a boon to heart-disease treatment that went way beyond the expected lowering of LDL cholesterol.

The Effects of Magnesium Compared with Those of Statins

Now let us compare the statin effects to those of magnesium, which is the natural inhibitor of HMG-CoA reductase. Here, magnesium and the statins are comparable. But magnesium also acts on two different enzymes, phosphatase reductase and phosphohydrolase, which reactivate HMG-CoA reductase. By its effects on these enzymes, which have contrasting activities, magnesium either stops cholesterol formation or allows it to continue, depending on the body's needs. Magnesium also affects another enzyme that has an impact on cholesterol, but in quite another way. Lecithin-cholesterol acyltransferase (LCAT) is an enzyme that converts LDL cholesterol into HDL cholesterol, and magnesium activates it. Through this action, magnesium actually increases HDL ("good") cholesterol while decreasing LDL ("bad") cholesterol.

With broader effects on cholesterol than the statins have, how does magnesium perform in providing the clinical benefits that the statins unquestionably achieve? Let's compare the statin effects with those of magnesium. Table 5.1 compares the physiological effects of magnesium with those of statins; table 5.2 summarizes the results from several studies on statins and magnesium supplements. While statins definitely lower LDL cholesterol, magnesium lowers it while also raising HDL cholesterol, something statins do less consistently. Both treatments lowered mortality and morbidity rates, but magnesium has some advantages. Instead of inhibiting or "poisoning" this important enzyme as the statins do, magnesium inhibits it in a way that permits it to be reactivated by other (magnesium-dependent) enzymes, so the body can make the amounts of mevalonate and cholesterol it needs. And, after all, cholesterol synthesis is a natural process that is necessary to the body. Cholesterol is a neceessary building block for hormones such as testosterone, estrogen, and the adrenal cortico-

Table 5.1 A Comparison of the Physiological Effects of Magnesium and Statin Drugs

Magnesium is a natural regulator of HMG-CoA reductase, the enzyme that is inhibited by the statins. In addition to lowering LDL cholesterol, magnesium reliably elevates HDL cholesterol through its effect on LCAT. Like statins, it has a favorable influence on the tendency of blood to clot in blood vessels. Unlike statins, it prevents muscle damage, does not increase liver enzyme levels, and is free of other side effects.

Effect	Statin Drugs	Magnesium
Target enzyme	HMG-CoA reductase only	HMG CoA reductase and LCAT
Effect on enzyzme	Inhibits or poisons	Regulates and controls
Lowers "bad" cholesterol	Yes	Yes
Raises "good" cholesterol	Sometimes	Yes
Prevents clot formation	Yes	Yes
Reduces inflammation	Yes	Yes
Slows and prevents atherosclerotic plaques	Yes	Yes
Raises liver enzymes past normal	Yes	No
Can cause myopathy	Yes	Prevents myopathy
Many side effects	Yes	No

steroids. Surely we don't want to interfere with this natural process unless there is a real medical necessity.

Since statins are drugs, the body deals with them as it would a toxin. The body actively processes them to eliminate them, either directly, if they are water soluble, or by being changed in the liver to other chemicals that are then excreted by the body, if they are fat soluble. They are all a bit different in how they are processed, and so they are excreted from the body at various rates, anywhere from hours to a few days. Thus, in order to keep the benefits of a statin working, one must

Table 5.2 A Comparison of the Health Effects of Magnesium and Statin Drugs

Both statins and magnesium supplements lower the rate of death due to heart disease. The table below summarizes the results of sixteen research studies, eight on statins and eight on magnesium.

	Drop in overall mortality	Drop in heart disease mortality	Drop in heart disease events
Statin drugs	17–22 percent	24–28 percent	13–45 percent
Magnesium supplements	37–80 percent	71 percent	49–76 percent

continue to take it, day after day. Otherwise the HMG-CoA reductase will not be inactivated, and everything will go back to the way it was.

In contrast, magnesium is an essential nutrient. True, it must be taken every day in food and water, and if that supply is inadequate, in the form of supplements. But rather than trying to eliminate it, the body tries to conserve this vital nutrient, especially if intake or body levels are low. Magnesium does not have to be processed by the liver as a toxin in order to be excreted. Rather, it is lost from the body through a normal metabolic process. If there is too much magnesium in the bloodstream, the kidneys excrete it; if blood levels are too low, the kidneys retain it. That is why it needs to be replenished on a daily basis. Since it is a nutrient rather than a drug, it has almost no side effects when taken as a supplement (other than diarrhea, which can occur if you take too much at any one time). Remember, milk of magnesia is magnesium hydroxide—which has a time-honored position as a laxative, when taken in sufficiently large amounts.

The Issue of Side Effects

As is the case with any drug, statins can have adverse effects. These are few, affecting under 2 percent of those taking them, which makes them very safe as well as effective drugs.

But the adverse effects are not zero. What are some of them? They affect the liver, as indicated by higher than normal levels of transaminases (liver enzymes) in blood tests. But these generally have been found to be temporary and reversible. Stopping the drug generally reverses the trend and the liver shows no permanent harm. Most studies do not even count this effect unless the transaminase is at least three times the normal upper limit. They don't always report the number of people who have only slight increases or even those with increases to the above-normal range but less than three times the normal level. A similar situation exists for the second major adverse effect found with all statins, the elevation of creatine phosphokinase (CPK). This is an enzyme that is generally reported when it reaches five times above the normal upper level. But, again, this occurs in few of the people who take statins. Myopathy, or muscle pain and/or weakness, is a main adverse effect that can be serious. Most cases occur when statin drugs are taken in conjunction with other drugs that use the same detoxification system in the liver as do the statins. This explains why cerivastatin (Baycol) caused fifty-two deaths worldwide and was voluntarily taken off the market by the manufacturer. It was too often prescribed with other drugs, such as gemfibrozil, or prescribed in high doses, which made it dangerous.

Other effects that have been reported but not seen as serious enough clinically to forgo the beneficial effects of statins are adverse drug reactions relating to the nervous system, intestinal tract, skin, and cardiovascular organs. Psychiatric disorders represented 15 percent of the reactions to statins in one data collection, and these reactions included aggression, nervousness, depression, anxiety, sleeping disorders, and impotence. Also, neuropathy (abnormal changes in the functioning of peripheral nerves) has been reported, as has inflammation of the lung and hepatitis. We want to emphasize that these effects are rare. But the main thing is that magnesium does all that a statin does without the adverse side effects, and without covering up a nutritional deficiency.

Other Issues

Finally, statins are not cheap. Depending on the brand and dosage prescribed, these drugs can cost anywhere from $35 to over $225 per month. Cost is the main reason people stop taking these drugs or fail to take them as prescribed. Sixty-seven percent of those who discontinue statin therapy do so because of the cost, while only about 2 percent stop using them because of side effects.

The statins are clearly breakthrough drugs, and we can expect to see them prescribed for many conditions besides cholesterol and heart disease in the future. They have been shown to decrease the incidence of death due to stroke and may turn out to be beneficial for osteoporosis. But they should not be used to replace or compensate for proper magnesium nutrition. For one thing, the cost would be prohibitive. Imagine if we were to go along not recognizing our low magnesium epidemic and try instead to find ways to get statins to every man, woman, and child. Certainly this would be neither a cost-effective nor a smart way to go. Besides, magnesium sufficiency is the logical alternative. Not only does it inhibit HMG-CoA reductase and therefore the synthesis of cholesterol, but it activates the enzymes that allow for cholesterol synthesis to resume as necessary. Magnesium is also crucial for the activity of LCAT, which converts bad LDL cholesterol into beneficial HDL cholesterol. Statins do not affect LCAT or the enzymes that reactivate HMG-CoA reductase. In addition, magnesium is necessary for the activity of another enzyme, desaturase, that is important for the production from fatty acids of other important substances that affect the cardiovascular system in other ways.

Omega-3 and Omega-6 Fatty Acids and Magnesium

The omega-3 and omega-6 fatty acids (also known as essential fatty acids or EFAs) need magnesium in order to be processed properly. These essential, delicate fatty acids, which are known to help heart disease in some cases, are processed by the bodies' cells into hormonelike substances called *prostaglandins* via a series of reactions, the first of which is achieved by the enzyme desaturase. Without adequate magnesium, desaturase cannot do its job.

There are two types of prostaglandins: prostacyclins and thromboxanes. These are very active chemicals that turn on and/or turn off a host of cell processes. Some of these processes protect against heart disease, and some promote it. Prostacyclins, which originate from the omega-6 essential fatty acid linoleic acid (LA), tend to keep blood platelets from sticking together and thus help prevent heart attacks and strokes caused by blood clots in the arteries. In contrast, thromboxanes, which originate from the LA derivative arachidonic acid (AA), promote platelet stickiness and clotting. When you have a cut, you want thromboxane to go into action and, temporarily, inhibit the anticlotting actions of prostacyclin. There is another prostaglandin that is derived from the omega-3 essential fatty acid linolenic acid (LNA). It has an inhibiting effect on the release of thromboxane from its dormant state in cell membranes. The interaction of these prostaglandins with one another and with the body's physiology is complex, but in a healthy body that is receiving adequate amounts of both essential fatty acids and magnesium, a balance of prostaglandins is achieved, naturally. Proper prostaglandin formation also requires vitamins C, B_3, and B_6, as well as zinc.

Desaturase is the first enzyme to work on LA and LNA in their biochemical pathway to becoming prostaglandins. Without adequate magnesium, desaturase cannot do its job, the essential fatty acids cannot get past the first biochemical step in their pathway, and the biochemical production of prostaglandins is blocked. People who are getting adequate amounts of magnesium (as well as zinc and vitamins C, B_3, and B_6) but inadequate intakes of essential fatty acids can be helped by increasing the amount of omega-3 and omega-6 essential fatty acids they consume. But without adequate magnesium (or other nutrients necessary for prostaglandin synthesis), we cannot expect these essential fatty acids to be beneficial—they cannot be processed properly. For optimal regulation and control via balanced prostaglandin synthesis, you must have an adequate intake of both magnesium and the essential fatty acids, along with vitamins C, B_3, B_6, and zinc.

Improving Your Magnesium Status to Reduce the Dangers of Fat and Cholesterol

A new picture of fat, cholesterol, and heart disease begins to emerge: adequate magnesium allows the body to properly control and regulate cholesterol synthesis. In one way, by inhibiting cholesterol synthesis, magnesium acts like a statin—a natural one. But in addition, magnesium acts on other enzymes that are crucial in fat biochemistry. Two are enzymes that permit the reactivation of the enzyme responsible for cholesterol production. Others are the enzyme that converts "bad" cholesterol to "good" cholesterol and the one that allows omega-3 and omega-6 fatty acids to be converted into prostaglandins.

This is all fine and helps us to understand some of the complexities that have muddied the picture of how the nutritional modification of fat metabolism functions in the prevention of heart disease. But what, then, should we eat? The diets advised by the American Heart Association? By Dr. Ornish? Or by Dr. Atkins? High-fat, low-fat, no-fat? Really, *all* these are right—as long as you get enough of all essential nutrients, especially magnesium. With enough magnesium—which many of us lack without knowing it—fats can be properly processed. Cholesterol synthesis is properly regulated and controlled, and LDL cholesterol is converted to HDL cholesterol and removed from the bloodstream in a healthy way, without robbing the body of its necessary cholesterol. Essential fatty acids (omega-3 and omega-6) can be properly converted to the right blend of prostaglandins. Delicate blood-vessel linings do not tend to tear as much; if blood vessel damage occurs, cholesterol deposition, overclotting, and the rushing in of calcium do not occur, and plaques do not form.

With magnesium sufficiency, HMG-CoA reductase is optimally regulated and controlled. As a result, mevalonate levels are not excessive. As with statins, the chance of death drops and the likely outcome of heart disease procedures is improved. The big difference is that proper magnesium nutrition is free of statin's adverse side effects, and the cost is minimal.

. . .

We believe it is best to concentrate on how to correct your magnesium status. Read on to find the situation that most closely matches your own, and follow the step-by-step directions. Give yourself time, select what will work for you on a long-term basis, work with a doctor to monitor your progress with laboratory results, and find out what your body needs to stay healthy and in optimal magnesium status.

Hyperlipidemia

You have hyperlipidemia if:

- Your total cholesterol is above 200, and/or
- Your HDL ("good") cholesterol is below 40, and/or
- Your LDL ("bad") cholesterol is above 125, and/or
- Your HDL:total cholesterol ratio is above 9:1, and/or
- Your triglyceride level is above 150 to 190 (this is treated separately below)

If this applies to you, carefully follow the steps below:

1. Make an assessment of medications you are now taking. Do any "waste" magnesium? (Consult Appendix H: "Common Medications That Affect Magnesium Status"; also consult your physician.) If you take any magnesium-depleting drugs, discuss this with your doctor and see if these might safely be changed.
2. Fill in the Magnesium Questionnaire in appendix A to help decide on initial supplement levels.
3. If your magnesium risk as determined by the questionnaire is low, and you are not taking any magnesium-wasting medications, start by using a high magnesium salt in all your cooking and at your table (see Appendix D: "Magnesium in Salt Substitutes"). This is a simple, healthy move that provides both magnesium and potassium. After three months, have your cholesterol values checked. If there is no improvement, go to the next step.
4. If using magnesium salt has not normalized your cholesterol values, start taking a magnesium supplement. You can take any-

where from 200 milligrams per day (if your questionnaire determines your risk to be low) to 700 milligrams per day (if your risk is high). Start at a lower dose and build up to your tolerance, which is the amount you can regularly take without having uncomfortably loose stools. If you do not like to take pills, try a magnesium supplement that dissolves in water and is taken as a drink or one of the liquid magnesium supplements. After three to six months, have your cholesterol values checked again. If there is still no improvement, go to the next step.

5. If the salts and supplements together do not work to your satisfaction, or if you would rather use food than pills to increase your magnesium intake (our recommended approach), look at your diet. Write down *everything* you eat for one to three days (the more days you list, the more accurate your assessment will be). After compiling your list, look up the foods in Appendix B: Common Foods Classified by Magnesium Content and mark them as high, medium, or low magnesium foods, as appropriate. (If a food is not listed, consult the USDA database as directed at the end of appendix B.) Now, ask yourself how you can change your diet, realistically, to include more high-magnesium foods. Could you eat more nuts? We know that nuts have been off-limits for people on low-fat diets, but eating nuts regularly has been shown to decrease the incidence of heart disease by 30 to 50 percent and the risk of death due to heart disease by 25 to 35 percent. Could you substitute soy counterparts for some dairy foods such as milk and cheese? Could you eliminate refined flour products, pasta, and refined rice and stick to whole-grain and brown rice instead? Could you cut down on the sugar? This is hard for some people to do, as sugar can be addictive (see chapter 4). If you just can't make yourself go without sweets, could you make your own using brown sugar plus some extra molasses? How about emphasizing fruits and vegetables, including legumes, and/or replacing some red meats with fish?

Using these principles in a vegetarian diet can also raise your magnesium and lower your cholesterol. Substitute legumes, nuts, and seeds for fish and meat; eat lots of fruits and vegetables;

and stay away from processed foods, refined sugar, and flour. Some people can do this, some cannot. For those who can, it is a great way to go, and if you use a high-magnesium salt, you and your family have a good chance of beating the magnesium deficit.

These are changes only you can make for your lifestyle and it will take effort, but should become easier as time goes by. If you need to have lunch out with colleagues and it's always a low-magnesium meal, try to make up for this at other meals or with a supplement. Take a look at your snacks. Could you switch from pastries to nuts? If done consistently (six out of seven days per week) this could mean a big improvement in your magnesium intake. Do what you can to increase the amount of magnesium in your diet. Don't worry so much about dietary fat as you look to keep your magnesium in the safe range. The improvement will be gradual as your dietary changes become habitual.

6. Learn more about omega-3 and omega-6 fatty acids and gradually try to integrate these essential nutrients into your diet. A good start is *Omega 3 Oils: A Practical Guide* by Donald Rudin and Clara Felix (Avery, 1996). If a diet that provides these essential fatty acids does not work for you, take a close look at your intake of magnesium, zinc, and vitamins C, B_6, and B_3.
7. If you switch to a magnesium salt, take supplements, and change your diet, and your cholesterol is *still* out of whack and/or you still have heart disease, you may be a "magnesium-waster" or you may have familial hypercholesterolemia.

Magnesium-Wasting

Magnesium-wasters lose much of their needed magnesium in their urine. This problem can be innate or a result of taking certain drugs. If your diet and supplements are more than adequate in magnesium and you are not taking any medications that cause magnesium loss in the urine (such as digitalis and diuretics), and you still have high cholesterol values, you may be a waster. The best way to find out is to do a magnesium retention test or other magnesium assessment with your doctor's guidance. (These will be discussed in chapter 10.) Some magnesium-wasters can do well with intramuscular magnesium sulfate or chloride shots. Work with your doctor and use the guidelines in Appendix F: Guidelines for Magnesium Injections.

Poor Magnesium Absorption

Like magnesium-wasting, poor magnesium absorption can be an innate problem or a result of taking various medications. A rare condition in infants is the inability to absorb adequate magnesium from food. This condition can interfere with normal development and even survival past childhood, so it is rarely found in adults.

Some drugs, including tetracyclines, some other antibiotics, and some hormone therapies interfere with magnesium absorption. If taken for short periods, this need not be a problem. Consult with your physician.

Familial Hypercholesterolemia

Familial hypercholesterolemia is a rare genetic disorder. If you have familial hyperlipidemia and have very elevated cholesterol, it is not known whether magnesium supplements can help you. A study in which individuals with this disorder were using 450 or 600 milligrams per day of supplements containing magnesium-pyridoxal-5'-phosphate glutamate (MPPG) resulted in no changes in cholesterol values. It is possible that higher amounts of magnesium might be effective.

High Triglycerides

If your blood triglycerides are too high, you need to make sure you are getting adequate magnesium. Magnesium lowers triglyceride levels. Statin drugs can lower a high triglyceride level if it is not above 300. You may also need to lower your refined carbohydrate intake. Steve's triglyceride level was 480 when he went on Dr. Atkins's very low-carbohydrate ketogenic diet. Within six months, his high triglycerides had dropped to 220—still too high, but quite an improvement. To get off refined carbohydrates is not easy. You may want to get help with a support group such as Overeaters Anonymous, Food Addicts Anonymous, Compulsive Eaters Anonymous-HOW, or other diet support group. (See Resources.)

The forms of magnesium that have been shown to work on dyslipidemia have been magnesium chloride, magnesium hydroxide, magnesium oxide, magnesium aspartate hydrochloride, magnesium citrate, magnesium gluconate, magnesium pidolate and magnesium-pyridoxal-5'-phosphate glutamate (MPPG). If you do not like to take pills or they don't work for you, we suggest that you try one of the magnesium-containing salts listed in appendix D at your table and in your cooking.

Coronary Artery Disease

If you have coronary artery disease, magnesium supplements can help your high-cholesterol values as well as the heart disease. Follow the supplement and dietary guidelines on page 148.

Statin Medications

If you are taking statin medications, before going off them (with your physician's guidance) you should be taking magnesium supplements or have made changes in your diet. Taking both a statin and magnesium will not further lower your LDL cholesterol, but since these both work on the same enzyme, before going off statins you should have the proper amount of magnesium in your body to regulate and control cholesterol synthesis. But, again, do not change any drugs without working with your doctor. Going off statins can have adverse effects, and changing statins can lessen their LDL-cholesterol–lowering effect.

Diabetes

If you are diabetic, you may be more likely to be low in HDL cholesterol and high in triglycerides. Read carefully the information on metabolic syndrome X in chapter 2 and follow recommendations in chapter 11 on how to increase your magnesium intake. Repleting your magnesium and reducing your refined carbohydrate intake should help your cholesterol and triglyceride values as well as type II diabetes.

6

Magnesium, Stress, and the Type A Personality

Joe was sixty when his doctor told him he needed a bypass operation. Terrified by hospitals, Joe hated the prospect. But his family was confident and grateful that medical science could and would extend his life, and his doctor was sincere in picking this particular procedure for Joe's case. "It'll give him years more," said the doctor, knowing that Joe was not a great candidate for lifestyle changes. Into the hospital Joe went, literally clutching the rails on his hospital bed. He was incredibly relieved upon awakening from the successful procedure and gratefully went home to rest and heal. He felt weak and barely able to cope, but he and his family were assured that rest would take care of him. Within ten days, Joe was recovering

> nicely, beginning to cope with the lessening pain and the changes he was facing. Suddenly, a loud, crashing car accident occurred in front of his house, shattering Joe's newly acquired calm. Within hours he was in the emergency room with severe chest pains, and he died in spite of the very capable doctors' best efforts.

How could this happen? The bypass operation was not a failure. It had successfully replaced Joe's severely narrowed coronary artery. Blood again flowed freely to Joe's heart muscle, and there was no infection. But the stresses caused by the operation, hospitalization, and anxiety before and after the surgery were so severe that they depleted Joe's magnesium—to an extent that the sound of the noisy crash induced enough of a stress reaction that Joe died of a heart attack in spite of his newly restored heart circulation.

We must look closely at this vague-sounding concept—stress—and find out how, when, and why it impacts our hearts.

Stress and Magnesium Requirements

Stresses can be emotional, such as fear, sadness, anger, or even great joy and excitement. Stresses can be caused by competition—mental or physical. They can be environmental, such as heat, cold, forced immobility, imprisonment, flashing bright lights, and loud noise, whether continuous or sudden. There are also physical stresses, such as extreme exercise, hunger, pain, illness, injury, medical operations, and invasive medical tests. Although stresses differ markedly, our bodies respond to them similarly, with a literal cascade of responses at the molecular, cellular, tissue, organ, and organ-system levels. Such responses are stimulated by increased secretion of the stress hormones adrenaline and adrenal cortisone, which are often called the *fright, flight, or fight hormones* because they help animals and people to survive during threatening situations.

Stress hormones cause a sudden rise in magnesium-dependent reactions. Energy production, nerve-impulse transmission, increased muscle function, and responses of heart and blood vessels all require magnesium. There is an immediate increase in the use of magnesium, so our need for magnesium soars as we respond to stress. Thus, our reactions to acute stress really put our magnesium status to the test. During stress, magnesium is mobilized from available sources (stores) that are not life-maintaining—for example, as part of bone-surface minerals. The mobilized magnesium enters the blood, which carries it to the heart, where it helps provide the energy needed by the heart to pump more rapidly and strongly. It also supplies the increased magnesium our voluntary muscles require, for a short time, during times of stress. However, these temporarily elevated blood magnesium levels signal the kidneys that there is too much magnesium in the body. In response, they decrease reabsorption of the magnesium from the blood as it circulates through the kidneys, with the result that more magnesium is eliminated in the urine and less is restored to the circulating blood. This reduces the amount of magnesium in the entire body. If magnesium nutrition has been adequate, the body magnesium stores are sufficient to meet this sudden, usually short-lived, increased need. But if the body's magnesium stores are too low, and the stress persists, the stress hormones begin to mobilize magnesium from even the vital tissues, such as the heart, and the response to acute stress can become dangerous.

With prolonged stress-inducing conditions, the need for magnesium remains abnormally high during the body's response to the sustained stress. Suboptimal magnesium stores can be exhausted. Even with seemingly adequate magnesium nutrition, there can be decreased resistance to chronic stress. It is possible to adapt to a condition of chronic stress, and once you achieve this, everything seems just fine for a while, sometimes for a long while. Such periods of adaptation to a stressful way of life can go on for years, and can delude a person into believing that living an extremely demanding and/or exciting life need not endanger his or her health or even survival. But the ability to adapt to stress can diminish, and if it does, irreversible damage can ensue.

Magnesium's Role in the Stress Reaction

The instantaneous rises in the body's heart rate, blood pressure, and energy needs for the fright, fight, or flight reaction necessitate a good

The stress reaction requires magnesium.

supply of magnesium. It is required to activate adenosine triphosphate (ATP), a substance that acts as the battery that powers life. (See chapter 1.) It is also required to burn glucose and fats to meet the sudden need for extra energy. Protein synthesis and heightened nerve-impulse transmission also demand magnesium. Magnesium is needed every time a new high-energy ATP molecule is produced, and magnesium is needed every time an ATP molecule gives up its energy for a needed cell reaction. These ATP batteries just won't work without magnesium. The batteries and their magnesium are necessary at all times in life, but when stress hormones are circulating, these molecular batteries have to work with extra intensity and speed. In a healthy body that has ample magnesium stores, enough is available to enable all these varied simultaneous reactions to speed up in response to circulating stress hormones, and to remain combined with ATP to keep it functional during the increased demands of stress. But with low stores of magnesium, acute or prolonged chronic stress reactions demand so much that blood magnesium can fall to dangerously low levels.

The Effects of Low Magnesium Combined with Stress

If stress hormones cause blood magnesium to fall to levels that are so low (hypomagnesemic) that the cells are abnormally low in magnesium, an indication of magnesium depletion, arterial spasms can result. How? In studies in which a volunteer was slowly infused with the stress hormone adrenaline for a period of three hours, there was decline of plasma magnesium, as well as of calcium, potassium, and sodium. Since adequate magnesium levels in arterial muscle cells cause the arteries to relax, or dilate, arteries constrict when magnesium levels are low. This is a consequence of calcium moving into the cells of the arteries to replace the missing magnesium; calcium causes arterial muscle contraction. If this occurs in the coronary arteries, the chest pain of angina pectoris can ensue as a direct consequence of magnesium loss. The angina pain is an alarm signal saying:

Stress hormones lower blood magnesium.

"Stop! Unwind! Relax! Pop a pill!" In experiments such as the one mentioned above, when the infusion of adrenaline is stopped, the level of that hormone in the blood drops after only five minutes, but it takes the heart half an hour to slow to its normal rate. The blood potassium level rises to normal again in that same half hour, but the level of the magnesium in the blood can remain lowered even longer. Thus, if magnesium stores are low when an acute stress reaction develops, the heart is endangered. Severe, unremitting stress can deplete magnesium, creating a substantial risk of injury to the heart—its muscle and its control of how fast or regularly it beats.

Magnesium deficiency exacerbates these physiological reactions to acute stress, while a mildly high blood magnesium tones them down. In addition, in a magnesium-deficient body, stress elicits a greater hormonal response than it would if that body were adequate in magnesium—quite a bit greater. The stress response is thus even more intense, making the magnesium requirement even higher and less likely to be met.

How Adrenaline Release and Magnesium Deficit Reinforce Each Other

Stress stimulates the secretion of excess adrenaline. This initially mobilizes magnesium from the body's stores, temporarily raising the level in the blood as it is transported to the cells of organs vital to the fright, flight, or fight response. When stress persists, more cellular magnesium is drawn into the blood to prevent circulating levels of magnesium from falling as a result of the kidneys' elimination of magnesium. (The kidneys filter out and excrete magnesium when blood concentrations are above normal.) This continues as long as there is sufficient cellular or stored magnesium. When these stores run out, blood falls below normal. This condition, called *hypomagnesemia,* by itself creates stress and directly initiates more adrenaline release. The result is a downward spiral for the body's magnesium availability that, in a person with marginal or low magnesium intake, can intensify the loss of cellular magnesium, with a risk of causing magnesium depletion and hypomagnesemia. If the body's magnesium stores are adequate, this

The Effects of Adrenaline

Adrenaline is one of the body's major stress hormones. When adrenaline is released into the bloodstream, it has simultaneous, rapid, and widespread effects on the body. These include the following:

- It has widespread effects on circulation, muscles, and sugar metabolism.
- It increases the heart rate.
- It increases heart output.
- It increases rate and depth of breathing.
- It increases the metabolic rate.
- It increases the force of muscle contraction.
- It delays muscle fatigue.
- It reduces blood flow to the bladder (muscle walls relax and sphincters contract).
- It reduces blood flow to intestines (muscle walls relax and sphincters contract).
- It increases blood pressure.
- It increases the level of glucose in the blood.
- It prompts an increase in the metabolism of glucose for energy especially in muscle cells. This process requires magnesium.
- It causes a release of free fatty acids. This process requires magnesium.
- It causes more oxidation of fatty acids. This process requires magnesium.
- It causes more ATP to be produced. This process requires magnesium.
- It causes blood vessels to constrict.

So much magnesium is needed for these heightened responses that magnesium leaves the blood and goes into cells.

potentially dangerous vicious circle does not occur. But if magnesium is borderline or deficient, the stress response can result in a dangerously low magnesium state that can produce magnesium depletion, with the risk of its severe effects such as heart attack and even sudden death from arrhythmia. When a magnesium-deficient person is stressed, the only ways to prevent a potentially catastrophic loss of magnesium are to:

- Reduce the adrenaline response (with beta-blockers)
- Replace the body's magnesium quickly by means of intravenous or intramuscular injection, followed by immediate and sustained supplementation with oral magnesium, to repair the deficit
- Provide supportive antioxidant nutrients that counteract the oxidative effect of the fall in magnesium (more about this later in this chapter)

When body stores of magnesium are dangerously depleted, these are the only ways to counteract the adrenaline flow and its lowering of magnesium stores and availability. No wonder a high dietary magnesium intake or oral magnesium supplementation before a traumatic event can help the body withstand a stressful episode. No wonder magnesium therapy during the ultimate stress event, a heart attack, lowered the death rate substantially in several studies (see chapter 1).

Damage to Magnesium-Deficient Cells Caused by Stress

Cell membranes are made of fats and proteins that are held together with magnesium ions. The membranes may be weakened, or made unstable, by magnesium deficiency, and may allow for inappropriate entry and exit of magnesium and other minerals. This is especially so in a high-stress situation, when adrenaline and other stress hormones are flowing, nerves are firing, and ions such as calcium, potassium, and sodium are flowing rapidly into or out of cells. Important for cell integrity, the precious magnesium, which is so important to the cell at this time, flows out of the cells through the faulty membranes. Calcium then moves in, replacing the magnesium, causing injury. This compromises the integrity of the cells, just as they must respond at their maximum capacity. If the magnesium that leaks out of cells even temporarily raises the blood magnesium level above the level that signals the kidneys to excrete it, the body loses it at the very time it is badly needed. This is how, when magnesium is suboptimal, stress can suddenly convert a slight deficiency into a severe one. And this is how stress, coupled with a magnesium deficiency, can precipitate a life-threatening heart attack or stroke.

The Effect of Magnesium Supplements in Stress Conditions

Deaths of livestock during the extreme stress of transportation under crowded conditions have been found to be less likely to occur if the animals are given magnesium supplements before the trip. Animal studies tell us that stressed animals that are not given magnesium supplements secrete more than twice as much the amount of stress hormones as do animals supplemented with magnesium for as little as three days before being subjected to exactly the same stress. Without adequate magnesium, stress can cause the body to overreact to stress, releasing excessive levels of stress hormones that can deplete magnesium stores, with the resulting risk of damage to cells, blood vessels, and heart muscle. In the case of transporting pigs, those given extra magnesium attacked one another less and died less than half as often as pigs getting the regular amount of magnesium. And the effect was even greater for piglets: among those not given extra magnesium, there were seven times as many deaths as compared with those given extra magnesium.

Can this knowledge be translated into the prevention of human deaths from stress? We know that magnesium supplements can reduce the severe effects of stress in people who are low in magnesium to begin with. A person with adequate magnesium stores can handle acute stresses without undue harm. But one can expect that a time of acute stress will lower the body's stores of magnesium. If these stores are not restored, the next stressful event can be expected to lower

Too low blood magnesium is a stress: It initiates the release of stress hormones.

them even more. After the stress reaction has subsided, temporarily elevated blood levels of magnesium—which normally represent less than 1 percent of total body magnesium—will go back to normal, and the body can appear healthy. But a person with inadequate magnesium stores, when confronted with acute or chronic stress, is in danger of not having enough blood-borne magnesium to be able to mount an appropriate immediate response to stress, or to prevent damage to both heart and blood vessels, even to the point of sudden death. Magnesium supplementation during and after periods of acute stress can prevent an overreaction to stress that can cause the magnesium depletion that endangers life.

How Stress Depletes Magnesium in Everyday Life

Major crises obviously can instigate the stress reaction and, along with it, losses of magnesium. But even the common irritations, anxieties, and competitions in life—such as seeking a new job or taking exams—are stresses that can cause magnesium loss. Money and job worries, illness (whether one's own or that of family members or friends), and grief at the death of a loved one are other examples of stresses that increase our magnesium needs. The following are discussions of some of the ways in which the theoretical information about stress and magnesium affects people in the real world.

Stress of Surgery and Hospital Procedures

Imagine now someone with adequate magnesium going into the hospital for an operation. A very stressful event. Fear and anxiety can be expected to induce an adrenaline response before, during, and after such an event, using up magnesium at a rapid rate. If the person has enough magnesium, he or she will heal, recover, and go on—probably with lower stores of magnesium, but in no serious danger caused by low magnesium. If the dietary magnesium intake has been and remains adequate, the drop in the body's magnesium stores will be temporary, as the body restores its reserve supply of this element.

Stresses Associated with Magnesium Loss

A body under stress requires much more magnesium than does a calm body. The stress reaction also results in a depletion of the body's magnesium. The following stresses have been shown, under experimental conditions, to promote the loss of magnesium:

- Noise
- Hunger
- Cooling
- Heating
- Immobilization
- Poisoning/exposure to chemicals
- Oxidative stress
- Trauma
- Injury
- Medical procedures
- Surgery
- Hospital stays
- Emotions (fear, anxiety, anger)
- Psychological problems
- Political intolerance and friction
- Racism
- Awareness of potential military attacks
- Permanent standby duty
- Mortal danger
- Childbirth
- Rage
- Aggression
- Violent action
- Listening to fighting

But what if the person going into the hospital for an operation is borderline or low in magnesium? If this is not recognized and replenished, the stress of preparatory procedures, surgery, the immediate recovery phase, and the demands of the repair processes of convalescence have a good chance of so depleting the individual's already low magnesium stores that recovery is slow and might be unsatisfactory. As a result, the postoperative and convalescent patient feels generally weak, with a poor sense of well-being. Adding to the problem is the likelihood that the nutritional support supplied in the hospital, including intravenous fluids given during recovery to postoperative patients, is not infrequently inadequate in magnesium.

A person with even a moderate magnesium deficiency who undergoes surgery is in danger of magnesium depletion as a result of adrenaline release. Continuous administration of intravenous saline, glucose-and-water, and other magnesium-free solutions may intensify this. In such a case, sudden death can result from arrhythmia (irregular heartbeats) as a result of low magnesium that in turn causes losses of potassium, with its adverse effect on cardiac rhythm (see chapter 1).

After surgery, people, including infants, often go through a period during which their magnesium blood level is below normal. Some excrete large amounts of magnesium and other nutrients in the urine after an operation. Women in labor show a drop in blood magnesium, too. This is because the amount of magnesium needed by cells goes up dramatically in response to the great stress of an operation or childbirth. This is also true of emergency-room and critical-care patients. Procedures less severe than an operation also can be occasions of acute stress. For example, heart patients who have undergone cardiac catheterization have higher cardiac death rates than do those not subjected to this stressful procedure. One study showed tracheal intubation (insertion of a breathing tube) to cause very high rises in blood pressure, except in people who had been treated with magnesium beforehand. Once again we see how adequate magnesium reduces the adverse effects of stress.

Magnesium supplies from the stores in bone and muscle must be drawn upon to bring the body back into health and balance after the stress of an operation or postoperative procedures. Only in this way can the stress hormones subside and magnesium balance and stores be regained. If body stores of magnesium, or other essential elements such as zinc, are low, convalescence can be protacted and full recovery delayed.

Maybe you've heard of people who underwent an anxiety-ridden angioplasty procedure or heart surgery that was followed by a heart attack. How can such carefully designed high-tech medical procedures make things worse? The interaction of stress and magnesium answers this question. A person with heart disease is likely to be low in magnesium. Such a person is susceptible to the adrenaline/magnesium interactions that cause profound magnesium losses when faced with a highly stressful situation. Angioplasty and cardiac surgery such as a bypass operation provide such a situation, as do other highly invasive medical procedures.

When such procedures are not accompanied or preceded by replenishment of the magnesium, they can cause severe enough magnesium depletion to precipitate a heart attack or, at the very least, worsen the chronic low-magnesium state that caused the trouble in the first place. This is what happened to Joe, whose story opened this chapter. His terror at the thought of the prospective operation plus the severe stress reaction to the bypass procedure so lowered his magnesium stores that a sudden terrifying noise could evoke his sudden, unexpected death. Had his magnesium stores been replenished, Joe might have enjoyed the "years more" promised by the bypass procedure.

Critical Illness and Injury

People who are very ill—whatever the cause—usually suffer the stresses associated with hospitalization, as well as stress from the discomfort of the disease and, possibly, anxiety about the possibility of death. Low magnesium, which is associated with increased risk of mortality, is common in such individuals, and magnesium therapy may improve their prognoses. People who have suffered severe burns and other types of trauma also have substantial magnesium losses and need it to be replenished.

The stress of pain can lower serum magnesium, and again, the extent of depletion is greater with more severe pain. When we couple these facts with the fact that low serum magnesium is common in hospital patients, we see that the stress of illness or injury has an impact on magnesium status. People who are injured or critically ill can often be low in magnesium due to the stress brought on by their condition, so much so that they show deficiency signs ranging from muscle weakness to heart arrhythmia and worse. Once again, low serum magnesium implies a rise in cellular magnesium requirements and can indicate magnesium depletion due to stress. And we know that stress hormones lower serum magnesium as part of the stress response.

Brain Injury

People who have sustained severe brain injuries, whether as a result of physical trauma, or interference with the supply of blood to the brain (as happens during a stroke and cardiac arrest) have low plasma magnesium levels. The more severe the brain injury, the longer the depression of magnesium lasts.

Drs. Robert Vink of Adelaide University in Australia and Ibolja Cernak of Georgetown University found that there were also low brain magnesium levels in humans who had suffered either blast injury or penetrating brain wounds, and suggested that magnesium therapy might have promise for reducing the loss of mental and physical function in people who had suffered brain trauma. This premise was based on their demonstration that administering magnesium to rats before inducing experimental trauma reduced the degree of permanent brain damage.

Professors Burton and Bella Altura of Downstate University in New York, who have contributed substantial knowledge, both experimental and clinical, of the protective role of magnesium in cardiovascular disease, have demonstrated that people who have suffered strokes experience a drop in both serum and brain-cell magnesium levels. They also showed that people who have suffered brain damage in car accidents that occurred while they were driving under the influence of alcohol suffer more permanent loss of brain function than do sober accident victims. Alcohol consumption causes substantial losses of magnesium.

At the Henry Ford Health Sciences Center in Detroit, Michigan, Dr. Joseph A. Helpern and his colleagues showed that in people who had had strokes, the area of the brain with poor blood supply had significantly lower levels of magnesium than did the brains of normal control subjects. Dr. Yair Lampl and coworkers at Tel Aviv University in Israel have found that the lower the cerebrospinal fluid magnesium level was, the larger was the area of infarct (brain damage) in patients with strokes.

Dr. K. W. Muir of the Institute of Neurological Science, in Glasgow, Scotland, reported that magnesium chloride and magnesium sulfate infusions had a significant protective effect on nerve cells in standard animal models with induced strokelike brain lesions. In these studies, benefits were evident at serum and cerebrospinal fluid magnesium levels that are attainable in humans. Small clinical trials have reported benefit in humans, and a large ongoing trial is to be reported in 2003–2004.

The possibility that magnesium might prevent permanent loss of brain function in people who have had strokes was suggested by an unexpected finding in a randomized placebo-controlled cardiology study from Duke University, reported in 1997 at the annual meeting of the American College of Cardiology. The researchers had hoped that giving intravenous magnesium to people who had successfully undergone cardiopulmonary resuscitation (CPR) after cardiac arrest would improve the survival rate, as it had in people who had had heart attacks. (See chapter 1.) Sadly, it did not; only 21 percent survived in both the magnesium-treated and the placebo group. However, Drs. Mark Thel and Christopher O'Connor and their colleagues found that 69 percent of the surviving patients who had received magnesium escaped brain damage and were able to return home. Of those not given the magnesium, three times as many patients had functional impairments that made it necessary for them to have skilled assistance or go to nursing homes.

Type A Behavior

The type A personality—characterized by driving ambition, impatience, restlessness, competitiveness, a near-constant sense of urgency, and a tendency toward aggression and quick anger—can be described as a state of self-maintained stress. Type A people are more sensitive to stress than are those who have the calmer type B personality. In any given stress-inducing situation, type A people make more stress hormones than do type B individuals, and so respond with a greater fight-or-flight reaction. Under exactly the same stressful experimental conditions, type A subjects have been shown to lose cellular magnesium more readily than do type B people. Since stress causes magnesium loss, which in turn adversely affects cardiovascular health, type A people are more at risk for heart disease than are those who are type B.

Low magnesium and stress reinforce one another.

Type A people require more magnesium than do type B people and in the long run are more apt to develop magnesium deficiency, which makes them more prone to heart and blood-vessel problems. Type A people, as a result of their heightened reaction to stress, and as a result of being in a state of more or less constant self-induced stress, can display an intermittent virtual magnesium deficiency state that can lead to high blood pressure, coronary artery spasms, heart attacks, and coronary infarcts (areas of cell death in heart tissue). To remain healthy, people who have type A dispositions should have higher magnesium intakes than people with type B personalities. Studies have shown that the blood cells of those who are type A have less magnesium than do those of type B individuals. Furthermore, people with a particular gene (known as HLA-Bw35) have low blood cell magnesium values. When tested for personality type, many of the carriers of this gene are found to display type A behavior.

Chronic Stress

We have seen how stress damage to the heart and blood vessels is made worse by a coexisting magnesium deficiency. Chronically, high levels of stress hormones can be the consequence of prolonged stress. In the healthy individual with adequate magnesium, the initial physical signs of stress will disappear as the body moves from the "alarm" into the "resistance" phase of chronic stress. At the resistance phase, the person is successfully adapting to the stress as the ability to resist reacting to stress stimuli increases. Many of us can adapt like this, to varying degrees. And our doctors tell us constantly to take time out with stress-reducing activities. For if sustained stress persists for too long, the pathological signs reappear; they can become irreversible as they lead to death. The exhaustion phase of chronic stress has been reached. Does this occur when the body's magnesium has been depleted as a result of the demands of the stress reactions in the presence of inadequate magnesium? More study is needed.

Noise

In both experimental animals and humans, noise has been shown to be a stress-inducing factor that causes magnesium loss. In fact, noise stress can induce a magnesium deficiency even in well-fed rats provided with plenty of magnesium. And exposing already magnesium-deficient rats to noise stress intensifies the deficiency to the extent that convulsions ensue. Other studies have shown that a magnesium deficit, in both experimental animals and humans, can increase the adverse effects of trauma created by too much noise, which has caused hearing loss. Conversely, magnesium supplements have been shown to protect soldiers against degrees of deafness caused by the noise of shots being fired close by. Aviators in training with noisy aircraft experience the same beneficial effects.

In noise-stressed individuals, especially if they have low magnesium intakes, both magnesium and potassium are low in the heart muscle cells, which accumulate too much calcium, sodium, and the amino acid hydroxyproline. This amino acid is the main component of collagen (a protein that is a component of scar tissue), and magnesium-deficient animals under noise conditions develop considerable cardiac scarring. Either low magnesium or noise alone can produce such damage, but both together intensify the scarring. Taking supplemental magnesium can help. One study found that if magnesium is adequate, even high-volume noise fails to trigger the release of adrenaline, whereas if magnesium is deficient, the same intensity of noise increases stress-hormone release.

The exacerbation of noise-induced stress by magnesium deficiency is not to be underestimated, and is even associated with permanent hearing loss. At this point, it is worth speculating that people who play in bands that produce very loud music and dissonant sounds (or those who listen to music at high volume) might be vulnerable to deafness and more serious consequences. Their audiences (for example at rock concerts or discotheques) might also be at risk, as they are not only exposed to extremely loud sounds and flashing lights, but also often are drinking alcohol, which also causes magnesium loss, at the same time.

In healthy people, short-term exposure to a loud noise has been shown to increase urinary excretion of magnesium. Such noises can come, for example, from industrial sources or from low-flying airplanes, initiating a startle response in people that can increase heart rate, cardiac output, blood pressure, and magnesium metabolism. With repeated noise exposure, the reaction is often intensified and can be triggered by a lower sound level. On a practical level, women working in a Yugoslavian textile plant with high noise levels who were given magnesium-rich mineral water to drink showed less fatigue with more job satisfaction and better productivity. In the case of Joe, the cardiac patient who reacted fatally to the loud crash of an accident outside his window while recovering from bypass surgery, the reaction to noise stress was fatal.

Heat and Exercise

Healthy young American army men, subjected to exposure to 100°F heat for several hours a day over a period of sixteen days, lost 16 to 18 milligrams of magnesium a day in their sweat, totaling as much as a quarter of the total body's excretion of magnesium. The amount of potassium in their sweat exceeded that of magnesium. Another study with Indian air force men who were exposed to even higher temperatures for an hour and given pure oxygen to breathe showed that high oxygen exposure during heat stress decreased the amount of magnesium lost in sweat.

Young American men who were not adapted to heat were exercised on a treadmill in a hot, dry environment. They experienced a significant drop in serum magnesium that could not be totally explained by sweat loss. Nine healthy young Israeli men had their magnesium blood levels studied over ten days during which there were periods when they adjusted to heat exposure, and during which they exercised by walking on an inclined treadmill. Their serum magnesium fell, but their red blood cell and white blood cell magnesium levels rose by the fifth day, indicating a shift to the blood cells. By the tenth day, the red cell magnesium fell to the starting level, but the white cell magnesium remained elevated, even in the post-heat stress period.

Most outdoor athletic competitions are held under warm to somewhat hot conditions. Apart from the effect of environmental temperature, the influence of exercise on magnesium levels, and/or on metabolic changes, depends on a number of factors. The intensity and duration of the exercise, the degree of resulting exhaustion and/or dehydration, and prior training or lack of conditioning influence whether magnesium deficiency will develop as a result of the stress of the exertion. If an individual has an underlying magnesium deficiency, severe physical exertion can intensify it. However, the diagnosis of low tissue magnesium may be impeded by a temporarily increased serum magnesium. That increase might be caused by dehydration and a shifting of magnesium out of the cells and into the serum.

There have been many studies on the effect of subjects' magnesium status before exercise testing, and on the effect of supplementation with magnesium, for varying lengths of time, on athletes' endurance and performance. That, however, is not the subject of this book. Here we consider factors that might shed light on damage from exercise due to magnesium deficiency—extending even to the tragic sudden deaths of athletes in the prime of their lives.

Israeli researcher Gustawa Stendig-Lindberg has attributed sudden cardiac death in sports to magnesium deficiency that is associated with increased blood lipids and blood glucose. This is based on her earlier work with colleagues that showed that young Israeli soldiers exposed to the stress of forced long marches developed hypomagnesemia that persisted, on testing, several months later. Additionally, these soldiers' lowered serum magnesium, which persisted when it was tested ten and eleven months later, was accompanied by elevated cholesterol, triglyceride, and glucose levels. It is of interest that in another study, high-intensity exercise without the undue heat exposure that made the serum magnesium fall and the blood cell levels rise, had little effect on serum magnesium, but did induce a rise in red blood cell magnesium. Running is a stress that elicits stress-hormone secretion, but when they take supplemental magnesium, runners release less stress hormone in response to the stress of running.

If a person exercises excessively, he or she uses up oxygen rapidly. Both inadequate oxygen in heart cells and the stress of the exertion trigger the release of adrenaline-related stress hormones that are made, stored, and released by the heart. A comparable response can occur if there is constriction or blockage of the coronary arteries that limits the supply of oxygen to the heart, just as when blood oxygen levels are lowered as a result of oxygen being utilized by the muscles during heavy exercise. The result is the same; there is loss of magnesium and potassium from the heart.

Emotional and Psychological Stress

Exposure to emotional stress causes significant rises in blood pressure, even in people taking antihypertensive medications. Both heart rate and blood pressure rise as part of an emotional response. The physiological response to mental stress differs from the response to infused adrenaline, even though adrenaline is released at the beginning of the mental stress. Even so, people with heart disease have been found to be as much as six to ten times more likely than healthy controls to be anxious due to a psychological disorder. We can easily speculate that mental, emotional, and psychological stress can have an impact as a chronic, unyielding fire that burns up huge amount of magnesium, making anyone in such a state more likely to be deficient in magnesium and thus more prone to heart ailments.

Oxidative Stress

The formation of free radicals in our cells can damage vital molecules such as proteins, essential fats, and even genetic nucleic acids such as DNA. Since such free-radical formation goes on all the time, these chemicals build up, and a high level of free radicals has been associated with aging and vulnerability to illness and injury. Many doctors have recently started prescribing antioxidants—substances that neutralize harmful free radicals—for their patients, including the antioxidants vitamins A, C, and E, to help cells resist this ongoing oxidative stress. One natural biochemical we make that protects naturally against this oxidative stress is melatonin. Since magnesium stimulates the biosynthesis of melatonin, thus helping to preserve the internal rhythm of melatonin formation, magnesium has a protective effect against oxidative stress.

Studies have shown that magnesium deficiency increases susceptibility to oxidative stress and that free radical formation, which is higher in magnesium-deficient tissue, causes part of the damage associated with magnesium-deficiency injury. What's more, oxidative stress has more than once been shown to be less if magnesium is amply supplied and greater if the magnesium supply is low. In one study on fifty patients who were accidentally exposed to acute oxidative poisoning (they were exposed to aluminum phosphide, a pesticide), those who received intravenous magnesium therapy showed much less oxidative damage than those who did not. In addition, the death rate among the magnesium-treated group was half that of those not given magnesium. Antioxidants enhance the protective effect of magnesium.

Keeping a healthy level of magnesium in our cells is thus a primary protection not only for times of adrenaline-induced stress, which makes magnesium need soar, but also against both ongoing and acute oxidative stress. An adequate supply of magnesium protects the vital cellular components from oxidative damage and resulting injury.

Stress Ulcers

The stress associated with hospitalization for major surgery, trauma, and other serious conditions and procedures has been found to cause stress ulcers—bleeding, painful ulcers in the upper gastrointestinal tract that can cause significant blood loss. This is an important complication of severe stress. For example, as many as 80 percent of people who are hospitalized for aortic surgery such as bypass operations develop stress ulcers. In animal models, magnesium deficiency has been shown to intensify the severity of the ulcerations, and magnesium treatment has been shown to protect against the development of stress ulcers. In people, treatment with magnesium-containing antacids has a long record of efficacy in the treatment of ulcers predominantly because they inhibit stomach acid. We have yet to learn through research whether the amount of magnesium in antacids would be sufficient to inhibit the formation of stress-induced ulcers in chronic ulcer patients.

What to Do if You Have a Lot of Stress

The first thing you need to do is to honestly assess the level of chronic stress in your life. Do you live in the city or the country? How much traffic do you have to cope with each day to shop, work, and play? How difficult are the politics at your workplace, clubs, and/or social settings? How violent or peaceful is your home? Do you have to cope with addictions, whether to alcohol, drugs, gambling, food, or other behaviors that lead to imbalance? We are not going to suggest ways to change these situations—they are topics for other books, and there are many resources. But we do suggest that you give yourself a realistic idea of how much stress your body needs to withstand on a regular basis.

If you live in an urban area, making meditation and/or relaxation exercises a basic part of your routine can help to lower your adrenaline level and preserve your magnesium. Yoga, meditation, laughter, exercise that you enjoy, listening to music that you love, spending worry-free time with loved ones and good friends all can and should be an important part of your life. But sometimes we cannot get away from the noise or a very stressful lifestyle in general, and we all have to pass through acutely stressful periods at some time in our lives. In such cases, magnesium supplements can make quite a difference in how well our bodies cope with the stress and how healthy we are when the stress is over. For a healthy person in a temporary high-stress situation, taking 200 milligrams of magnesium per day can replace short-term magnesium loss. Add this amount to whatever else you are taking as a magnesium supplement as dictated by your general magnesium requirements. If you have a chronically stressful lifestyle, you may need more magnesium, depending upon the results of your Magnesium Questionnaire (see Appendix A) and other risk factors.

Take some time to assess your needs by reading the general information in chapter 10, as well as other pertinent chapters. Be sure to list all medications you take and compare them with the list in Appendix H: Common Medications that Affect Magnesium Status. Assess your diet using Appendix B: Common Foods Classified by Magnesium Content to see if you are getting a high, medium, or low level of magnesium in your diet. Then determine how much of your magnesium requirement is met by food and how much you should add in the form of supplements. If you live in a very noisy urban environment, or if you are a drummer, constantly sounding the cymbals next to your ear, or you work or live in a high-noise, high-stress area, add anywhere from 200 to 500 milligrams of supplemental magnesium, depending upon the amount of stress you encounter as a general rule. Choose the form of supplement best for you, be it a magnesium-containing salt, a liquid, or a tablet. If you take too much, your stools will loosen and you may get diarrhea. If this happens, reduce the amount you are taking until your stools are comfortably soft.

Be aware that stress has a substantial impact on your health if you are low in magnesium, and that magnesium can protect you against the stress of noise, trauma, oxidative stress, hospital stays, medical procedures, and emotional stress. It will not take away the stress nor your need to deal with it, but it can compensate for the effect of stress on your magnesium stores, preventing a weakened state when the stress subsides.

You may be living a high-stress life and feel just fine about it. You are coping. You are healthy. You seem resistant to the negative aspects of a modern, stressful life. As stress expert and author Dr. Hans Selye has so well pointed out, *be careful*. You may be in the resistance stage of stress and feel as though you could go on forever without making any changes. But this is a false notion. If the stress is really excessive and if you are truly in the resistance stage, sooner or later you will move into exhaustion and permanent damage will be done to your body and health. We speculate that magnesium adequacy can prolong the resistance stage of chronic stress and maybe even lessen the impact of exhaustion. But this has not been tested and should not be relied upon. We recommend that you use magnesium supplementation carefully and diligently, but do *not* use it as a way to avoid making necessary changes in a life filled with too much stress.

If you need to undergo a stressful medical procedure such as angioplasty, bypass surgery, or some other invasive test or procedure, talk with your doctor about using magnesium therapy before, during, and after the procedure. It has been shown to be effective in preventing adverse heart episodes and recurrences, as well as sudden death. The therapy consists of either an intravenous magnesium infusion or intramuscular injections, and must be administered by your doctor. The references for this chapter that pertain to how magnesium therapy prevents bad outcomes with stressful procedures might be of interest to your doctor. (See the References section at the end of the book.) At this time, enlightened cardiologists often use magnesium therapy in treating their heart-surgery patients, in cardiac care units, and in treating stressed emergency room patients who have developed arrhythmias or chest pain, even before an electrocardiogram confirms a heart attack.

7

Magnesium and Genetics: Family History and Sex Differences

Let's compare two friends—same age, same sex, same lifestyle. They run together, work together, snack together, and commute together. They shop at the same grocery stores; they eat similar foods. Each has a good family life and a satisfying job. One gets heart disease and the other does not. Why?

Studies of genetic differences provide clues into this enigma.

Genetics and Nutrition in Disease Prevention

Genetics and nutrition are closely interrelated, in many complex ways. Individual genetic makeup provides the basic blueprint for each person's bodily structure and function. But how these genetic blueprints express themselves is greatly affected by nutrition. Our individual genes contain the codes for the enzymes that power the chemistry of life and structures of each cell and the entire body. Using the nutrients we get from food or supplements, human cells make many organic chemicals necessary for life, such as enzymes, cholesterol, adrenaline and other hormones, proteins, sugars, amino acids, fats, and much more. Nutrients the body cannot make, which are thus called *essential*, include magnesium and other minerals, vitamins, and some of the fatty acids (the basic building blocks of fats) and amino acids (the basic building blocks of proteins). (See Appendix J: The Essential Nutrients.) These *must* come from food or supplements. If the supply of any one or several of the essential nutrients is insufficient to meet its needs, the body must adapt as well as it can to compensate for the deficiency. If the need exceeds the body's ability to adapt to reduced supplies, dysfunction or illness—or, if the deficiency is severe enough, death—inevitably results. The genes themselves need essential nutrients to replicate properly and to house themselves in chromosomes. The interaction of genes and environment is largely the interaction of genes and nutrients because what we eat (or do not eat) is a large part of the human's daily environment that keeps us alive and relatively well or unwell. All humans are alike nutritionally in that they need the essential nutrients on a regular and balanced basis to maintain the optimal health afforded by their genes.

Think of it this way: The best architects could draw perfect sets of plans and hire the very best carpenters. But if they couldn't get lumber, nails, and other essential materials, they could not construct their building. The genes are like the architect's plans and the cellular apparatus is like the carpenter's. In the cells, the building materials are the essential nutrients. The body cannot make them from other substances. It has to get them from what we eat.

We can use the same metaphor for an injury or illness: Imagine that you have a fire that destroys a part of your home. You need to repair the damage to bring your life back to normal. If you cannot obtain the requisite supplies, no building or repair can take place. This image is akin to living with a nutritional deficit—if it is not corrected, it is a time bomb threatening your future health.

Genetic Variability in Nutritional Needs

Every person has a genetically programmed need for each essential nutrient. Any given individual might need more than the officially recommended daily intake of magnesium but less than the recommended intake of vitamin C, an average amount of vitamin E, and so on for all essential nutrients. Our nutritional needs are like a fingerprint in this respect—unique for our specific genetic composition, environment, and history. This individual variability, like other traits, can be hereditary and is often reflected in familial trends. Patterns of eating behavior also tend to run in families, but habit and cultural differences also strongly influence our familial food preferences.

Genetic Studies and Health

We have heard of Nobel prize–winning genetic research, from the discovery of the structure of DNA up to the current focus on the human genome mapping. The genetic revolution is in its early stages as regards practical applications for the treatment and prevention of disease. In the foreseeable future, individual genetic profiling might become cost-effective and tests might be developed that tell doctors who will benefit from a particular drug and who is likely to have an adverse reaction to it. Even prior to this genetic revolution, though, traditional medical genetics discovered hereditary patterns for a few severe congenital diseases, some of which are caused by abnormal handling of a nutrient. Such discoveries have enhanced our ability to cope, individually and as a society, with the problems such diseases present.

Genetics and Cardiovascular Disease

What have genetic studies taught us with regard to differences in the utilization of nutrients that are needed to prevent and manage cardiovascular diseases, which collectively are the largest cause of illness and death among Americans? That there is a genetic component of heart disease has long been acknowledged. If someone related to you has had a heart attack, both you and your doctor are aware that this increases the chance that your health might similarly be compromised. Likewise, being male, which obviously is something controlled by one's genes, carries with it a greater risk for heart disease than does being female, at least before menopause. Researcher Herbert Schuster, M.D., a pioneer in the field of cardiovascular genetics, tells us:

> Although some people inherit an altered gene that rearranges the heart's architecture or disturbs its rhythm, most heart disease is caused by the stealthy work of several gene variations that subtly alter cholesterol levels, blood pressure, fat storage, homocysteine metabolism, and other factors. Left unchecked, these can evolve into high cholesterol, high blood pressure, obesity, and set the stage for a heart attack.

We believe that this "stealthy work of several gene variations" is in part due to gender and family differences in responses to magnesium, and in the amount required to maintain cardiovascular health. Direct evidence for this has been provided by the French researcher Jean-Georges Henrotte and his coworkers, who discovered that there are genes that control cellular magnesium levels that reflect interrelationships among the intestinal absorption, utilization, and excretion (through the kidneys) of magnesium.

Familial Differences in Cardiovascular Disease and Genetic Handling of Magnesium

Family histories of cardiovascular disease, and the study of familial diseases that are associated with a high likelihood of developing cardiovascular complications, provide clues that link magnesium and familial risk of heart disease. Magnesium is often ignored as an essential nutrient that is required for cardiovascular health. Along with other essential nutrients, magnesium helps to maintain normal fat metabolism (which assures a normal lipid profile), normal utilization of sugar, and an appropriate response to salt. These basic

Magnesium needs vary with lifestyle and genetics.

activities maintain normal blood pressure and other aspects of cardiovascular health, such as maintaining a normal, healthy heart rhythm and integrity of the heart muscle, heart valves, and blood vessels. If magnesium intake is, and consequently the cellular levels of it are, consistently low, the genetic blueprint (with the cellular apparatus) cannot "build" its optimal, healthy cardiovascular system.

The application of research to maintaining health by enabling physicians to detect the genetic variants that alter requirements for essential nutrients has begun. There are familial diseases that have been proven to be (or are suspected of being) associated with abnormalities in utilizing magnesium. Most of the studies have dealt with genetic alterations responsible for extreme abnormalities in magnesium utilization—its absorption from the intestines after it is consumed, and its retention by the kidneys after it is absorbed.

Here we will consider some common conditions that run in families and thus are genetically linked, that affect the heart and arteries, and that may be linked to abnormal utilization of magnesium.

Type A Personality

Dr. Henrotte and his colleagues found that type A people—those who are driven by ambition and competitiveness, and who are particularly prone to cardiovascular complications—have lower levels of magnesium in their red blood cells than do the more laid-back type B people. In addition to the lower cellular magnesium levels, Dr. Henrotte found that these type A people tested positive for a substance designated human leukocyte group A (HLA-Bw35; this is an identification code used to identify a specific genetic subgroup.) This was not true for the type B people. In one of the reports of this group of French investigators, they describe the different responses of type A male students and type B male students before and after exposure to the stresses of noise and assigned work. After the stress, the type A group secreted more adrenaline than the less tense type B students. They had a slight increase in plasma magnesium, but a more significant *decrease* in red blood cell magnesium, which suggests that the adrenaline mobilized magnesium from the cells to move into blood plasma. These findings suggest that type A individuals are more sensitive to stress than are type B subjects and lose their intracellular magnesium more readily. These people are not sick; but their bodies hyperreact to stress, and they are more likely than less driven people to have high blood pressure and, as a result, strokes, as well as spasms of the coronary blood vessels, with resulting angina or heart attacks.

Diabetes

That diabetes tends to run in families has long been known. More than half a century ago, Dr. Helen E. Martin of UCLA and her colleagues described the abnormal handling of magnesium in their diabetic patients—before and during the treatment that was then available—for the acute complications of their disease. It took another quarter-century for research to provide some understanding of how important magnesium is for insulin to work properly. The past fifteen years have seen the development of knowledge of the role of magnesium in preventing the cardiovascular complications of diabetes and of other clinical conditions characterized by insulin resistance (see chapter 2).

Now that we have the tools to discover what genetic components are responsible for the hereditary nature of diabetes, it has been shown that both types of diabetes (type I and type II) are linked genetically. It has been discovered that there are several chromosomal sites involved, but that a subdivision of the HLA group (a genetic group with low cellular magnesium) is the major genetic locus for diabetes. It is different from HLA-Bw35, which is associated with the low cellular magnesium seen in type A individuals (see page 167), but like the type A subgroup, it is characterized by low cellular magnesium levels.

Mitral Valve Prolapse

Although only found in about 5 percent of the total population, mitral valve prolapse is the most common disorder of heart valves. In people with this condition, the heart valve between the two left chambers of the heart billows abnormally into the left atrium (the upper chamber) when the ventricle (the lower chamber) contracts. It often causes no disturbing symptoms, but some people experience fatigue, shortness of breath, palpitations, and chest pain, and a doctor may detect a murmur (an abnormal sound that is heard through the stethoscope when the upper and then the lower heart chambers contract, pushing the blood forward) when listening to the heart. Mitral valve prolapse is hereditary, and several genetic types have been identified, the most frequent being the form that is associated with the HLA-Bw35 antigen—the same antigen found in type A individuals—who have been shown to have low cellular magnesium. HLA-Bw35 is found most frequently in individuals who have chronic fatigue syndrome (known in Europe as latent tetany syndrome) that is characterized by magnesium deficiency, and who also have a greater incidence of mitral valve prolapse than the general population. So it is not surprising that people with mitral valve prolapse have low cellular magnesium levels, and that magnesium supplementation for long periods of time has been somewhat helpful in relieving some of the symptoms and signs—cardiac as well as nervous—of this disease, in up to half of the people in whom it has been tried.

Everyone Is Different

A unique combination of environment and genetics for every individual makes each of us different. All of us come into being with a one-of-a-kind combination of chromosomes from a sperm and an egg. Identical twins arise from a split that occurs after this original combination, but even identical twins are exposed to different environments, so by the time they are out in the world—even as children, but certainly as adults—they are no longer absolutely identical. Sisters and brothers are very similar genetically, but they are certainly not identical.

Everyone is different.

Unquestionably, all human beings share identical genes—those that make us human—and we even share many genes with the rest of the biological world. But despite these shared genetic characteristics, there is substantial individual uniqueness. We are all oh so different.

Genetic Control of Magnesium Requirements

A very important way in which we differ from one another is in how much magnesium our bodies need to be healthy. There are genetic differences in how well we absorb the magnesium from the food we eat and from the water we drink, in how well we retain it, and in how we distribute it to the cells of different tissues in our bodies. In other words, we differ genetically in how well our bodies utilize the magnesium we ingest. While, admittedly, the environment plays a role in magnesium requirements, so too do less compromising individual genetic variations that can exist in essentially normal people.

There are a few genetic diseases that specifically interfere with the absorption or retention of magnesium. These are fortunately rare. They prevent normal growth, development, good health, and even survival. We will discuss them here to provide examples of how serious severe magnesium deficiency is.

Genetic Intestinal Magnesium Malabsorption

Occasionally, infants who have failed to thrive, and who have had severe recurrent convulsions, have been found to have a markedly reduced ability to absorb magnesium that is not associated with the inability to absorb other nutrients. We have found no reports of gene studies done with families of children with this disease, but more than one child in a family has been reported, pointing to a hereditary nature. Very few such children survive to adulthood.

Malabsorption of magnesium is associated with very severe magnesium deficiency, usually requiring high-dosage magnesium infusions to manage seizures. Sometimes, the disorder can be managed with over six times the normal oral magnesium requirement. One child who developed bone and joint disease from the deficiency died of congestive heart failure before he reached his teens, despite having been intensively treated with oral and intravenous magnesium. One young man who was unable to absorb enough magnesium for his needs when he took it by mouth, required the continuous subcutaneous administration of magnesium by means of a mechanical pump to control convulsions. Another individual was enabled to survive for twenty-one years by the continuous administration of magnesium salt solution by means of a tube threaded through his nose and reaching his stomach.

Renal Magnesium Wastage

An innate inability of the kidneys to retain magnesium is another disorder that causes severe magnesium deficiency, as well as losses of potassium, in which genetic abnormalities have been identified. Although a renal defect in handling magnesium, or both magnesium and potassium, may allow for longer survival than does the intestinal inability to absorb magnesium, it causes lifelong electrolyte and metabolic disorders. The numerous tiny tubules of the kidneys of such individuals lack the capacity to increase reabsorption of one or both of these essential minerals from the fluid filtered from the blood when the blood levels are too low. Too much magnesium is thus excreted in the urine. High-dosage magnesium and potassium therapy can partially control some of the manifestations of these disorders.

There are several genetic disorders that are associated with such renal magnesium wastage. The two best known are Gitelman's syndrome and Bartter's syndrome, named after the physicians who first described their characteristics in the 1960s. The genetic abnormalities differ in these two conditions and affect the absorption of magnesium in different portions of the renal tubules. The loss of potassium in Bartter's syndrome is correctable by replacing magnesium. People with Gitelman's syndrome require both magnesium and potassium supplementation.

One of two sisters with renal wasting of magnesium described by Gitelman in a 1966 paper suffered profound weakness and low magnesium and potassium levels. She also had abnormal heart rhythm, associated with electrocardiographic (ECG) tracings called long QT intervals, or LQT (see chapter 1). A more recent study of twenty-nine people with Bartter's syndrome whose electrocardiographic tracings had been taken reported that eighteen had LQT.

Magnesium is the treatment of choice for LQT. There is a highly fatal arrhythmia called *torsade de pointes,* also characterized by LQT, that is caused by severe acquired magnesium deficiency. The use of certain medications, alcoholism, and other factors that cause magnesium and potassium loss have caused *torsade de pointes*. It responds better to treatment with intravenous magnesium than to any drug.

Different Magnesium Needs in Healthy People

We do not know whether the genetic flaws of magnesium absorption and retention considered above are an all-or-nothing phenomenon, or whether there can be degrees of abnormality that might explain why seemingly normal individuals can differ so much in their magnesium requirements. The evidence showing the high variability in the magnesium needs of healthy normal men and women comes from what are called metabolic balance studies.

Ideally, metabolic balance studies are done in a controlled setting, in which healthy volunteers are given meals containing measured amounts of magnesium. Each subject's magnesium intake and magnesium output (excretion via urine and feces) are carefully measured. A few studies have even analyzed the amount lost through sweat, tears, saliva, menstrual blood, and semen. When each subject's output is subtracted from intake, that person's magnesium balance is calculated. A positive balance means intake is greater than output. This takes place under several conditions. There might have been a prior magnesium deficiency, and the retained magnesium might be correcting that insufficiency. Or it might be that extra magnesium is needed for growth, development, or repair, or is stored, usually in bone. A negative magnesium balance means that its output exceeds its intake. This can occur under conditions of illness, such as those that cause chronic diarrhea, or as a result of treatment with diuretics (water pills) or other drugs that cause magnesium loss, or as a result of severe stress or a too-low magnesium intake. If a negative balance persists, body stores of magnesium are mobilized and a subclinical (not apparent by observable signs or symptoms) magnesium deficiency can develop. If the negative balance continues for a long time, the body draws upon func-

The Concept of Magnesium Balance

Magnesium balance studies measure the amount of magnesium ingested and the amount eliminated by the body, and compare the two. Such studies provide a reliable indicator of whether an individual is getting adequate magnesium to maintain health and to allow for growth, development, and repair. The following table summarizes factors that affect the body's magnesium balance.

Daily Intake	**Daily Output**
Magnesium taken in via:	Magnesium lost via:
• Diet	• Urine
• Water	• Feces
• Supplements	• Sweat
	• Menstrual fluid
	• Semen

Positive "+" Balance	**Negative "–" Balance**
Intake greater than output	Output greater than input
Body retaining magnesium to:	Body losing magnesium, leading to:
• build up stores of magnesium	• depletion of magnesium stores
• correct a deficit	• magnesium deficiency
• growth and development	• abnormal growth and development
• repair after illness or injury	• slower recovery from illness and injury
	• development of metabolic syndrome X or other illness

tional magnesium from the liver and the muscles, even heart muscle, and signs of magnesium deficiency can become detectable.

Even small daily losses of magnesium can mean a large cumulative loss of magnesium. Any time a person's intake of magnesium is less than the amount lost each day, that person is in negative balance, which means there is a net loss of body magnesium over the course of that day. Figure 7.1 summarizes the results of metabolic balance studies that show how individual requirements for magnesium can vary.

Figure 7.1 Balance Studies Showing Variations in Magnesium Requirements

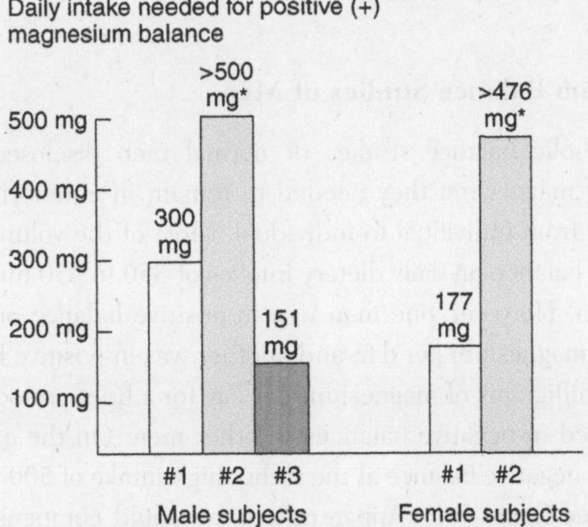

*Positive balance still not reached at this intake

Magnesium balance studies show that even healthy, normal individuals vary quite a bit in their magnesium requirements. These are reflected in the graph, above. We believe that this variability in magnesium need is at least partly genetic, and is partly responsible for the "family history" risk factor for heart disease.

The daily losses reported in the studies used to compile this table range from 10 to 216 milligrams of magnesium per day for those in negative balance. The range is wide. At the extreme, a person losing 216 milligrams of magnesium per day experiences a substantial cumulative loss of magnesium rapidly, in less than one year if such daily losses continue. But even small daily losses of magnesium, if sustained over long periods, can lead to a significant deficit. So even among those in negative magnesium balance, the severity of magnesium deficiency varies widely, as does the time it will take to develop clinical manifestations. A person is in metabolic balance or equilibrium when the magnesium eliminated is replaced by the amount that is consumed, absorbed, and retained. Individuals whose magnesium status is thus being maintained so as to meet their needs can expect to remain free of magnesium deficiency–induced impairment of their health. We discuss men and women separately since the balance studies indicate that their requirements differ.

Magnesium Balance Studies of Men

The metabolic balance studies of normal men disclosed that the amount of magnesium they needed to remain in equilibrium differs quite a bit from individual to individual. Most of the volunteers were in positive balance on daily dietary intakes of 350 to 450 milligrams of magnesium. However, one man was in positive balance on 300 milligrams of magnesium per day, and another was in positive balance on only 151 milligrams of magnesium per day for a brief period, amounts that resulted in negative balances in other men. On the other hand, one was in negative balance at the rather high intake of 500 milligrams per day (see figure 7.1). Apparently, some could compensate better than others for a short-term low intake of magnesium. Possibly, those who could tolerate low intakes, even for short periods of time, had a better capacity to absorb and/or retain minimal amounts. The study was not continued for long enough to indicate just how long such a compensation might last. Did the man in negative balance on 500 milligrams per day have a genetic or a temporary need for large amounts of magnesium, or did that high requirement for the duration of the study merely reflect an existing deficiency or a temporary condition of increased need, perhaps due to alcohol consumption? We do not know.

Among the metabolic magnesium balance data analyzed in the survey of worldwide metabolic balance studies of men, reported in 1964, were findings from East Asia that provided a new dietary explanation of the much lower heart disease death rate there than in the West. A widely held belief was that the greater consumption of vegetable oils in Asian countries, instead of saturated animal fats as in the industrialized West, had a protective effect. Analysis of the magnesium balance data, however, provided additional insight. Instead of the average 2.2 milligrams of magnesium per pound of body weight (about 5 milligrams per kilogram) of the American men, the magnesium intake of the Indian, Ceylonese, and (prerevolutionary) Chinese men was almost twice as high. Not quite half of the American men, on their customary low-magnesium intakes, were in balance; the rest were in negative balance. In contrast, among those consuming as much magnesium as was customary in the East, over three-quarters of the men were in positive balance. In fact, for the Asian men studied, positive magnesium balance was the rule. Since magnesium had been shown, in numerous animal experiments, to have protective effects on the cardiovascular system—even with animals fed high-cholesterol diets or otherwise challenged—I [M.S.S.] proposed that high magnesium intake was the protective factor.

Data from Japan support this premise, but from another perspective. As in the rest of eastern Asia, the rate of heart disease in Japan was lower than in the West, but strokes were more frequent. The high salt intake of the Japanese has long been accepted as a contributor to their susceptibility to high blood pressure and strokes. But now that the American-type diet has taken hold there, the heart attack rate has risen, and efforts are being made to induce the Japanese either to return to their original (high-magnesium) diets, or to increase their magnesium intake by taking supplements.

Based on the findings from the metabolic balance studies, both in the United States and in the East, how much magnesium should healthy men consume daily? Keeping in mind that individual variability is great, 2.4 milligrams per pound (6 milligrams per kilogram) of body weight should be adequate for the majority of men who are not very active. As activity or stress rises, so should magnesium intake, to about 4.5 milligrams per pound (10 milligrams per kilogram) of body weight.

Magnesium Balance Studies of Women

Analysis of the figures from the magnesium metabolic studies with women indicate that women tend to maintain their equilibrium on less magnesium per pound of body weight than do men. The women in these studies were in balance on 2.1 to 2.3 milligrams per pound (4.5 to 5 milligrams per kilogram) a day. As women's activity level increases, the magnesium requirement rises to about the same level as that of active men. The same is true for pregnant women and nursing mothers.

Individual women also differ in their magnesium requirements. Balance studies on women showed that some were in positive balance on such low magnesium intakes as 177 milligrams per day. Other healthy women were still in negative balance on intakes as high as 476 milligrams a day. (See figure 7.1.) Remember, these are all "normal" women. These are not women with asthma, heart disease, leukemia, cancer, diabetes, or even the flu, any of which would affect their need for magnesium in one way or another. Judging by their weights, these women were neither abnormally tall nor short, nor abnormally fat nor very thin. Because they were selected as "normal," we can assume they did not have any symptom-causing abnormalities in utilizing magnesium resulting from identified genetic states that affect magnesium, nor did they have any other metabolic diseases. The observed variations in the amounts of magnesium they needed might merely indicate the limitations of metabolic balance studies in determining absolute requirements. In the early extensive metabolic balance studies of young men and women, it was found that short-term studies might yield inaccurate findings, since the ability of the body to adjust to new intakes takes time.

Differences between the Sexes in Utilizing Magnesium

While individuals vary widely in their magnesium needs, when taken as a whole, women seem to need less magnesium than men do. In a summary of several balance studies on men and women, fewer than half of all participants on a low daily intake could maintain magnesium equilibrium, or balance, if the daily intake was low. About three-quarters of the men and four-fifths of the women were in magnesium balance at intermediate intakes; over 90 percent of the men and all of the women were in balance on high intakes (see table 7.1). These results tell us that higher and higher daily intakes of magnesium bring more and more people into positive balance, and that women do slightly better than men at each intake level.

Estrogen and Magnesium Retention

There is evidence that the female sex hormone estrogen plays a role in how magnesium affects cardiovascular disease. It is likely that the

Table 7.1 Summary of Magnesium Balance Studies on Healthy Men and Women

The table below shows the percentages of men and women who could achieve magnesium balance on low, medium, and high intakes of magnesium. Note that more women than men were able to achieve a positive balance at each level of magnesium intake. This is because women can utilize low intakes of magnesium more efficiently than can men.

Magnesium Intake	Percentage of men in positive magnesium balance	Percentage of women in positive magnesium balance
Low intake—less than 2.3 mg per lb (5 mg per kg) of body weight	45%	50%
Medium intake—2.3–4.5 mg per lb (5–9.9 mg per kg) of body weight	78%	81%
High intake—4.6–10 mg per lb (10–22 mg per kg) of body weight	92%	100%

greater female ability to maintain magnesium equilibrium on lower intakes than the amounts that are needed by men is a factor in the sex differences to vulnerability to heart disease.

For one thing, young women have heart disease less often than do men. It has long been known that young women are less susceptible to heart disease than are young and middle-aged men—or than elderly women, in whom cardiovascular disease, such as coronary artery disease and strokes, far outnumbers other causes of illness and death. The protection against cardiovascular disease of young women gradually disappears after their estrogen secretion ceases at menopause. By age sixty-five, the rate of death from cardiovascular disease is about the same for women and men, except, possibly, for women on hormone re-

Women use magnesium more efficiently than men.

placement therapy (HRT), although that possibility has become controversial (more about that later in this chapter).

The balance studies cited earlier showed that young women tend to remain in magnesium balance on lower magnesium intakes than is the case for young men. At each level of magnesium intake—low, medium, or high—women did better than men in retaining magnesium. This is not only due to their lower average body weight, because the trend still holds if you calculate the intake on a per-pound basis (see table 7.1). Perhaps the fact that young women have less body muscle mass than men offers at least a partial explanation. For whatever reason, young women seem to be able to get by on less magnesium than men can. In addition to needing less magnesium overall per pound of body weight, they are also better than men at conserving magnesium if their intake is low, and as a result can stave off magnesium deficiency longer than men if on a low-magnesium diet. On high-magnesium intake, women are able to store more of the excess magnesium than men can. Is this due to a genetic ability to use magnesium more efficiently than do men? We believe that these genetic differences in magnesium need, utilization, and conservation explain why being a young female helps to protect against cardiovascular disease, while being male increases the risk of developing it.

It occurred to me [M.S.S.], back in 1964, that the lesser magnesium requirement of young (nonpregnant) women as compared with that of young men explained gender differences in vulnerability to heart disease.

Estrogen and Blood Clotting

It may be that women are protected from cardiovascular disease by the influence of estrogen on the internal distribution of magnesium. There is evidence that estrogen causes magnesium to shift from the circulating blood to the tissues, where it is less available to the kidneys for excretion—hence better magnesium retention. As the magnesium level in the cardiovascular tissues increases, under the influence of estrogen, it may well function to protect these vital tissues from damage inflicted by magnesium deficiency. However, the shifting of magnesium out of the circulating blood in women whose magnesium intake is marginal or low creates a situation that, paradoxically, increases the risk of a different type of damage within the blood vessels. Estrogen increases the tendency of blood to clot, whereas magnesium has anticoagulant effects. It may be that the procoagulant (proclotting) effect of estrogen occurs because it lowers blood levels of magnesium, which removes that protection against the formation of thrombi in the blood vessels.

More than thirty years ago, oral contraceptive agents with a high estrogen content were in common use and were associated with such clot-associated complications as strokes and heart attacks. It was then suggested that taking magnesium, which prevents platelets from sticking together—an important step in thrombus formation—could protect women taking oral contraceptives from this dire complication. Twelve years ago, I [M.S.S.] published a review of the literature that clearly showed that postmenopausal women taking estrogen and calcium supplements to prevent osteoporosis were at increased risk of clot formation in their blood vessels—which could cause thromboses, heart attacks, and strokes—if they did not also take magnesium. I then pointed out that not only did magnesium prevent the platelets from clumping, it also inhibited other aspects of blood coagulation—those that are increased by high calcium levels. (See chapter 2 for a discussion of the role of the cellular calcium-to-magnesium ratio in heart disease.)

The fact that postmenopausal women are now routinely urged to take substantial amounts of calcium to protect against osteoporosis makes the role of calcium in blood clotting especially pertinent. A large, controlled study, as part of a Women's Health Initiative (WHI) of the National Institutes of Health (NIH), tested the generally accepted premise that hormone replacement therapy for menopausal women could protect not only against osteoporosis, but against heart attack. Menopausal and postmenopausal women took estrogen plus progestin, a synthetic form of the sex hormone progesterone. This is the form of HRT most commonly prescribed. The study verified that HRT protected against osteoporosis. However, because of the unexpected finding that the women taking the hormones had more cardiovascular events than did those given placebo, the study was terminated earlier than had been planned. These unanticipated complications were

Figure 7.2 Influence of Gender on Magnesium Balance at Different Intakes of Magnesium

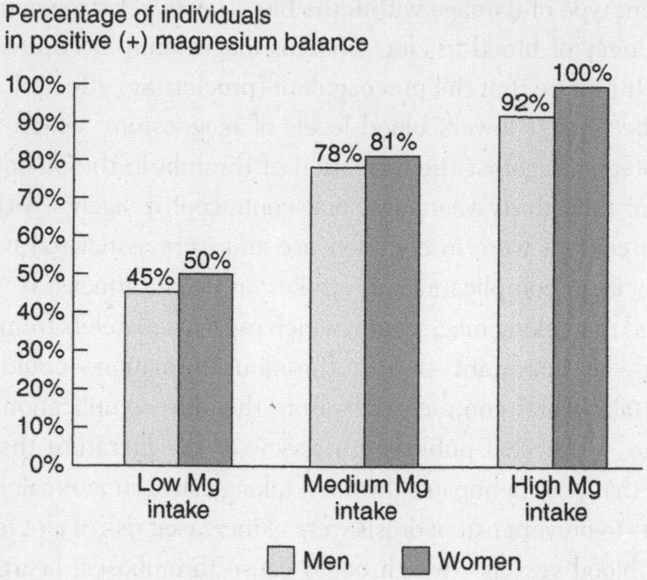

Percentage of individuals in positive (+) magnesium balance

	Men	Women
Low Mg intake	45%	50%
Medium Mg intake	78%	81%
High Mg intake	92%	100%

The graph above shows that at all levels of magnesium intake, more women than men are in positive magnesium balance. This is due in large part to the fact that women in general lose less magnesium than do men.

caused by increased clotting in arteries or veins and were manifested as 29 percent more heart attacks, 41 percent more strokes, and twice the rates of blood clots in the lungs and legs as compared with women taking the inert placebo. It is noteworthy that in the published design for the study that was stopped, subgroups were included who also were using nutritional modifications such as a reduced-fat intake or supplementation with calcium plus vitamin D in addition to the estrogen and progestin. No subgroup was given magnesium supplements. Not reported in the paper on the early termination of the study was the effect of HRT on the level of magnesium in the blood or urine.

Individual Differences in Utilizing Magnesium

The people in balance studies absorbed anywhere from 0 to 90 percent of the magnesium in the food they ate. This is a huge range. They excreted anywhere from 8 percent to 78 percent of the ingested magnesium in their urine. Another huge range. In addition, some of those in negative balance lost only small amounts daily, while others excreted as much as 216 milligrams of magnesium per day. Those in positive balance retained anywhere from small amounts daily to as much as 450 milligrams of magnesium per day. These ranges are very large, especially when they occur on relatively similar daily intakes.

We have considered the importance of normal intestinal absorption of magnesium, and normal renal reabsorption of magnesium in light of the severe illness that genetic abnormalities of these functions cause. In a healthy person, the kidneys are the safety valve for the handling of magnesium. They limit its excretion by increasing its reabsorption from kidney structures called renal tubules when blood levels are too low, and increase its excretion when blood levels are too high. Because the absorption and excretion of magnesium are so important in meeting our needs, genetic variations in intestinal and kidney function are important in controlling magnesium metabolism.

We are not all alike when it comes to magnesium nutrition. We vary widely in how we handle our magnesium intake, as well as in how much our bodies need. Thankfully, very few of us have genetic mutations that are devastating in that they prevent utilization of this vital nutrient. Whether some of us have small genetic changes that can interfere to some degree with how we absorb or retain magnesium is something that requires further study. A few people can maintain magnesium health on a low daily intake—possibly as little as 200 milligrams daily, at least in the short term—but most of us need between 300 and 650 milligrams of magnesium daily to maintain magnesium equilibrium or to store enough for repair or emergency (stress) needs. Some people need even more on a regular basis. All of us can be healthy as long as we have magnesium adequate to our needs, but it is clear that our needs for magnesium differ. A lot of this—not all, but a lot—is due to our genes.

Living in the industrialized world, with its generally meager dietary magnesium supply, people with a genetically high requirement for magnesium are more likely to suffer from marginal intakes than are those with hereditarily low magnesium needs. As a result, families with high genetic magnesium requirements are more likely to have members who develop heart disease than are families with a lower genetic need for magnesium. This, we believe, is an important explanation of why heart disease tends to run in families. Since men regularly need more magnesium than women, they are more prone to heart disease than are women. Anyone with very high genetic requirements for magnesium, male or female, could go on a low-fat diet, stay calm, exercise regularly, and *still* have heart disease if his or her magnesium intake is below what is needed. We propose that, until we routinely assess the magnesium status of people, the individual susceptibility to heart disease will remain essentially unpredictable.

Individual Differences in Manifestations of Magnesium Deficiency

Another genetically determined difference, beyond the difference in magnesium requirement, is in how magnesium deficiency is expressed. Infectious diseases such as the flu tend to cause similar symptoms in all people and therefore can be easily identified and diagnosed. This is not true of magnesium deficiency. In early human nutrition studies in which researchers induced magnesium deficiency alone, without any other illness or nutritional shortages, the subjects' symptoms were not uniform. Some developed neuromuscular symptoms, and others developed cardiovascular changes. Loss of appetite, nausea, apathy, and persistent fatigue or weakness occurred in some, while personality changes, muscle spasms or cramps, pain, or tremor occurred in others. The signs of magnesium deficiency differ in different individuals. Some people develop high blood pressure with a magnesium deficit, others do not. In some people, total cholesterol levels rise while "good cholesterol" falls (see chapter 5), but this doesn't happen in everyone. Some people get type II diabetes or metabolic syndrome X, others do not. Some have angina or heart arrhythmias and others do not. Some experience no symptoms at all until there is a heart attack or sudden, unexpected cardiac death. This genetic difference in people is one reason

Our genes and past history tell how and when a magnesium deficit will manifest.

why magnesium deficiency can be so hard to diagnose. Unlike the measles, which gives anyone who gets it spots and a high fever, a magnesium deficiency does not show up in everyone in the same way. So it is difficult to determine by symptoms or signs that we are not meeting our unique daily magnesium requirement. The genetics of magnesium utilization is a potentially rewarding field waiting to be tapped, that should pay benefits in the prevention of disease.

How to Use Magnesium if Your Family Has a History of Heart Disease

If you have a family history of heart disease, you may have a higher genetically determined requirement for magnesium than the general population. If so, you can benefit from raising your magnesium intake daily. In order to help yourself determine your magnesium need, do the following:

1. Start with a family tree of heart disease. Make a pedigree of your family—your parents, brothers and sisters, aunts and uncles, cousins and grandparents. Under each person's name, indicate any aspect of heart disease of which you know. Hypertension? High cholesterol? Angina? Palpitations? Heart attack? Sudden death with no other symptoms? And so on. For each case, list the age at which it began. If there was some alcoholism or drug addiction, mark it. Alcohol abuse can cause severe magnesium loss. So can cocaine abuse. So if the only heart attack in your family was in the alcoholic or drug-addicted relative, and if you are not drinking to excess or abusing drugs, you may not have a high family need for magnesium. Analyze the pedigree you have made and decide if there is a good chance that people in your family have a higher magnesium need than people in most families.
2. Assess your own health. Are you generally healthy or do you have manifestations of heart disease risks such as high cholesterol, high blood pressure, heart palpitations, arrhythmias, and so on?

3. Estimate your magnesium need. If many members of your family have had heart disease, we suggest that you take in the higher amounts of magnesium daily, even if you are generally healthy (unless you are very healthy and over age seventy). But remember that older adults lose some of their capacity to absorb and retain magnesium. If you have made it this far in good health, your habits are probably pretty good. But if you are young, you could be accumulating a magnesium loss that will manifest itself as heart disease later in your life. You can prevent this by taking care of your magnesium needs now. If you suspect you may have been accumulating a magnesium deficit for some years, recognize that you will first need to correct that deficit with high doses of magnesium supplements each day, and that when the deficit is corrected you may maintain your magnesium health with smaller daily doses or with diet alone.
4. Use appendix B to figure out the level of magnesium in your diet. Then consult appendix C to assess the amount of magnesium you are getting in your water and appendix H to determine whether any medications you may be taking might be altering your magnesium status.
5. Adjust your current magnesium intake accordingly, then add enough supplements to be in the following range, as appropriate:

    - For men: Most normal, healthy men can maintain magnesium balance on 2.7 to 4.5 milligrams of magnesium per pound (6 to 10 milligrams per kilogram) of body weight per day. If you are a man with a family history of cardiovascular disease, you should assure an intake starting at the higher limit of the range given for normal men.
    - For women: Most healthy nonpregnant women can maintain magnesium balance on 2.3 to 2.6 milligrams of magnesium per pound (5 to 5.9 milligrams per kilograms) of body weight per day. If your magnesium intake each day falls above this range, you can, hopefully, put yourself into positive magnesium balance even if your genetically determined need is

high. If you are pregnant or nursing, it is wise to increase your intake to about the upper limit for men.

Start on the low side and increase to the maximum, letting your supplement amount vary until your stools are comfortably soft. This daily amount of magnesium should be enough. If you are magnesium-depleted, you will be able to take high doses comfortably until your depletion is corrected. Then, all of a sudden, you may notice diarrhea. If this happens, adjust your dose downward until your stools are, again, comfortably soft.

If you eat a lot of dairy foods or take calcium supplements, use the higher magnesium range as your target. If your diet changes to add more high-magnesium foods, reassess your magnesium supplement. You may be able to tolerate magnesium pills easily. But some people do not. This is another manifestation of our genetic differences. If pills do not work for you, consider the liquid forms of magnesium supplements or seriously consider a magnesium-containing salt. Some people will have to get their magnesium from foods only, while others may show allergies to the highest magnesium foods—nuts. Everyone is different. You will need to find out how best your body can get its precious daily magnesium.

6. If a particularly stressful period arises in your life, add a supplement containing 100 to 200 milligrams more daily of magnesium during the time of excess stress.

8

Magnesium and Other Heart Disease Risk Factors

There are a number of addicting or habit-forming behavior patterns that can intensify the problems caused by dietary magnesium deficiency, by increasing losses of magnesium, or by exacerbating the effects of a lack of adequate magnesium in the body. Chronic alcohol abuse, leading to what we know as alcoholism, is primary among these. It was one of the conditions that was recognized as causing severe magnesium depletion. The relationship of smoking to problems associated with magnesium inadequacy is less certain, because there has been little research into its effects on magnesium. However, the fact that heavy smokers are at high risk of developing cardiovascular disease, metabolic syndrome X, diabetes, and other complications to which magnesium deficiency contributes, suggests that smoking might interfere with the utilization of magnesium. Also, the use of cocaine, which has increased substantially in the last decades, has been associated with high blood pressure, heart attack, and sudden death from arrhythmias, mostly in young people, in whom these conditions are uncommon. Each of these serious cardiovascular problems is known to be related to loss of magnesium. Animal studies have shown that cocaine causes losses of magnesium, so it is not far-fetched to relate the cardiovascular diseases seen in abusers of cocaine to magnesium loss.

Another risk factor for cardiovascular disease is a condition known as *hyperhomocystinemia,* or abnormally high blood levels of the amino acid homocysteine. This results from an inborn metabolic error rather than from behavior or lifestyle choices. Although high homocysteine is a genetic risk factor for arteriosclerosis, high blood pressure, and strokes, as well as heart disease, it was not included in the preceding chapter because our current understanding indicates that magnesium has an indirect rather than a direct role in causing homocysteine production; vitamins that are directly involved depend on magnesium for their activity. But recent research shows us that high levels of homocysteine in the blood are associated with lower cellular levels of magnesium.

Alcohol

Chronic alcoholism has long been known to cause magnesium loss, with resulting symptoms of magnesium depletion. Edmond B. Flink, then Chairman of the Department of Medicine of the University of Minnesota and a pioneer in the clinical identification of disorders caused by magnesium deficiency, first reported magnesium depletion in patients with the delirium tremens (DTs) of chronic alcoholism in the mid 1950s. He and his staff, both then in Minneapolis and later in West Virginia, showed that magnesium infusions rapidly corrected the delirium, tremors, delusions, convulsions, and other neurological signs of alcoholic DTs. This finding was reported about half a century ago. Excessive ingestion of alcohol results in markedly increased excretion of magnesium through the kidneys. In addition, alcoholics tend to eat poorly and often suffer bouts of vomiting and diarrhea. They thus consume and retain insufficient amounts of nutritious food to provide enough magnesium to meet normal needs, let alone to make up for losses. The physical consequences of alcoholism are many, including damage to the liver, brain, and bones, but we will limit our consideration to the cardiovascular damage caused by magnesium depletion.

Cardiovascular Diseases of Alcoholics

In the mid 1960s, a disease of heart muscle called cardiomyopathy, which was detected in many alcoholics on autopsy, was noted to resemble very closely the condition caused by experimentally induced magnesium deficiency in animals. The hearts were flabby and had many areas with small scars, and the coronary arteries had clots along their linings. Examination of the clinical records of people who had such abnormal hearts disclosed that they had had abnormal electrocardiograms, some even showing the long QT (LQT) associated with magnesium deficiency (see page 184). Some of these people had died of heart attacks, some had died after a siege of congestive heart failure, and some had died suddenly of lethal arrhythmia, particularly ventricular fibrillation or torsade des pointes, the types of arrhythmia associated with LQT. (See chapter 1.)

High blood pressure and angina that develop as a result of the type of constriction of arteries that has been shown to be caused by low magnesium-to-calcium ratios can also be complications of alcoholism. And strokes, both the form caused by increased coagulation and thrombi and those caused by cerebral arteriosclerosis (rupture of rigid blood vessels in the brain), also are causes of death and long-term disability of alcoholics. Yet more alcoholics die from suicide, liver disease, and accidents, or from the poisoning aspects of alcohol at an unusually young age (the mean age at death from cardiovascular disease for alcoholics is fifty years) while the nonalcoholic population has a higher incidence of death from cardiovascular disease but at a later age (a mean age at death of seventy-four years).

Moderate Drinking and Cardiovascular Disease

People who drink just a little actually have low rates of the cardiovascular diseases that cause serious problems and death in heavy drinkers. Can magnesium nutrition explain this unanticipated relationship between alcohol and heart disease?

Light to moderate alcohol consumption, on a daily basis, has a beneficial effect on cardiovascular health. But the extreme health risks that accrue from heavy alcohol drinking are so severe that many health-care professionals fear recommending a drink or two each day to protect against cardiovascular disease since it might be risky for people with a genetic susceptibility to alcoholism.

Some research tells us that having two to four drinks per day if you are male and one to two per day if female may be more conducive to good health than abstaining. One drink (12 ounces of beer, 4 ounces of wine or 1.5 ounces of 80-proof spirits) each day has been reported to lower cardiovascular risk by 30 to 50 percent. Some studies suggest that anywhere between four and a half to seven glasses of wine a week provide this health benefit, but that beer or spirits do not. Others suggest that any type of alcohol, as long as it is consumed in moderate amounts, is beneficial even for older adults (up to age seventy-five) and people with diabetes. Even people with left ventricular dysfunction (those with a left ventricle that is weakened due to the stress of high blood pressure or scarred due to a prior heart attack) are less likely to have a new (fatal) heart attack if they take one to two drinks per day than if they consume no alcohol at all.

Moderate Alcohol Use and Magnesium Status?

There is evidence that having a relaxing drink at the end of the day can reduce stress and enhance relaxation. Perhaps this daily practice can reduce magnesium losses due to stress. (See chapter 6.) It is only as a regular habit that mild alcohol consumption is beneficial. In modest amounts, alcohol raises HDL ("good") cholesterol, lowers LDL ("bad") cholesterol, and interferes with the aggregation of blood platelets—just what we would expect from improved magnesium status. But having a couple of cocktails before or with a meal can increase the excretion of magnesium via the urine. So if the alcohol helps the dinner go down, make sure that that dinner is a meal rich in magnesium, or that it is followed by a magnesium supplement.

In addition to offering the relaxing effect of alcohol, red wine seems to have an additional benefit over white wine, beer, and spirits. It has been speculated that this benefit comes from compounds known as polyphenols, which are antioxidants, relax the blood vessels, and have anticlotting properties. It has also been speculated that levels of the polyphenol resveratrol, which has special properties good for the heart, are high in grape skins, which are present only in red wines. We extend another speculation: that red wine is a minor source of magnesium. Red wine has more magnesium than white wine, rosé wine, or beer. Rum, gin, vodka, and whiskey have no magnesium at all.

Tobacco Smoking

Smoking cigarettes increases the chance of developing heart disease, but how it does this is not entirely clear. Obviously, smoking coats the lungs with foreign substances that are sticky and thick, so the exchange of carbon dioxide in the blood for the oxygen in the inhaled air is not as efficient as it is in lungs without the smoke-derived coating. Thus, it seems reasonable that the heart has to work harder to bring oxygen to the body's cells. Your heart rate goes up if you smoke, down if you quit. Day after day, year after year, the heart of a smoker has to beat more than that of a nonsmoker.

The traditional view goes beyond the extra work a smoker's heart must perform. Smoking brings nicotine and other toxic substances from cigarettes into the bloodstream, where they injure the lining of coronary arteries, causing them to constrict and also causing clots to form. But if we are to understand how smoking can damage the heart and blood vessels by impacting magnesium status, we must consider other aspects of smoking.

The Thermogenic Effect of Smoking

Smoking a cigarette causes the body's metabolic rate to go up for a while. This is called the *thermogenic* effect of nicotine. The effect occurs each time a person has a cigarette, occurs only in response to smoking a cigarette, and is completely reversible. When you stop smoking, the temporary rise in metabolism caused by smoking ceases.

When the metabolic rate and all life reactions accelerate, the need for magnesium increases, because it is required for the enzymes that keep these reactions going. We cannot expect people to get any more magnesium because they smoke—in fact, smokers may get less magnesium than nonsmokers because they tend to eat less. Therefore, smokers can be expected to become magnesium-deficient more readily than nonsmokers, and one of the ways this can express itself is in damage to the cardiovascular system.

Smoking's Impact on Magnesium Status

There is little direct research on the effect of smoking on magnesium status. One study showed that heavy smokers had significantly lower plasma levels of magnesium, as demonstrated by the finding that among nonsmokers, only 8 percent had low levels, but among smokers, more than twice as many had low magnesium levels. Among smokers who also drank fairly heavily, 24 percent had low plasma magnesium. Although a normal plasma magnesium level is not a good index of adequacy of magnesium, consistent low levels are fairly reliable indicators of magnesium insufficiency. (This will be discussed in detail in chapter 10.) Another study showed smokers to have lower hair magnesium levels than nonsmokers, but the significance of hair magnesium is controversial.

It is known that people who smoke have more of the risk factors for metabolic syndrome X than do nonsmokers, including higher triglycerides, more insulin resistance, and lower HDL ("good") cholesterol. Among healthy people, smokers have more insulin resistance, higher glucose levels, and much higher insulin levels as determined by glucose tolerance tests than their healthy, nonsmoking counterparts. Healthy smokers also have almost twice the levels of triglyceride-rich VLDL ("bad") cholesterol and 30 percent lower HDL cholesterol than do healthy nonsmokers. In addition, it is known that insulin resistance, a characteristic of metabolic syndrome X that is caused by low cellular magnesium, improves when smokers stop smoking. Although these are not direct measurements of magnesium status, these facts imply that smoking lowers cellular magnesium levels.

Nicotine, the principal drug in tobacco, is a stimulant that causes the release of adrenaline. This means that people who smoke will need more magnesium than nonsmokers. (See chapter 6.) Also, oxidative damage goes up with smoking, and this increases the amount of magnesium needed to maintain optimal health.

Smoking and Weight

Often, people with heart disease or risk factors for cardiovascular disease are told to both stop smoking *and* lose weight. To do either of those things is difficult, and many people who have tried to stop smoking know only too well that they face gaining weight in the process. If a person regularly smokes, say, twenty or so cigarettes a day, the thermogenic effect occurs with each cigarette smoked. Simply smoking a cigarette results in more calories being burned. This is one reason why smoking is associated with lower body weight. When people stop smoking, they often gain weight—partly because of this lower run on calories and partly because they tend to eat more.

Smoking is never good for anyone's lungs, and we believe that quitting is always good. But, if you cannot or will not quit, taking magnesium supplements might lessen the impact on your body's heart and vascular system. It will not protect your lungs from smoking-related disease, nor your body from the toxic effects of nicotine. It will only replace magnesium lost due to the impact of smoking on your metabolism. And if you do quit and tend to gain some weight, making sure that your magnesium status is up to par will help to compensate for any adverse effects of a moderate weight gain on your cardiovascular system.

Cocaine

Cocaine has been used for thousands of years in South America, in the lands of the Incas. Its use has increased dramatically over the last decade, especially in United States, with resulting adverse cardiovascular reactions.

The first report of acute myocardial infarction (heart attack) due to cocaine use was in 1982. Since then, more than 250 cases, predominantly in young men, have been documented in the literature. In a study of a large series of cases of myocardial infarction, the risk was found to be 23.7 times higher in cocaine users in the sixty minutes after cocaine use as compared with nonusers. The elevated risk decreased rapidly thereafter. The use of cocaine has been associated with a large, abrupt, and transient increase in the risk of heart attack in people who are otherwise considered to be at relatively low risk. About one of four nonfatal myocardial infarctions among 10,085 adults aged eighteen to forty-five years was found by the Third National Health and Nutrition Examination Survey to be attributable to frequent cocaine use.

But heart attacks are not the only cardiovascular complication of cocaine abuse. Cocaine is a powerful vasoconstrictor (a substance that causes the blood vessels to contract), which explains the high blood pressure, and strokes in young users.

When given to experimental animals, cocaine has been shown to lower tissue magnesium levels in the blood vessels and the brain. Severe spasms and rupture of blood vessels in the brain has resulted in hemorrhagic stroke in cocaine-injected rats. Treatment with magnesium lowered the death rate in the cocaine-injected animals from 40 percent to 13 percent. In a study of treatment of very dangerous arrhythmias of patients who had taken cocaine, calcium-channel blockers—including magnesium—were found to protect against ventricular fibrillation, a type of arrhythmia that is highly lethal. Another highly fatal arrhythmia that has been seen in cocaine users and that can cause sudden unexpected death, is torsade des pointes, the same arrhythmia that can develop with LQT. This is an arrhythmia that develops with magnesium deficiency—for example, from alcoholism—and that responds best to magnesium infusions.

Homocysteine

A disease caused by a genetic "mistake" is *homocystinuria*, meaning "homocystine in the urine." It is so called because when blood levels of the amino acid homocysteine are too high, it is excreted in an altered form (homocystine) in the urine. That would be just a strange, interesting fact, except that high blood homocysteine levels have serious consequences.

Homocysteine is an amino acid that is produced as a result of the metabolism of methionine, an essential amino acid (a building block for the formation of protein).

During the 1960s, a genetic condition was recognized that led to high amounts of homocysteine in blood and homocystine in urine. People with this genetic abnormality died very young of atherosclerosis, or buildup of severe plaque in their arteries.

In the population as a whole, there are varying amounts of homocysteine in the blood. The level parallels that of some of the trends toward heart disease. In general, smokers have more blood homocysteine than nonsmokers and men have more than women, although after menopause, women begin to build up to the level of men. High levels of homocysteine are strongly associated with an increased risk of heart disease and stroke, as well as death from these conditions. High levels correlate generally with the number of major heart artery blockages in patients with coronary artery disease.

These facts and other evidence present a good case for high homocysteine in the blood as an independent risk factor for heart disease. It seems to pose a level similar to that associated with smoking and high cholesterol. But the association is not total; not all people with heart disease have high homocysteine levels, and not all people with high homocysteine levels have heart disease.

Several of the B vitamins—folic acid, vitamin B_{12}, and vitamin B_6, all of which depend for their activity on the presence of adequate magnesium—can lower high levels of homocysteine in the blood. But it is not yet known whether reducing homocysteine levels can prevent or reverse heart disease. Nor is it known whether taking magnesium, which is needed by the vitamins that are helpful for homocystinuria, would improve the body's response to these vitamins.

High Homocysteine and Low Cellular Magnesium

If there is too much homocysteine in a cell's environment, cellular magnesium levels drop, especially if the cell's magnesium level is low to begin with. It does not alter the calcium level. The B vitamins that lower homocysteine in the blood—folic acid, vitamin B_{12}, and vitamin B_6—stop homocysteine from lowering the level of magnesium in the cells. But all three of these B vitamins have to be together for this to happen, and the cells' magnesium level must be adequate. If the cellular magnesium is too low to begin with, these vitamins, even if together, cannot stop the drop in cellular magnesium that homocysteine evokes.

Studies on metabolic syndrome X tell us that low cellular magnesium causes abnormal functions that lead to atherosclerosis and associated conditions. We see these same conditions in people with elevated homocysteine, including thrombosis, platelet aggregation, and endothelial damage, as well as early-onset coronary artery disease and heart attacks at young ages. It seems plausible that high homocysteine levels produce these atherosclerotic conditions by lowering the cells' magnesium content.

Homocysteine and the Controlling Enzyme for Cholesterol

There is also indirect evidence that homocysteine reduces magnesium in cells. High homocysteine levels in cells cause an increase in the activity of the enzyme HMG-CoA reductase by 130 to 190 percent. This is the enzyme, controlled by magnesium, that sets up the synthesis of cholesterol. If magnesium is low, this enzyme "turns on" and too much cholesterol can be produced. The statin drugs inhibit this enzyme, and that's how they lower cholesterol. Homocysteine, by lowering cellular magnesium, turns this cholesterol synthesis enzyme on and works like an antistatin. (See chapter 5.)

If you and your doctor find that you have high homocysteine levels, be sure your magnesium nutrition is adequate. Also be sure you are getting enough folic acid, vitamin B_{12}, and vitamin B_6. If you are a vegan, be aware that a vegan diet can be very healthy, but is low in vitamin B_{12}, which is found almost exclusively in foods of animal origin, although there are vegetarian B_{12} supplements available. And remember that if your magnesium is too low, these three B vitamins cannot protect against high homocysteine.

Over the years (over thirty for M.S.S., eighteen for A.R.), we have been following the research on magnesium and heart disease, we have repeatedly uncovered evidence that each new risk factor announced for heart disease seems to have a connection to low magnesium. As the research unfolds and closer scrutiny becomes possible, these links to magnesium only become stronger. We are convinced that the explanations for the major risk factors for heart disease—high blood pressure, high cholesterol levels, a high-fat diet, gender, family history, the type A personality, stress, and all the others—start to make more and more sense only when you consider the magnesium factor that connects them all.

9

Are We Really Low in Magnesium?

Many medical and nutritional professionals believe that, in general, our diets have plenty of magnesium, and that unless you have specific medical problems, your magnesium status is undoubtedly just fine. This is the conventional wisdom of our time.

But in reality, the diets many of us eat do not provide the recommended daily allowance (RDA) or the daily recommended intake (DRI) for magnesium.

A close look at modern processes for food and water show why. They take magnesium out and do not put it back in.

Table 9.1 Magnesium in Refined versus Whole Foods

The table below shows the calorie and magnesium contents of some whole (unrefined) foods and their refined counterparts. Notice that, in general, refined foods have more calories and less magnesium than do the whole foods from which they are refined.

Food Item (per 100 grams [3.5 ounces])	Number of Calories (in kilocalories [calories])	Amount of Magnesium (in milligrams [mg])
OILS VERSUS WHOLE FOODS		
Avocado:		
avocado oil	884	0
whole avocado	161	39
Corn:		
oil	884	0
whole cooked corn	108	32
Olive:		
oil	884	0
whole olives	115	4
Peanut:		
oil	884	0
whole peanuts	318	102
Safflower:		
oil	884	0
whole seeds	517	353

The Modern Diet: Low in Magnesium

As we saw in chapter 4, magnesium is often removed from foods during processing, and is not replaced. Table 9.1 shows exactly how modern refined foods compare with original whole foods as sources of magnesium.

As you can see from table 9.1, oils have no magnesium. Safflower

REFINED VERSUS WHOLE-GRAIN FLOUR		
Wheat flour:		
All-purpose white flour	364	22
Whole wheat flour	339	138
REFINED VERSUS UNREFINED SUGAR SOURCES AND SUGARS		
Cane:		
granulated white sugar	387	0
cane syrup	279	4
brown sugar	376	29
molasses	235	215
Maple sugar	354	19

Source: U.S. Department of Agriculture (USDA) Agricultural Research Service, 2001. USDA Nutrient Database for Standard Reference, Release 14. Nutrient Data Laboratory Home Page, www.nal.usda.gov/fnic/foodcomp.

seeds, a common source of oil, have a lot of magnesium—680 milligrams per 1,000 calories. After the seeds are processed into oil, that value goes down to zero. The same happens with peanuts made into peanut oil and corn into corn oil. These are not the only nutritional changes, but in general we can see that eating 100 grams (about 3½ ounces) of safflower seeds is very different from eating 100 grams of safflower oil—the same amount of oil (by weight) has many more calories and lacks magnesium, among other differences. The same is true for nuts and nut oils, olives and olive oil, avocados and avocado oil, and so on. Whether it ends up as plain oil or hydrogenated or partially hydrogenated oil, the process of separating oils leaves magnesium behind. These zero-magnesium oils are used in many processed foods as well as in home cooking.

Refining wheat flour is not quite so bad, because refined white flour is not completely lacking in magnesium. But it has only one-sixth the magnesium of whole wheat flour. Refined wheat flour is a basic staple of the industrialized world's processed food. When wheat is processed into white flour, the bran and germ of the grain are removed, along with most of the fiber, protein, and fat, and 80 percent of the

Processed foods have magnesium separated out but not put back in.

magnesium. This leaves the white, starchy endosperm to be milled into the flour that is used to prepare the white breads and rolls, pastries, pasta, baking mixes, muffins, crackers, cookies, gravies, ready-to-eat cereals, and numerous snack foods we so love. Enrichment adds back iron, niacin, thiamine, riboflavin, and folate, but not magnesium. So white flour has much less magnesium than does whole-wheat flour milled from unseparated whole wheat. Look at the lists of ingredients in your processed foods. How often do you see "enriched flour"? This is the white flour we are discussing, the one with 80 percent less magnesium than whole wheat, and the flour that is in many of our foods.

Sugar has zero magnesium. Molasses and fiber are removed from sugar cane to produce the pure granulated white sugar that has no magnesium. Molasses is very high in magnesium, so once again we see how basic processing separates out and removes magnesium. Nutritionally, eating sugar cane is really different from eating pure white sugar. Granulated sugar has the sweetness we have learned to love and cooking properties that sugar cane could never hope to achieve, but it is a purer and less nutrititious commodity that is higher in calories and lower in magnesium, as well as lower in fiber and many other nutrients. Sugar is used a lot in processed foods, sometimes under other names. (See Appendix I: Alternative Names for Sugar for a list of the names under which sugar may appear in food product ingredient lists.)

These staples of the modern diet—oil, sugar, and white flour—have wonderful cooking and storage properties. They can be shipped long distances and stored for longer times than the whole foods from which they are created. This is why they are used, with other processed staples, to make the bread, desserts, cake mixes, snacks, cereals, and other processed foods that we buy at the supermarket. They are among the staples used by restaurants and bakeries. We store and use them in our homes. But they are low in magnesium, and they make up a large part of the food supply available to us.

Saturated fat lowers magnesium absorption.

If a processed food product has oil (hydrogenated, partially hydrogenated, or otherwise), enriched flour or sugar as one of the first three ingredients, it is most likely a low-magnesium food.

Beyond not providing enough magnesium in the first place, the modern industrial diet is high in both saturated fats and refined sugar, which can actually worsen magnesium status. A diet high in saturated fats reduces the absorption of magnesium from the intestines. High levels of sugar increase the excretion of magnesium in the urine. These two food elements do not help our low-magnesium intakes.

But I Take a Multivitamin Supplement Every Day!

Because magnesium and calcium are both bulky minerals, they are not routinely added in significant amounts to one-a-day type vitamin and mineral supplements. If they provided amounts near the RDA or DRI, the pills would be so big that no one would want to take them. As a result, people and physicians who rely on this type of supplement "insurance" need to know that they are not getting magnesium and calcium in the amounts they need from most multivitamin and mineral supplements.

Most multivitamins do not provide the RDA for magnesium.

Water Supplies: Low in Magnesium

Current drinking water habits are not helping our magnesium status.

One big change over the last century has been the municipal "softening" of water supplies. Soft water is great for making soap lather and leaving no soap scum, but it is low in magnesium. Hard water is made soft by taking out the magnesium and the calcium. The process also adds sodium. Thus, during the last fifty years or so, an important source of nutritional magnesium for some geographic areas has been wiped out.

Adults consume an average of two liters (about two quarts) of water per day, including the water in their coffee, tea, reconstituted fruit juices, sodas, milk, beer, soup, and other liquids. Some natural drink-

Hard water is made soft by taking out the magnesium and calcium.

ing waters are very high in magnesium and contain enough magnesium to supply all of the adult RDA or DRI given this two-liter intake. That is if the water has at least 175 milligrams of magnesium per liter of water (also expressed as 175 parts per million [ppm] of magnesium). But most municipal drinking waters have much less magnesium—0.1 to 60 ppm—which supplies anywhere from zero to one-third of an average adult's magnesium need. (See Appendix C: Magnesium in Drinking Water for a list of the magnesium levels in the water in selected U.S. cities.)

Many people have turned away from drinking municipal water to bottled water. They want to ensure pure, healthy water without chlorine and other products of municipal processing. Much of this water is deionized (demineralized) by a process called reverse osmosis, and as such has just about zero magnesium—less than 0.1 ppm. Most have sodium added for taste. Distilled water has no magnesium and no sodium.

Some bottled "mineral" and "spring" waters do have magnesium, European brands more often than American ones. But the levels vary considerably, and the magnesium almost always comes with varying amounts of calcium and sodium—from very high to quite low. There is a huge variability in these bottled waters, but if you choose carefully, a bottled spring or mineral water can supply up to 40 percent of an adult's magnesium requirement without overdoing the calcium and sodium (see appendix C for more information on this vast subject).

Many bottled waters have little or no magnesium, while others have plenty.

Medications

Many diuretics, which are commonly prescribed for high blood pressure, increase the loss of magnesium through the urine. Some antibiotics do the same, as does cisplatin (Platinol) and other anticancer drugs. Digitalis, long used for heart failure, can increase the body's need for magnesium. Estrogen, found in birth control pills and hormone replacement therapy (HRT), increases the secretion of adrenaline, which in turn increases magnesium requirements (see chapter 6; also see Appendix H: Common Medications that Affect Magnesium Status). It also lowers circulating levels of magnesium, increasing the risk of blood clotting.

Calcium Supplements

During the last decade, medical professionals have become convinced that many people, especially menopausal women, need calcium supplements to prevent osteoporosis and bone loss. With the aging of the population, this is a very important problem. Taking calcium supplements can be very beneficial—if magnesium nutrition is adequate. But if they are taken with a consistently low or suboptimal magnesium intake, calcium supplements can make matters worse. If magnesium levels are low, calcium cannot be properly utilized by the body; this includes absorption by the bone. Also, under conditions of magnesium deficiency, low blood calcium *cannot* be corrected with calcium supplements. Only restoring adequate magnesium will set things right. We strongly recommend getting adequate magnesium before starting calcium supplements, and then maintaining a balanced intake of both magnesium and calcium. This is the safe way to prevent bone loss using supplements.

Calcium supplements should be avoided if you are low in magnesium.

For both heart and bone health:

- Magnesium must be adequate
- The overall ratio of calcium to magnesium from all sources, including food, water, supplements, and medicines, should be about 2 to 1

When choosing supplements, select those with a calcium-to-magnesium ratio between 1 to 1 and 2 to 1, depending on your diet.

Since both calcium supplements and HRT increase magnesium need, we were not surprised by a recent study that showed women on HRT are more prone to heart disease than women not using such therapy. Adequate magnesium may be the answer for menopausal women who want the bone protection of HRT and calcium without increasing the danger of heart disease.

Study Results

Given the realities about our food supply, our water supply, modern medications, and current supplement recommendations, it is not hard to see how many of us could easily be low in magnesium—at least getting less than the RDA or DRI. And some researchers think that these values are too low anyway.

It has been estimated that the modern industrial diet is, on the average, about 170 milligrams low in magnesium per day. Since this is an average and we are a highly varied population, this means that some people are getting plenty of magnesium while others are short by hundreds of milligrams per day. How can we assess our individual magnesium needs? The next chapter tries to answer this question.

10

Do You Need More Magnesium?

We wish we could tell you that assessing your magnesium status is easy, but it is not. We have designed a questionnaire to help you assess your "possible" magnesium status. (See Appendix A: Magnesium Questionnaire.) Let us emphasize the word "possible" since this questionnaire has not been scientifically tested. It is only a guide, designed to help you gather pertinent factors in your life that can affect magnesium status. Take this questionnaire and then read on for information about other research and laboratory tools that may be available to help you determine your true magnesium status.

Why Can't I Just Get a Blood Test for Magnesium?

There are blood tests that measure magnesium levels, but these have limitations as ways to assess your true magnesium status. The magnesium tests currently available to your doctor measure total magnesium concentrations in red blood cells, whole blood, serum, or plasma. *Whole blood* refers to blood samples as drawn from the body. *Plasma* is the blood fluid without the blood cells, obtained from whole blood by separating out the cells without allowing the blood to clot. *Serum* is the fluid portion of the blood that remains after the blood clots. All three have electrolytes, including magnesium, dissolved in them.

Most blood tests for magnesium do not reflect true magnesium status.

Total magnesium values in blood fluids have been shown to be the least sensitive of all magnesium values. The level of magnesium in the blood can remain stable even with long-term low magnesium nutrition. If your blood magnesium is deemed by these tests to be much above or below the normal range, you are probably in the hospital or very ill. But if it falls within the normal range, this total magnesium blood value cannot tell you or your doctor much, if anything, about your overall magnesium status.

Most of the body's magnesium is found either in the bones (about 60 percent) or inside muscle and other cells (about 40 percent). Less than 3 percent is found in extracellular fluids like serum or plasma. Magnesium in the blood's noncellular fluid is kept within strict bounds—2 to 2.5 milli-equivalents per liter (mEq/L) of serum or plasma, although the low limit is controversial (levels as low as 1.85 mEq/L are listed as normal in laboratory manuals). If there is enough magnesium in the diet, the blood magnesium is replenished and any extra (above the upper limit) is removed by the kidneys and excreted in the urine. If a person's daily magnesium intake is insufficient to keep the blood level in the normal range, magnesium can be moved out of the bone and muscle cells and into the blood to keep the blood values relatively constant. Thus, the body can be low in magnesium—that is, the bones and/or muscle cells can become magnesium-depleted—while blood values look completely normal.

Knowing this, researchers first found valuable magnesium measurements, ones that truly reflect the body's overall magnesium status, by measuring levels inside cells. Unfortunately, at this time, these sensitive measurements of magnesium status are not widely available to doctors. What are they, and how can we get to them?

How Magnesium Researchers Assess Magnesium Status

Magnesium researchers have worked hard to develop a reliable test for magnesium status that is both easy to use and sensitive enough to detect disease states that are short of catastrophic. This is important. One researcher, Lawrence M. Resnick, M.D., of the Cornell University Medical College, observes that although magnesium research has generated excitement in the medical community, interest has waned because a reliable, meaningful blood test is not readily available.

Cellular-Free Magnesium via NMR

Working with laboratory animals, researchers have found that levels of cellular-free magnesium—that is, the unbound magnesium inside brain, heart, muscle, and other cells—is closely correlated with heart health. For example, raising the level of free magnesium in the cells of working rat hearts can increase blood flow by one-third while lowering heart rate by one-third. After extensive work in animals, this finding was confirmed in humans. Free magnesium within cells (Mgi for short) is measured using nuclear magnetic resonance (NMR). It correlates with blood pressure and insulin-response measurements plus other aspects of cardiovascular health in humans.

Getting brain, muscle, or heart tissue for such a test is certainly not convenient, let alone noninvasive. Muscle samples have been taken from patients in a few countries, but it is not a procedure that is likely to find general acceptance in the United States. Taking brain or heart samples from living subjects is sure to be a most uncommon procedure, except possibly during surgery.

Thus, magnesium research was greatly advanced when researchers found this NMR technique could measure free Mgi in red blood cells (as opposed to the total red blood cell magnesium measured by tests available to your doctor). This less invasive measurement was found to reflect brain, heart, and muscle tissue Mgi. Researchers can depend upon this more convenient measurement and with it have found that people with hypertension, type II diabetes, and other disease states have low Mgi. The trouble is that only fresh blood will produce accurate results, and the NMR equipment is expensive and not widely available in clinical laboratories. Although this test is seen as the gold standard for magnesium research, it seems impractical for development into a widely used clinical test.

Magnesium Load Testing

In the magnesium load test, the subject is injected or gradually infused with a controlled amount of magnesium (after collecting a preinjection twenty-four-hour urine specimen). Starting immediately after the injection, a second twenty-four-hour urine specimen is collected. The magnesium in this sample is measured and used to calculate the percentage of the injected dose that was excreted. If a large proportion of the injected dose was excreted, it is assumed that the body was adequate in magnesium; it could let most of the dose be eliminated in the urine. If only a small proportion of the dose was released in the urine, it is assumed that the body's cells needed the injected magnesium and retained most of the amount that was provided. This test is reliable except for people who are taking diuretics or other drugs that cause magnesium loss, and for genetic magnesium-wasters—people with magnesium deficits who nonetheless excrete much of any magnesium available to them. Such individuals will excrete a high proportion of the magnesium dose even while they are short on magnesium. (See chapter 7.)

Magnesium load testing has been used in research studies, but if you are not in a hospital, it requires discipline to collect your urine over a twenty-four-hour period, store the urine correctly, and transport it to a facility where it can be analyzed. Thus, this test does not lend itself to widespread use.

Other Magnesium Tests

Are any reliable tests for magnesium status available to the public now? There are several tests that can help people determine if they need to begin a magnesium supplement regimen and can give information on how well the regimen is working.

Magnesium status is difficult to assess.

Ionized Magnesium

Magnesium researcher Dr. Bella Altura, her husband, Dr. Burton Altura, and their coworkers have searched for a sensitive laboratory test for magnesium in serum that could be developed for wide clinical use. Using what is known as the ion selective electrode (ISE) technique, developed by Nova Biomedical of Waltham, Massachusetts, the Alturas measure ionized magnesium (Mg^{2+}), rather than total magnesium, in serum. Mg^{2+} levels correlate with measurements of Mgi and have been shown to be accurate in detecting magnesium deficiency in people with type II diabetes and in finding other magnesium deficiencies that measuring total serum magnesium does not detect. It can also reflect a large magnesium intake that total serum magnesium measurements cannot detect. Dr. Altura calls this method the I Mg^{2+} test, and it is promising for wide clinical use. But its development is still in process. There are three commercially available electrodes for this test, and unfortunately they all give somewhat different values. Dr. Altura has found that several details in the methods of collection, transport, and storage of blood samples are crucial if one is to get accurate values using I Mg^{2+}. Temperature, timing, the type of collection tube stopper, whether the patient has been fasting—all of these can have an impact. Nevertheless, the Alturas have patented a protocol that will give reliable, reproducible results if followed to the letter and if the protocol-specified electrode is used. They have said that they will be glad to give your physician the protocol and to run your test. It is not inexpensive, but it includes the magnesium:calcium ratio. The Alturas can be reached as follows:

Dr. B.M. and B.T. Altura
Department of Physiology—Box 31
SUNY Health Science Center at Brooklyn
450 Clarkson Avenue
Brooklyn, NY 11203-2056
718-270-2194

Exatest

There is a commercial test available for determining cellular magnesium status that is a bit more costly than the Altura's I Mg^{2+} test, but is covered by Medicare and several insurance providers. It is Exatest and is offered by Intracellular Diagnostics, Inc. of Foster City, California. This commercial laboratory provides a kit to your doctor, who takes a light swab of cells from under your tongue, puts it on a slide, allows it to dry, and sends it off to the laboratory. They use a technique called energy-dispersive X-ray analysis to measure the magnesium and other elements inside these sublingual cells. The sublingual cells analyzed by this test have been shown to have magnesium levels comparable to that of heart cells (as determined by testing patients undergoing bypass surgery) and to that of magnesium in muscle tissue. It is a noninvasive test that measures the total magnesium within cells. Only one laboratory performs this analytic method, so it is not commonly used in magnesium research. But it is readily available and a lot easier than the magnesium load test or NMR tests used in research.

The laboratory can be reached as follows:

Intracellular Diagnostics, Inc.
553 Pilgrim Drive #B
Foster City, CA 94404
800-874-4804
www.exatest.com/minerals.htm

A Final Word

The tests discussed in this chapter can help you to determine your magnesium status. It is a good idea to have evidence of your actual magnesium status, so that you can have your need for and response to treatment evaluated objectively. But if you have certain risk factors for heart disease, trying magnesium is a good bet, as previous chapters have shown. Remember, doctors do not wait for blood tests to assure them as to blood levels of blood-pressure medications. The symptoms call for the medications. These same symptoms call for enhancing your magnesium nutrition. Give it a fair try. And as long as you do not have kidney failure, it can't hurt. See if your symptoms improve.

We suggest you use the Magnesium Questionnaire, the information in Appendix E: Problems Associated with Low Magnesium Levels, and an assessment of your general health to determine whether you need to add magnesium to your diet. The next chapter will show you how.

11

Making Sure You Have Enough Magnesium

How did your magnesium questionnaire come out? Is your risk of a magnesium deficit low or mild, or is it moderate to very high?

How is your health? Are you generally healthy, or do you have too many low-energy days and too many muscle aches or pains? Do you have any of the many symptoms of magnesium deficit? (See Appendix E: Problems Associated with Low Magnesium Levels.) Do you have symptoms of heart disease such as high cholesterol, high blood pressure, or heart palpitations? Are you using medications that add or waste magnesium? (See Appendix H: Common Medications that Affect Magnesium Status.) Does your health history include a severe illness or particularly stressful period in which you may have gotten low in magnesium?

Use your answers to these questions to determine if:

- You need only to fill a daily magnesium gap to prevent a deficit
- Your magnesium gap is a deficit that must be corrected

Closing Your Daily Magnesium Gap

The officially established RDA/DRI for magnesium ranges from 310 to 410 milligrams per day for teenagers and adults. For children aged nine to thirteen, it is 240 milligrams per day. Low-magnesium diets and soft water mean that many of us have a daily magnesium gap. We may not yet have a deficit or any clinical symptoms, but each day we are getting less magnesium than we need to stay healthy. The average shortfall or gap has been estimated to be 170 milligrams per day. This means that some people are getting plenty of magnesium while others are falling short by anywhere from 1 to 10 milligrams to several hundred milligrams a day. You will want to close your magnesium gap to ensure your future health.

If you are very healthy and over age seventy, your diet has probably been adequate in magnesium during much of your life. However, you may now need to pay special attention to your magnesium nutrition. Your ability to absorb magnesium (and other essential minerals) can go down as you age past seventy. But even if you are very healthy and young, a daily magnesium gap can build into a magnesium deficit that could manifest itself as heart disease later in your life. You can prevent this by closing your daily magnesium gap now.

If you have no symptoms or risk factors for heart disease and scored in the low to mild risk categories for magnesium deficit according to the Magnesium Questionnaire in appendix A, you may assume your magnesium stores are adequate, especially if you are living a relatively stress-free life. You should be able to prevent heart disease, maximize your health, and maintain your energy by maintaining this good magnesium state as you age. This means closing any daily magnesium gap, which is probably small or nonexistent. We recommend that you increase your

The average daily magnesium gap is about 170 milligrams.

magnesium intake by 100 to 250 milligrams per day. You can do this with diet (our recommendation) or use any of the other methods described in this chapter. Choose the method or combination of methods most comfortable for you. If you choose to use magnesium supplements to do this, we suggest that you start with a dose of 100 to 200 milligrams of magnesium per day.

If a particularly stressful period arises in your life, add 100 to 200 milligrams more magnesium daily during the time of excessive stress, or starting as soon after it as possible. If you eat a lot of dairy products or take calcium supplements, use the higher end of the range as your target. If your diet changes and you increase your consumption of foods high in magnesium, reassess any magnesium supplement you may be using.

The Importance of Nutrient Balance: Food or Supplements

The delicate balance between calcium and magnesium nutrition discussed in chapter 1 points out a general principle of nutrition: All essential nutrients serve you best when you get them in balanced amounts. If a slight deficiency in one essential nutrient occurs, taking supplements of another can worsen the situation. Just as extra calcium can worsen a low-magnesium state, if your calcium intake is very low, taking large amounts of supplemental magnesium can intensify a calcium deficiency. Keep in mind, however, that vitamin D needs magnesium to help it absorb calcium. Too much sodium can worsen low potassium. Zinc supplements can make a slight iron deficit in a young woman worse. This is why getting essential nutrients from foods is always preferable. If a deficiency in one nutrient, such as magnesium, develops, it is likely that other nutrient intakes also have been less than optimal. A balanced, safe regimen of nutrient replacement may be necessary for a time, but nothing can replace the healthful value of a nutritious diet rich in vegetables, whole grains, fruits, and nuts, with protein from either a balanced combination of legumes and whole grains or animal sources such as eggs, fish, meat, and dairy products.

So many processed foods provide calories without balanced micronutrients. If your diet currently contains a lot of processed foods, please remember that relying on lifelong supplements is a difficult balancing act and, we suspect, never as good as a diet of whole foods.

Correcting a Magnesium Deficit

If your questionnaire results showed you to have a moderate to very high risk of magnesium deficit, or if your health assessment leads you to believe that you may have been accumulating a magnesium deficit over some years as a result of a daily magnesium gap, recognize that you will first need to correct that deficit, most likely with magnesium supplements. When the deficit is corrected, you may maintain your magnesium health with smaller daily supplement doses, with a magnesium-containing salt, or with diet alone.

Persons with specific risk factors for heart disease, such as high cholesterol, high blood pressure, or a family history of cardiovascular disease, will need to add to their program the strategies described for their condition in the appropriate chapters of this book.

If you scored at moderate, high, or very high risk of magnesium deficiency, if you have any symptoms of heart disease or any risk factors for it, you will probably need to build up your magnesium stores with more than 200 milligrams of extra magnesium per day. Supplement doses of 400 to 700 milligrams per day are common. Read the appropriate risk factor chapter(s) to decide on a good starting point for your magnesium replacement program. You may need to use supplements before you can rely on dietary changes alone to keep you in good magnesium health. Read the chapters pertaining to the risk factor you are experiencing and follow the guidelines as you work with your doctor. Keeping close tabs on your risk factor will help you assess how your magnesium program is working. If possible, use a test such as the Ex-atest or the Alturas I Mg^{2+} test before and during your program.

Remember, building up magnesium stores is different for everyone. For some the process is rapid, as it was for Jack, whose story appeared in chapter 1. Some, however, can take magnesium supple-

Over time, a daily magnesium gap can become a deficit.

ments for as long as two or three years before their magnesium stores are replenished. Be patient. Do not compare your results with anyone else's. We are all different.

In this chapter we are going to present three main ways to close the magnesium gap:

- Diet
- Magnesium-containing salts
- Supplements

Using the results of your Magnesium Questionnaire, choose your program. If you are shown to be at low or mild risk of a magnesium deficit, you can choose either the diet, salt, or supplement approach to bridge any magnesium gap. If you have a moderate to high risk of a magnesium deficit, you will probably need to use supplements, at least for a while, though you can taper off once you have built up your magnesium stores or after making dietary and/or lifestyle changes. If you have a very high risk, you will need to do both until your magnesium status becomes adequate. This may take time, care, and some attention to detail, but the benefits will be a true lowering of your risk of cardiovascular disease, including heart attack and stroke, plus the vitality you can achieve when you get enough of this life-giving, energy-boosting mineral.

Maximizing Magnesium in the Diet

There are two elements of your daily diet that can serve as sources of magnesium: the water you drink and the food you eat. Here we will consider each in turn.

Getting Magnesium from Water

Drinking water can account for as much as 10 to 20 percent of your daily magnesium requirement. It is a good way to get magnesium because magnesium in water is easily absorbed by the body.

If you mainly drink bottled water that is distilled or deionized, you may be getting little if any magnesium as you drink. But if you also drink coffee, tea, soups, reconstituted juices, and other liquids and do not go to the trouble and expense of using such highly purified bottled or filtered water for these beverages, you may be getting magnesium from your tap water. Appendix C lists the magnesium content of municipal water from selected locations in the United States. Use this to see if you live in an area with high-magnesium water. If your city or town is not on the list, find out what you can by calling your local water company and asking them if they can tell you how much magnesium is in the water. Some water companies measure it, some do not. If not, they might be able to tell how hard the water is, but hardness can represent any combination of magnesium and calcium. If they have measured hardness and calcium, you can get a rough calculation of the magnesium using the formula in appendix C.

If you want to drink bottled water, make the effort to choose one that is moderate to high in magnesium while moderate to low in calcium and sodium. Use appendix C as a starting point for your search. There are some good mineral and spring bottled waters on the market, and some very good ones from Europe. But there are also many that are low in magnesium or very high in calcium and/or sodium. Be choosy. Stay away from drinking distilled or deionized waters that have no magnesium, or consider fortifying your water with one of the mineral supplements now available for this purpose. Information about these also can be found in appendix C.

If you live in a high- or medium-magnesium water area and wish to maximize this source, all you have to do is drink and cook with the tap water. If you filter your drinking water, be sure the filter you are using does not remove magnesium. If you are worried about other aspects of your tap water, or if your area's water is low in magnesium, you will have to close your magnesium gap using other sources. Maximizing magnesium in your foods is a good way.

Maximizing Magnesium from Foods

Maintaining a good magnesium status through diet and lifestyle includes the wide use of high-magnesium foods, especially if your water supply is not rich, or at least adequate, in magnesium.

Consult Appendix B: Common Foods Classified by Magnesium Content. This may look simple, but it is a quick guide to maximizing the magnesium in your food. Foods listed in the first of the three columns are very high magnesium foods. Those in the second or middle column are midlevel when it comes to magnesium. Those in the right-hand column are low-magnesium foods, which should be minimized or avoided. Additionally, foods in each column are listed in descending order, from the greatest to the least magnesium content. Thus, any food in any column has more magnesium than any food listed underneath it or to the right of it. Use this resource to assess your diet for magnesium content. How many high-magnesium foods are you eating each day? How many medium-magnesium foods? How many low-magnesium foods?

If you cannot find a particular food on the chart, use the instructions following the table in appendix B to look it up in the United States Department of Agriculture Agricultural Research Service (USDA ARS) food database, and place it in its proper location as you expand the chart to fit your diet.

If more than one-third of your food is coming from the third column, or if less than one-third comes from the first column, you need to make some changes if you wish to close the magnesium gap with food. Consciously turn away from the foods listed in the last column and eat more foods listed in the first column. If this turns out to be unrealistic for you on a regular, ongoing basis, seriously consider using a high-magnesium salt or a magnesium supplement.

If less than one-quarter of your food is from the low-magnesium column and you scored low to mild risk in the Magnesium Questionnaire, you are probably doing pretty well in consuming magnesium. You can also maximize the magnesium in such a diet by lowering your saturated fat intake, lowering your sugar intake, cutting out soft drinks made with phosphoric acid (see Appendix G: Soft Drinks Made with and without Phosphoric Acid), drinking little or no alcohol, and lowering the level of stress of your daily life. A vegetarian diet is both low in fat and high in magnesium, which is probably why there are lower rates of heart disease among vegetari-

Careful food selection can close the magnesium gap.

ans than among the general population. People who meditate regularly and/or follow relaxing regimens such as yoga can lower their need for magnesium, which soars with stress. These last two strategies combined are the basis of Dr. Dean Ornish's program.

Supplementing with Magnesium-Containing Salts

The simplest solution to low magnesium is to use supplements, and the easiest way for some people to do this is with a cooking/table salt that contains magnesium. Some of these are discussed in detail in Appendix D: Magnesium in Salt Substitutes. Two of these supplements have been shown to lower the risk of heart disease and, if you use salt, using a magnesium-containing salt instead of standard table salt requires you to make only a minimal change in your daily life. Using such a salt in cooking and at the table can give you a significant, simple source of magnesium. They also can cut sodium intake and add potassium.

The typical American diet includes about 11 grams of table salt, sodium chloride, each day. A very simple way to add a consistent daily source of magnesium to your diet is to use a magnesium-containing salt in place of ordinary table salt. Be aware, however, that if you have kidney disease, you must not use any salt supplements containing substantial amounts of either magnesium or potassium.

Using Magnesium Supplements

We are lucky to have a wide variety of magnesium supplements available to us. Magnesium supplements come in several forms, including:

- *Magnesium oxide.* This is marketed as MagOx (usually found behind the pharmacist's counter but no prescription is necessary), and on the shelf under a variety of trade names.
- *Magnesium chloride.* This is marketed as SlowMag, in the form of a tablet that is coated to protect it from water in the atmosphere, which would cause this form of magnesium to dissolve.
- *Magnesium gluconate.* This is available, mixed with magnesium oxide, as a product named Magonate.

- *Magnesium lactate.* This is marketed as MagTabs.
- *Magnesium aspartate* (and other magnesium amino acid chelates). Magnesium aspartate hydrochloride is marketed in the United States as Maginex, both as coated tablets and as a soluble powder that can be dissolved in water or fruit juice. This form is good for people who need large doses because it does not generally cause diarrhea.
- *Magnesium-containing laxatives,* such as milk of magnesia (which is magnesium hydroxide), epsom salts (which is magnesium sulfate), and liquid magnesium citrate. These can be taken in small amounts, such as a teaspoonful one to three times a day, which is usually not enough to cause diarrhea.

These various forms of magnesium come in tablets, capsules, gelcaps, and wafers with dosages ranging from 65 milligrams to 400 milligrams of magnesium in one tablet. Most of the manufacturers of these supplements recommend that you take enough tablets, capsules, or other type of supplement to get 400 milligrams of magnesium per day.

Correcting a magnesium deficit can require supplements.

There are liquid forms of magnesium for those who cannot handle pills. These range from 20 milligrams of magnesium per teaspoon all the way up to 500 milligrams of magnesium per teaspoon. These very concentrated forms are designed for fortifying deionized or distilled water with magnesium and other nutritional minerals. There is one product called Natural Calm, which is magnesium citrate powder. It is comparatively expensive for the amount of magnesium it supplies, but a teaspoon dissolved in hot water makes a relaxing cup of tea that provides 100 milligrams of magnesium, if you don't mind the somewhat sour taste.

Magnesium is often found in combination with other nutrients in several supplements. These primarily include:

- Calcium (sometimes calcium plus zinc). These have various calcium-to-magnesium ratios. Be sure to consider this aspect in your supplement selection. We recommend a 1:1 to no more than 2:1 calcium/magnesium ratio in supplements. Dolomite and bone meal are combinations of calcium and magnesium, as are cal-mag aspartate and cal-mag citrate.

- Potassium.
- Vitamin B_6, which increases magnesium absorption.
- Other trace minerals.
- Multivitamin and minerals. As a general rule, these do not contain much magnesium. Even those labeled "super" supplements rarely have more than 125 milligrams of magnesium per tablet. This can be enough to fill some people's magnesium gap, but is too low for others.

Magnesium is found in several antacids, both liquid and tablets, as well as laxatives. Be sure to count these sources when assessing your magnesium intake.

As a general rule, when taking magnesium supplements, start at a low dose and gradually build up. When you get diarrhea, you can back off until your stools are comfortably soft. This daily amount of magnesium should be enough to rebuild your magnesium status. If you are magnesium-depleted, you will be able to take high doses comfortably until your depletion is corrected. Then, all of a sudden, you may notice diarrhea. If that happens, adjust your dose downward until your stools are, again, comfortably soft. Maintain that dosage until things change again, then readjust. You can speed up your program by taking your magnesium supplement in two or three daily doses. This way you can take in more magnesium per day without diarrhea or loose stools.

Julee was in her fifties when a nutritionist suggested she take magnesium for her mitral valve prolapse condition. She had had rheumatic fever as a child, which may have helped deplete her of her magnesium, and years later, a cumulative low magnesium balance was bringing on clinical symptoms. She began with a daily dose of 700 milligrams of magnesium and found it quite comfortable for three to four months. Suddenly she developed diarrhea and, with the help of her nutritionist, realized that her magnesium deficiency might be gone. She could now find a lower daily dose of magnesium that was comfortable for her so that she could remain in positive balance for the rest of her life.

Oral magnesium supplement doses of as little as 120 milligrams per day and as high as 1,920 milligrams per day have been reported to safely control symptoms of magnesium deficiency, even in people who lose large amounts of magnesium for genetic reasons.

There are many good magnesium supplements. The trick is to balance magnesium with calcium. To forestall conditions such as osteoporosis, many of us are using calcium supplements, which are popular among both supplement producers and doctors. If you have enough magnesium, calcium supplements are fine. But if you have a low or marginal magnesium status, as many of us do, extra calcium can be dangerous.

For people interested in closing a daily magnesium gap to prevent heart disease, 150 to 250 milligrams of supplemental magnesium per day will probably be enough, along with not more than 1,200 milligrams of calcium from all sources—food, water, and supplements. For people who need to correct a magnesium deficit, most will do well on 400 to 700 milligrams of magnesium per day, along with not more than 1,000 milligrams of supplemental calcium, depending on how much calcium is in your diet. Those who need to reverse some aspect of heart disease may need more magnesium. Each of these special needs is discussed in the relevant chapters of this book.

You may be able to tolerate magnesium pills easily. But some people do not. If pills do not work for you, consider trying a liquid supplement or magnesium-containing salt. Some people will have to get their magnesium from foods only, while others may be allergic to the highest magnesium foods—nuts. Everyone is different. You will need to find out how best your body can get its precious daily magnesium. If you are pregnant or nursing, adequate magnesium is especially important, as your needs are higher. Know the magnesium RDA or DRI for your condition. Talk with your doctor about any special needs you may have beyond these levels.

While magnesium supplementation is generally quite safe, there are some circumstances under which you should *not* take magnesium supplements. For example, people on certain antibiotics should not take magnesium with the antibiotic. *If you have kidney disease (renal failure), you must not take any magnesium supplements.* People with kidney disorders need to work closely with a physician to correct a magnesium deficiency and not try to supplement on their own. There have also been some reports of magnesium toxicity—they are few, but specific. One report told of elderly people dying after taking large quantities of over-the-counter antacid medicine. The authors of this report assumed that it was the magnesium in the antacids or laxatives that became toxic with overdosage, causing the deaths. This may be true. Or it may have been the aluminum in the antacids or that such extreme overuse of these widely available medicines meant that these people had some undiagnosed underlying conditions that caused some of their deaths. At any rate, this source caused two deaths per year, an exceedingly low incidence.

12

Magnesium: The Silent Guardian of Our Hearts and Arteries

Magnesium is essential for life. It has prominent and varied functions that maintain the integrity and functioning of each component part of the cardiovascular system, and of the blood it carries. We think of this dynamic system mostly in terms of the heart that beats and the arteries that carry the blood from the heart to the lungs to pick up the oxygen we need and eliminate the carbon dioxide that results from life processes. The capillaries, where the exchanges of the gases and nutrients between the blood and the constituent cells of the tissues take place, and the veins that carry the blood back to the heart are also part of the cardiovascular system. All the parts of this system, which keeps our body functioning, depend on an adequate supply of magnesium. Although it is not considered in this book, we should remember that magnesium is necessary not just for the cardiovascular system, but for the health of all of our systems, for the health of our entire body.

Magnesium and the Heart

Magnesium is necessary to prevent damage to the muscles of the heart so that it can contract and relax as required. It is also necessary for maintaining the enzymes that keep the cells working properly—to utilize nutrients and to maintain an appropriate electrolyte balance. Without optimal amounts of magnesium, heart muscle cells lose the ability to produce the energy they need to contract—for each beat of the heart. They also lose the ability to keep potassium inside the cells and sodium and calcium outside. And the loss of potassium makes the heart beat irregularly, a condition, called arrhythmia, to which magnesium depletion predisposes. The other side of the electrolyte imbalance that magnesium deficiency causes is abnormally high levels of sodium in the cells. If the heart cells cannot keep excess sodium out, the sodium attracts water, leading to edema (swelling due to fluid retention), which can occur in the heart and lungs as well as in the tissues where it can be seen—for example, as swollen ankles. The presence of increased amounts of calcium in the heart cells is an early sign of damage that develops in magnesium-deficient animals even before the cells break down, or become necrotic. Scarring then takes place, and the injured muscle fibers are replaced by fibrous tissue, further compromising the ability of the heart to do its work. The condition caused by these pathologic changes in the heart is called *cardiomyopathy* (which means "damaged heart muscle"), and it leads to heart failure, or the inability of the heart to pump blood adequately to meet the body's needs. Whether the cause of heart failure is inadequate energy to beat, leading to a tired and ultimately weakened heart, or whether the cause is replacement of cardiac muscle cells with fibrous scar tissue, magnesium inadequacy is a contributor. Conversely, adequate magnesium protects against both problems.

Another effect of too much calcium reaching the heart is arrhythmia. This was discovered in the 1930s when intravenous calcium given to milk cows caused arrhythmia that could be controlled by intravenous magnesium. Also, by the 1940s it was found that the arrhythmia caused by digitalis (which increases the level of calcium in the heart) could be controlled by magnesium injections.

Magnesium and the Blood Vessels

Magnesium is needed by the muscles of the arteries—large and small—for them to contract and relax (dilate) reversing constriction caused by calcium. Angina pectoris, or chest pain, is the heart's warning that the coronary arteries (the arteries that supply nutrients and oxygen to the heart) are not bringing it enough oxygen. That happens when the coronary arteries and arterioles (the small arteries of the heart) constrict too much. The arteries most prone to excess narrowing (for example, in response to stress) usually are already narrowed by arteriosclerosis. As a result, insufficient blood can reach the part of the heart that is supplied by one or more constricted, usually arteriosclerotic, coronaries. The normal constriction and dilation of the arteries—all arteries, not just those of the heart—is influenced by hormones, the secretion of which is controlled by the amount of magnesium present. Additionally, substances called prostaglandins produced by the endothelium (the cells that form the linings of blood vessels) play an important role in controlling constriction and dilation of the arteries, and their release also depends on magnesium. So magnesium's role in keeping the endothelium normal is important in preventing angina, and also in protecting against developing high blood pressure.

We think of high blood pressure as a result of arteriosclerosis. Here again we must consider the effect of magnesium on the endothelium. Without enough magnesium, the blood vessel linings become fragile. Even slightly damaged surfaces attract substances that build up plaques and calcify—the groundwork of hardened arteries, the arteriosclerosis that underlies many of the diseases of the cardiovascular system. Plaques form in the linings of the arteries, largely from deposits of fatty substances like cholesterol. And here, too, magnesium plays an important protective role. It limits excess cholesterol production and guards against formation of the "bad" fats—low-density (LDL) cholesterol and triglycerides—that form the plaques. It also does more. It activates the enzyme that is necessary to form high density lipoproteins (HDLs), the "good" cholesterol that carries the cholesterol away from the arterial linings.

If the endothelium is damaged, blood platelets stick to the injured areas and clump in little aggregations, the early phase of blood coagulation. Also part of the clotting process is a series of changes in proteins that in sequence is called the *coagulation cascade.* This entire process is increased by calcium and decreased by magnesium. Blood coagulation is essential to prevent us from bleeding too much when our skin is broken. When clotting occurs within a blood vessel, however, it contributes to plaque formation, and to the formation of thrombi (circulating clots), from which pieces can break off and be carried to other parts of the circulatory system and become lodged there as *emboli,* blocking blood flow. If this happens in the brain, it can cause a stroke; if in the heart, it can cause myocardial infarction, or heart attack. So here, too, magnesium is protective. It inhibits blood coagulation within the blood vessels, protecting against thrombosis and subsequent strokes and heart attacks.

Magnesium and Metabolic Syndrome X

Low levels of magnesium are related to metabolic syndrome X, which is characterized by many findings that accompany and/or predispose people to developing cardiovascular disease. There is strong evidence that metabolic syndrome X is associated with a cellular imbalance between magnesium and calcium. Instead of a normal state, in which the magnesium content of cells is high and the calcium content is much lower, in this metabolic disorder there is a tendency for the cellular magnesium to fall and cellular calcium to rise. Impaired glucose tolerance, with or without diabetes, and overproduction of insulin—to the action of which the cells are resistant—are major parts of metabolic syndrome X. High blood pressure, accompanied by insulin resistance—again, with or without type II diabetes—can also be present. Increased blood clotting within the blood vessels, dyslipidemia (an unhealthy balance of blood fats), obesity, and cardiovascular disease are all part of the picture of metabolic syndrome X. These manifestations can occur in various combinations or independently.

Why this constellation of abnormalities has become more prevalent in recent years is uncertain. It is possible that changes in our diet have contributed to the prevalence of magnesium deficiency, and that the widespread deficiency of magnesium is a major factor in the growing emergence of metabolic syndrome X as a problem. Its different manifestations give rise to a variety of miseries in themselves. And the metabolic disorders contribute greatly to the increasing severity of cardiovascular disease as a killer, not only among older adults but also, increasingly, among younger people.

Magnesium in the Treatment of Cardiovascular Disease

Although magnesium has long been accepted as an essential nutrient by nutritionists, physicians who have used high doses of magnesium as a drug that can control toxicities of "other" drugs, and that has striking therapeutic actions in its own right, often persist in considering it a medication rather than a nutrient. For example, cardiologists have long used it to correct arrhythmias caused by digitalis, diuretics, and other magnesium-wasting drugs. More recently, its efficacy against serious arrhythmias caused by nonsedating antihistamines, some antibiotics, and some drugs used in the treatment of depression or psychosis has attracted attention.

Its usefulness in controlling angina of coronary artery disease (ischemic heart disease) has been known for half a century, and its efficacy in helping to manage congestive heart failure for not quite as long. Many well-controlled studies of the use of magnesium in the treatment of acute heart attacks have shown it to reduce the death rate and especially arrhythmic complications. This has been particularly dramatic for older people and others for whom "clot-buster" treatment is often deemed inappropriate. Sadly, the failure of two large multi-institutional studies to confirm the lifesaving potential of magnesium in treating myocardial infarction patients has caused many physicians to look with a jaundiced eye at magnesium as a treatment for heart attack patients.

However, Dr. Michael Shechter, one of the cardiologists who has shown how useful magnesium treatment has been in the treatment of heart attacks, has gone on to show that long-term survival was also improved with magnesium therapy. His demonstration that taking oral magnesium supplements prevents platelet clumping, thereby helping to protect against new cardiac events in people who have had heart attacks or who are considered at risk for them, is important. He and his colleagues, both in southern California and Israel, have also shown that when such people take oral magnesium supplements, their exercise endurance improves. Magnesium's natural calcium-blocking activity has also found use in the treatment of ischemic heart disease.

Magnesium has been employed for many other therapeutic uses for almost a century—for example, against convulsions and hypertension of toxic pregnancies (preeclampsia and eclampsia). So potent a remedy has been hard to accept as a simple nutrient.

Can Magnesium Reverse Changes That Cause Cardiovascular Disease?

Much of the evidence for the efficacy of magnesium in the treatment of cardiovascular disease is actually proof that it reverses changes that cause the symptoms requiring treatment. Its usefulness in correcting arrhythmias reflects the fact that it reverses electrolyte abnormalities (low levels not only of magnesium but of potassium, as well as too-high levels of calcium). Its usefulness in the treatment of heart failure is, at the same time, evidence that it is reversing the cellular accumulation of sodium that leads to edema within cells, including those of the heart, and also that causes fluid retention and swelling of other parts of the body. Its protection against the harmful effects of too-high cellular levels of calcium—which occurs as an early element in beginning heart damage and as a manifestation of metabolic syndrome X—is evidence both of its value as a helpful medication and of its ability to reverse a damaging process.

Arteriosclerosis

As for structural changes that take place in arteries, early changes that might be reversible with magnesium supplementation are difficult to demonstrate in people with arteriosclerosis. In animals in which arterial or cardiac damage has been induced by cholesterol, salt, or excess vitamin D, phosphate, and/or calcium, there have been numerous studies showing that giving magnesium both prevents and reverses some of the lesions, whether the animals are subjected to low-magnesium diets or not. In the case of the arteries, in which formation of plaques—causing atheromas—has long been faulted in atherosclerosis (the fat-deposition form of arteriosclerosis), the effect of magnesium in promoting the formation of "good" HDL cholesterol might well reverse the process. HDL cholesterol has been shown to mobilize fat from the arteries in fat-loaded animals. It doesn't seem far-fetched to believe that a higher intake of magnesium than most of us are accustomed to might gradually lower the fat in atherosclerotic arteries. Since magnesium also mobilizes calcium from soft tissues, why not expect it to do the same for the arteries that calcium hardens?

Hardened arteries also lose their elasticity. It is interesting to remember that as long ago as 1938, magnesium deficiency was shown to cause damage to the elastic portion of the small and large arteries of calves. Those arteries became calcified and rigid as calcium was deposited in the fragmented elastin. (*Elastin* is the name of the protein that can stretch, and *elastica* is the name of the portion of the arterial lining that contains elastin). In 1950, another group of investigators, also working with magnesium-deficient calves, showed these changes also in the lining of the heart, with—additionally—fibrosis replacing some of the heart muscle, and the deposition of collagen, the protein that makes up scar tissue. Other animal species have developed comparable changes when made magnesium-deficient. The research group that showed how important magnesium is to raising "good" cholesterol levels, at the expense of the "bad" cholesterol, also showed that arterial damage and calcification were early changes in magnesium-deficient rodents. They also found that there was increased collagen formation in magnesium-deficient animals, and that magnesium deficiency interfered with resorption (breakdown and removal) of the collagen. Since repairing magnesium deficiency counteracts such changes, it is tempting to speculate that replenishing magnesium in people might be beneficial. It might even reverse some of the changes that our dietary patterns cause.

Mitral Valve Prolapse

That magnesium deficiency increases the deposition and interferes with the removal of collagen is pertinent to the most common heart valve disease in humans: mitral valve prolapse. This hereditary disorder has been shown to develop more often in people who have any or all of a number of neuromuscular signs of magnesium deficiency than in those free of these disturbances. These manifestations include anxiety, tension, hyperemotionality, fatigue, and headaches—sometimes migraine, insomnia, dizziness, and chronic fatigue. In the United States, this condition is commonly referred to as chronic fatigue syndrome (CFS). In continental Europe, it is commonly referred to as latent tetany of magnesium deficiency. Mitral valve prolapse has been shown to develop far more commonly in people with latent tetany, whose magnesium levels are low, than in people with normal handling of magnesium. Measurements of urine magnesium levels has shown that even though their blood levels are somewhat low, these people excrete large amounts of magnesium. Is the cause of their magnesium deficiency a variant of genetically determined renal magnesium wasting? This possibility has not been explored.

Several cardiologists have reported that high-dosage magnesium therapy, given for prolonged periods of time, has not only provided relief of the neuromuscular complaints, but also gradually produced some regression of the valvular abnormality, in half of the people with mitral valve prolapse they have treated with it. So even in this disease, with its structural heart damage, magnesium has been able to reverse the process, partially, at least in some. It is of interest that some of the investigators have advised people with latent tetany syndrome to take magnesium supplements faithfully to avoid developing mitral valve prolapse.

Epidemiologic Support of Magnesium's Value to Prevent/Reverse Cardiovascular Disease

Let us now consider some epidemiologic evidence that suggests that some reversal of cardiovascular disease may, indeed, be possible.

The Finnish/North Dakota Experience

When I [M.S.S.] returned, in 1979, from a lecture tour in Finland, a country with exceedingly high illness and death rates from strokes and heart attacks in youngish to middle-aged men, I met Dr. Enterline, an investigator of the U.S. Department of Agriculture, at a meeting we attended. He came up to me after I had reported the Finnish findings to tell me of something he thought I might find interesting. He had recently returned from North Dakota, where he had been sent to see if he could find out what it was there that was responsible for North Dakotans having unusually low heart attack and stroke rates and long life expectancies, despite their having many of the risk factors for cardiovascular disease. He told me that the families he surveyed were relatively recent immigrants from Finland. Their diets were rich in animal fat, salt, and calcium, and poor in magnesium and potassium. Moreover, they were heavy smokers and tended to be fairly heavy drinkers of hard liquor. These lifestyle factors were precisely the same as in Finland. The only difference Dr. Enterline could find was in their water, samples of which he took back to his laboratory for analysis. He said that he had never before encountered water that contained as much magnesium as was in the well water that they drank and used for cooking. At another meeting, I met an investigator who was stationed in Grand Forks, North Dakota. I told him this story, and he laughed and said that he was keeping a scrapbook of local newspaper clippings. His favorite was the report of a golden wedding anniversary party that was attended by both parents of the bride!

It seems that living in an area where the drinking water was very high in magnesium must have counteracted the adverse effects of their diets, smoking, and alcohol drinking, habits that they brought with them from Finland. It seems to have protected them from the high early death rates prevalent in Finland. Did it reverse the damage the older family members might have already experienced? That is speculative, but there is a little more evidence that it might be so.

Heikki Karppanen, the Finnish investigator who had invited me to give lectures in Finland, formulated a new salt that contained a magnesium salt, which he added to replace some of the sodium chloride.

He induced some of the food processors to use that salt in place of regular salt (even in the preparation of their very salty smoked fish and sausages) and has encouraged Finns to use the salt at home. It is difficult to ascertain how much his addition of magnesium to salt contributed to the drop in death rates from heart attacks and strokes in Finland between 1971 and 1995—by 73 percent in North Karelia, the area with the worst cardiovascular mortality, and by 65 percent in the country as a whole—but since 1971, there has been an intensive education program to induce the Finns to reduce the fat in their diets and to increase their vegetable and fruit intakes. It has been reported that fruit and vegetable consumption has gone up two- to threefold—a major factor in their increased intake of both magnesium and potassium. Although reduction of blood cholesterol has been credited for the lowered cardiovascular death rates and no attention has been paid to magnesium, it is plausible that the higher magnesium intake might be helping—at least to prevent further progression of heart disease, and maybe to reverse some of the damage already experienced. Several epidemiologists have commented that in people with insulin resistance (metabolic syndrome X), with or without type II diabetes, the mortality rates have actually risen. Maybe they had not eaten the fruit and vegetables or used the magnesium-enriched salt, but we do know that in people with metabolic syndrome X, cellular magnesium levels are low.

The drinking water is one of the reasons people are healthier and live longer in some parts of the United States, and in some parts of the world, than in others. Unlike North Dakota and other states in the upper Midwest, where cardiovascular health and life expectancy are better than average, parts of the southeast have been called the heart attack–kidney stone belt. The magnesium content of the water explains why. Water hardness comes from both magnesium and calcium, and some of the unwillingness to accept that it is the magnesium that is protective comes from England, where hard water is mostly due to calcium. However, we must consider another factor. Both magnesium and calcium make the water alkaline, while soft water tends to be acid, and thus leaches out of water pipes any toxic minerals in the metal of the pipes. Lead and cadmium are sometimes part of the pipe metal, and each has been implicated in cardiovascular and other damage. A word of advice is appropriate here. If you plan to soften the water coming into your house, exclude the pipe that brings water to the kitchen faucet, where you get your drinking water.

The Serbian Experience

From Serbia comes information that is of value in sorting out the difference between magnesium and calcium in drinking water. Investigators surveyed sixty-five municipalities for cardiovascular disease death rates, as related particularly to these two minerals. People living in hard-water areas where the water was rich in magnesium and poor in calcium were found to have very low death rates from cardiovascular disease. Those in other areas that also had hard water, but where the water was rich in calcium and poor in magnesium were found to have high rates of death due to heart disease.

The Japanese Experience

Moving away from the water supply and back to food, we come to the change in the incidence of heart disease in Japan. Like most people in the Far East, until fairly recently, the Japanese had not nearly the high heart disease death rates that are common in Western countries. As they adopted eating habits closer to those of most Americans, this advantage has been lost. Articles are appearing in Japanese professional journals that stress the need either to return to the earlier diet, which was high in vegetables and fish, or to take magnesium supplements to lower the growing heart attack rates.

Why the Importance of Magnesium Is Often Ignored

Medical Education

In most medical colleges, students are exposed to magnesium mostly in their biochemistry course. There they are introduced to magnesium as a factor that makes a large variety of enzymes functional. But after memorizing some of the reactions in which magnesium plays an important role, the students concentrate on more practical things, especially the things that will be on their tests. The classic subjects—anatomy, histology (the study of cells and tissues on a microscopic level), physiology, pathology, and endocrinology (the study of our hormones)—necessarily take a great deal of time. Microbiology, which involves not only bacteria and parasites but also varieties of viruses and how to diagnose and treat them, takes more time now that biological weapons are of increasing concern. Pharmacology courses introduce medical student to drugs—old and new—and how they act to cure, or to produce side effects. Here they get a little more information on magnesium, at least as regards the drugs that cause magnesium loss or interfere with its absorption. There have been so many new developments in medicine, including new surgical techniques, that have to be taught, that there is not enough time to devote much attention to nutrition. The vitamins are often taught as interesting medical history, and trace minerals and calcium receive much more attention than magnesium. Furthermore, the teaching of most of the professors and instructors reflects their own medical education, which was meager in the knowledge of magnesium's values as a protective nutrient.

Many years after I [M.S.S.] went to medical college and had become so interested in magnesium that I searched the literature for information that I lacked, I found that three of my former professors had published important studies on magnesium and the heart. Two had discovered that people with heart failure who developed serious arrhythmias when they were treated with digitalis could be kept on that lifesaving drug if they were also given magnesium injections. Another had reported that a poison that damaged the heart did so by causing magnesium to leave the heart. He went on to do basic work on how magnesium deficiency causes serious cardiovascular damage in experimental animals and found that giving them a high-magnesium diet prevented that damage. But their important work, some of which was done while I was one of their students, was not part of their course curricula. I didn't discover their contributions until I found that a drug on which I was working was the only one of that class of medications (diuretics) that did not cause magnesium loss, and I wanted to know whether the sparing of magnesium had any significance, so I looked for information on how magnesium worked.

Shortage of Research Funds

The major sources of funds to support scientific and medical research come from the government and from the pharmaceutical companies. Government support tends to be devoted to areas of research that have evoked a great deal of interest, at least by the staff responsible for making the grants. Today, investigation into specific genetic flaws seems to generate the most support. Perhaps the evidence we presented here concerning genetic defects in handling magnesium might stimulate interest in that area of genetics. But we are not holding our breath waiting for that to happen. Far more individuals suffer from nutritional imbalances that lead to magnesium deficiency than suffer from genetically determined magnesium malabsorption or magnesium-wasting.

Many of the major advances in the treatment of disease have come from the pharmaceutical industry, which has developed numerous lifesaving patented drugs whose sales can in turn fund further research, as well as providing salaries for employees and dividends for investors. Magnesium is not a patentable substance, and so has not attracted the interest of private industry, since they could not be assured that any money they spend on research would result in their selling enough of any magnesium product they might market to make a profit. The knowledge that would result would be published in journals available also to companies selling competitive magnesium products.

Despite the inadequacy of financial support for magnesium research, there are dedicated physicians and research scientists, including nutritionists, who have discovered how magnesium acts in cardiovascular and other tissues and want to apply that knowledge to improving health. It is from their work that the material in this book is drawn. More hope derives from the fact that there is an International Society for the Development of Research in Magnesium, which was organized thirty years ago by Dr. Jean Durlach and continues to be active today. In addition, the American professional organization that holds Gordon Research Conferences holds one on magnesium developments every few years, and the New York Academy of Science will be holding their second annual meeting on magnesium in 2004.

The Cost of Publicizing Magnesium's Value

The education of the public and the postgraduate education of physicians as to the importance of assuring adequate magnesium intake is expensive. It requires background searches, hiring medical writers, and producing and distributing the information. Companies that market magnesium products would want some assurance that they might earn a return on the cost of undertaking such a program by selling more of their product. Without patent protection, they risk providing information that can be used by other companies to sell competeng products. A few nutritional supplement companies have undertaken such efforts, in the hope that the important information they provide under their names will evoke enough customer loyalty to give them some added sales. They deserve credit for this action, which might well have significant public health benefits.

How Magnesium Deficiency and the Epidemic of Heart Disease Developed

Cardiovascular disease has run rampant in the Western world as the processing and marketing of foods has made it easier to get food products that we like to eat but that are often low in magnesium. Even though starvation continues to plague many parts of the world, due to natural and political disasters, we are now confronting another sort of malnutrition (the word which really means *bad nutrition,* not *undernutrition*). It is overnutrition of the wrong nutrients that has resulted in undernutrition of magnesium. It is a poor intake of magnesium that is at fault in the growing epidemic of cardiovascular diseases. And this problem is spreading to other lands with the globalization of our industrial society.

Our free-market legal and patent-regulatory system has permitted enormous medical benefits, with the development of drugs that have eliminated diseases that used to wipe out large segments of the population. New diagnostic and surgical techniques have further advanced doctors' ability to treat their patients, most of whom suffer from cardiovascular diseases. To keep us well, or at least to treat us when we become sick, our physicians have available to them many drugs and procedures—most of which are expensive.

These medications, along with intense coronary care, have reduced the incidence of death from heart attacks from 30 percent thirty years ago to 10 percent now. Medicine, the American Heart Association, the cardiology specialties, the pharmaceutical industry (which develops new drugs), and the National Institutes of Health (which establish and support research projects to resolve health problems) continue to whittle away at this number.

But preventive measures that are poorly supported, such as recommending dietary changes, have taken us in directions that have not notably decreased the prevalence of cardiovascular disease. Advising that we cut down on our salt and sugar intake, substitute unsaturated for saturated fats, and increase the amounts of vegetables, fruits, and whole grains in our diets are steps that have been helpful. But for many people, this means changing their diets more than they wish to do. At the same time, we are told we should harden our bones to prevent osteoporosis by increasing our calcium intake to as much as 1,500 milligrams per day. It is not mentioned that, if magnesium intake is left at little more than a fifth of that amount, that recommendation results in a calcium-to-magnesium ratio of 5 to 1. This exceeds the 4 to 1 ratio that was blamed, in large part, for Finland having the highest heart disease death rate in the world! At the time Finnish researcher Heikki Karppanen did his analysis of cardiovascular mortality as related to dietary intakes of calcium and magnesium in 1978 (summarized in figure 1.4), the country second to Finland, both in death rates from heart disease and in high dietary calcium to magnesium ratios, was the United States. The most recent data indicate that there has been a substantial decline in the Finnish cardiovascular death rates, except for those with metabolic syndrome X, that has followed the government's institution of an educational program directed at lowering fat consumption and increasing fruit and vegetable intake. In Finland, this program has, in fact, been successful in changing people's diets and in lowering the rate of death due to cardiovascular disease in men by as much as 73 percent. It is not possible to determine whether, and how much, Dr. Karppannen's creation of a salt product for table and cooking use that has had magnesium added, and his success in inducing food processors to use that salt, has contributed to the improvement in his country's cardiovascular statistics.

We have considered dietary indiscretions or abuses that can contribute to the imbalance between calcium and magnesium that leads to metabolic syndrome X. Extensive metabolic balance studies have indicated that the best absorption and retention of both minerals was achieved with an intake of no more than twice as much calcium as magnesium. Can the current overenthusiasm for putting calcium into our bones while disregarding our need for magnesium be contributing to our putting more into our cardiovascular tissues as well?

We can expect more and more pharmaceuticals to come out that help us, with the help of our physicians, to deal with our health problems. The research that stems from new drugs widens our knowledge—even our understanding—of how a magnesium deficit can damage the cardiovascular system. Finding out about the numerous enzymes that need magnesium to function properly has vastly increased our knowledge base. But medications that change the functioning of one enzyme can also affect another, then another, and possibly several others—often in unforeseen ways. In this book, we have considered some of the ways in which a drug can affect cholesterol production by altering a single enzyme's function. But the body must maintain complex interrelations among all enzymes, having them turn on and turn off at the right times. If you start to control one important enzyme with drugs, you can expect several other enzymatic and physiological actions and properties to be changed to some degree. It is partly from studying how drugs act that we have gained more insight into how magnesium acts. Such studies have also shown us new aspects of how low magnesium levels set up the very abnormalities that have necessitated the development of new drugs. When will we address ourselves to preventing magnesium deficiency, since magnesium is required by so many enzymes essential for bodily functions and integrity?

It is important that we recognize that this deficit is real and requires remedy. The controversy over magnesium—do we need to use supplements or not?—is not even on the table at this time. We hope this book will at least start the conversation.

The realization of our need to replenish magnesium should be followed by an educational program and research to determine how best to set things right. This is not easy. Even though hard water has been associated with lower cardiovascular disease and death rates, putting magnesium into our water supply would create practical problems. Consider all the water softeners that are in use to prevent the deposition of insoluble hard material inside the pipes, which raises the plumbing bills to clean them. Magnesium and calcium are what make water hard, and we soften water also so that we can get ample sudsing to wash our clothes and ourselves. Just a word of advice for those living in hard-water areas: Do not soften the water you drink.

Replenishing the magnesium in agricultural soil or adding magnesium to fertilizer is a good idea. Plants would grow better and be greener. Most gardening shops and supply houses stock cartons or bags of epsom salts (magnesium sulfate crystals) to be used for that purpose in soft-water areas, where the soil is likely to be low in magnesium.

Putting magnesium into some foods or drinks, such as putting magnesium citrate into orange juice, might prove acceptable. Replacing it in foods from which it has been removed, like white flour, makes sense, but it might create problems in some food properties, such as getting dough to rise. Some of these suggestions might be feasible, but if altering your diet is not to your taste, using supplements is more practical for the time being, and it is something that is under your personal control.

A Final Word

Magnesium is often ignored as an essential nutrient that is required for cardiovascular health. Perhaps its long-time use as a lifesaving medication for people with cardiac arrhythmias or heart attacks has resulted in its being considered a drug rather than a nutrient. Along with other vital nutrients, magnesium helps to maintain many facets of a normal heart and blood vessels. It helps in keeping potassium in the cells and sodium out, thus working to prevent arrhythmias. It also keeps calcium out of the cells, protecting against metabolic syndrome

X, and improves the response to insulin, preventing the insulin resistance that is also part of that syndrome that predisposes people to developing high blood pressure and heart disease, as well as type II diabetes. Magnesium participates in fat metabolism, helping to maintain a normal blood lipid profile. It plays roles in maintaining a balance between arterial constriction and dilation, thereby helping to keep blood pressure normal. It is important in keeping the linings of the blood vessels and the heart healthy, protecting against their tearing and providing the injured sites on which blood clots and fat aggregations can deposit—processes in plaque formation that start the hardening of the arteries. Magnesium also inhibits the formation of clots in blood vessels, thereby protecting against the thrombosis and embolus formation, which can cause heart attacks or strokes. It protects the heart from effects of temporary interruptions in its blood supply and prevents the abnormality of scar tissue formation and collagen deposition that is part of arterial and heart valve disease. It also protects the elastic component of our arteries from degenerating, which is important in keeping our arteries normally flexible, and also because the damaged elastic tissue is where early calcification of the arteries takes place.

All of these functions are accomplished with normal magnesium levels—levels that are provided by a magnesium-rich diet, which is what most of us do not get. Imagine if a drug could be synthesized that did all of these protective things! If harmful processes have already resulted in tissue damage and malfunction, such as arrhythmia, larger amounts of magnesium are required, given by injection.

At the higher levels, magnesium acts like a drug and has been lifesaving. With such damage as is seen in mitral valve prolapse, very high doses also seem to be necessary to reverse some of the damage. The question of how best to achieve whatever reversal is possible requires intensive investigation. Whether combining magnesium with antioxidant nutrients or drugs to enhance the antioxidant effect of magnesium itself would achieve this desirable end has not been proved. Perhaps the National Institutes of Health might be interested in demonstrating that this very inexpensive substance has activities that might markedly reduce the cost of health care—and, at least as important, improve the quality of life of those it benefits.

Appendix A: Magnesium Questionnaire

Use this questionnaire to help you assess your probable magnesium status. It is not rigorously scientific, but it is a guide that will aid you in identifying factors in your life that may be affecting your magnesium status. In conjunction with any cardiovascular risk factors you may have and, possibly, laboratory testing, it will help you to determine how likely you are to be magnesium-deficient and what steps you may wish to take to correct any deficit.

Part One

Circle the appropriate number beside each statement and total your score at the bottom.

Statement	Less than once a month	Once a month to once a week	2–4 times per week	4–7 times per week	More than once a day
1a. I take a calcium supplement with no added magnesium	0	1	2	3	4
1b. I also am on hormone replacement therapy or birth control pills	0	1	2	3	4
2. I drink distilled or deionized bottled water	0	1	2	3	4
3. I drink fruit drink, ade, or punch	0	1	2	3	4
4. I drink sodas containing phosphoric acid (see appendix G)	0	1	2	3	4
5. I eat candy	0	1	2	3	4
6. I eat pastries, cakes, pies, or desserts	0	1	2	3	4
7. I have sugar in my coffee	0	1	2	3	4
8. I eat white-bread products (including bagels, croissants, muffins, french bread, croutons, crackers, etc.)	0	1	2	3	4
9. I eat pasta, spaghetti, or noodles (including Chinese noodles)	0	1	2	3	4
10. My diet is high in saturated fat	0	1	2	3	4
11. I drink alcohol	2	2	1	0	15

Total, Part One ________

Part Two

How many total cup servings of nuts or vegetables (¼ cup of nuts or ½ cup of vegetables) do you eat each day? Include salads and legumes such as soy and other beans. Circle the score beneath the appropriate number of servings.

Average servings of nuts or vegetables eaten	**5–7 servings per day**	**3–4 servings per day**	**1–2 servings per day**	**less than 1 serving per day**
Score	0	3	5	10

Part Three

When you eat breads and cereals, how often are they whole-grain foods? Circle the score beneath the appropriate description of how often you choose whole-grain products over processed-grain products.

Occurrence	**Exclusively whole grains**	**Mostly whole grains**	**Sometimes whole grains**	**Rarely or never whole grains**
Score	0	3	5	10

Part Four

Circle the appropriate number beside each statement and total your score at the bottom.

Statement	**True**	**False**
1. I have high blood pressure, whether treated or untreated (see chapter 3)	15	0
2. I have high triglycerides, high LDL cholesterol and/or low HDL cholesterol (see chapter 5)	15	0
3. I have type II diabetes or a high fasting glucose level (see chapters 2 and 5)	15	0
4. I take a thiazide diuretic (see chapter 3)	15	0
5. I take digitalis	15	0
6. I am 70 years old or older	15	0
7. I have a family history of heart disease	25	0

Total, Part Four ________

Now add up your scores from all four parts:

Part One: ________
Part Two: ________
Part Three: ________
Part Four: ________

TOTAL: ________

Interpreting Your Results

Use the following general guide to assess your likely risk of magnesium deficiency:

0–12 points = Low risk of magnesium deficiency
13–20 points = Mild risk of magnesium deficiency
21–30 points = Moderate risk of magnesium deficiency
31–40 points = High risk of magnesium deficiency
41 + points = Very high risk of magnesium deficiency

Why Are Calcium and Phosphorus on the Questionnaire?

Getting too much calcium and/or phosphorus while in a suboptimal or deficient magnesium state may worsen the magnesium inadequacy. High-dose vitamin D supplements can have an impact on these minerals as discussed in the following section (page 260).

CALCIUM

When a magnesium deficit occurs, calcium levels in the blood go down, even if calcium intake is adequate. When the body is in such a state, the absorption of calcium can remain normal while excretion of calcium in the urine becomes low. Thus, even though blood calcium is low, the body tends to retain calcium when in a magnesium-deficient state. Extra calcium intake at such a time could cause an abnormal rise of calcium levels inside the cells, including the cells of the heart and blood vessels. If magnesium is replenished, the calcium level in the blood returns to normal, as does its excretion in the urine. Given the delicate balance necessary between calcium and magnesium in the cells, it is best to be sure magnesium is adequate if you are taking calcium supplements. This can be especially important if you are taking hormone replacement therapy or birth control pills (see chapter 7).

PHOSPHORUS

Experimental rats can be made magnesium deficient—enough to cause calcification of kidney tissue—by adding excess phosphorus and calcium to their diets. The amount of phosphate-containing additives in processed foods can be substantial (providing up to 1 gram per day, especially from baked goods and processed meats). Phosphoric acid–based sodas contain between 50 to 160 milligrams of phosphorus per serving, depending upon the size of the drink (see appendix G). Given these unintentional sources, people may be ingesting more phosphorus than a low magnesium intake can safely counteract, especially if calcium supplements are part of the dietary picture. However, if calcium intake is low and phosphorus intake high, the bone can be adversely affected. Once again, the proper balance is necessary. Studies on this interaction between calcium and phosphorus often do not include an assessment of the subjects' magnesium status, but the physiological parameters of excess phosphorus and calcium can be similar to those described in magnesium deficiency. This is a complex area of nutrition, but it is safe to say that adequate magnesium plus a proper balance between calcium, magnesium, and phosphorus intakes is desirable, and you should remember that the amount of phosphorus in processed foods that contain phosphate-based additives can be higher than you would expect. The DRI/RDA for phosphorus is around 700 milligrams for adults. An adequate intake for calcium for adults is 1,000 milligrams per day from all sources, 1,200 milligrams per day if you are over age seventy. At these intakes of calcium, keeping the recommended two-to-one (2:1) calcium-to-magnesium ratio requires daily magnesium intakes of 500 milligrams, an amount rarely consumed by Americans.

HIGH-DOSE VITAMIN D

Vitamin D is necessary for calcium absorption. When vitamin D levels are low, not much calcium is absorbed from the intestines into the bloodstream, even if there is plenty of calcium in the diet. However, doses of vitamin D higher than the amount necessary to achieve normal calcium levels can have negative effects. If magnesium status is low or suboptimal and vitamin D is very high, and especially if calcium is also high, calcium absorption can be high enough to make the magnesium deficiency worse and to worsen the risk of calcium moving abnormally into cells and soft tissues, including those of the heart and arteries. The amount of vitamin D people need varies with age, skin pigmentation, exposure to sunlight, the latitude at which they live, and even their individual genetic makeup, all of which can limit the amount that can be safely consumed without causing excess calcium levels. Vitamin D nutrition is a complex subject that is difficult to quantify or generalize about. It does play a role in magnesium, calcium, phosphorus nutrition. The adult adequate intake for vitamin D ranges from 200 to 400 international units per day, 600 international units per day for people over age seventy. The upper limit has been set at 2,000 international units per day.

Like most nutrients, calcium, phosphorus, and vitamin D have a range of optimal intakes. An intake below this range means deficit; an intake above it means that the otherwise beneficial nutrient can become toxic. If you are low in magnesium, it is easier for calcium, phosphorus, and vitamin D to become toxic or, conversely, for resistance to vitamin D to develop.

We are not suggesting that you forgo calcium supplements to prevent osteoporosis, to do without phosphorus and vitamin D, or to avoid vitamin D–fortified milk. We *are* suggesting you get adequate magnesium so that a high level of these nutrients will not exacerbate a deficient or suboptimal magnesium intake. If you are told that you need unusually high doses of any vitamin, keep in mind that magnesium activates vitamin D, and that lower doses of vitamin D are needed when inadequate magnesium is corrected.

Why Are Fruit Drinks, Ade, and Punch on the Questionnaire?

These sweetened drinks are quite high in sugar. A 12-ounce serving of fruit drink contains roughly 12 teaspoons of sugar, whereas the same amount of cola has 9 teaspoons and a piece of white layer cake with chocolate frosting has 6 teaspoons. A high intake of refined sugar can lead to magnesium loss in the urine, and these drinks can really add a lot of sugar to one's life, even though their fruit flavor leads some people to believe they are healthy. Look for pure fruit juices rather than fruit drinks or ades. Fruit drinks, ades, and punches have added sugar.

Why Are Other Common Foods on the Questionnaire?

The reasons for including some of the other elements of the questionnaire can be summarized as follows:

- *Candies and desserts* are usually made with refined sugar. Refined sugar has not only had all the magnesium removed from it, it increases the excretion of magnesium in the urine (see chapter 9). There is one bright spot to this restriction. If you must break your diet with a little candy, take a piece of chocolate, preferably dark semi-sweet. Chocolate contains magnesium.
- *White breads and pastries made with white flour* are low-magnesium foods (see chapter 9). These products can also be a significant source of phosphate-based additives. A steady diet, year after year, of white bread or baked products made with white flour can easily be low in magnesium, especially if it does not include several servings of vegetables each day.
- *Alcohol,* especially the excessive consumption of hard liquor, promotes the excretion of magnesium, enhancing the risk of cardiovascular disease, while moderate, regular use of alcohol may spare magnesium (see chapter 8).
- *Certain types of bottled water* may have all the natural magnesium removed (see chapter 9 and appendix C).
- *Saturated fats* impede the absorption of magnesium through the intestine (see chapter 5).

Appendix B: Common Foods Classified by Magnesium Content

To increase the magnesium content of your diet, emphasize food items listed in the left-hand and center columns of the table below, and minimize those in the right-hand column. Foods are listed in subcategories (grains, vegetables, and so on), and within subcategories are, in general, listed by relative magnesium content, with the highest-magnesium foods listed first.

High-Magnesium Foods	Medium-Magnesium Foods	Low-Magnesium Foods
DAIRY PRODUCTS		
	Hard cheeses	Eggs Milk Butter Cream
FISH AND SEAFOOD		
Periwinkles Conch Shrimp Whelks Clams Cockles Crab	Lobster Prawns Oysters Sardines (canned) Mackerel Bluefish Salmon Herring Haddock Flounder	
FRUIT		
Dried figs Dried apricots Dates Coconut (fresh or dried)	Dried peaches Dried prunes Avocados Bananas Raisins Blackberries	Raspberries Cantaloupe Cherries Strawberries Plums Peaches Oranges Pineapple Grapefruit Apricots Apples Pears Cranberries Grapes
GRAINS, FLOURS, AND GRAIN/FLOUR PRODUCTS		
Bran (all types) Raw oats Whole barley Brown rice Cornmeal, whole Whole-wheat bread Rye flour	Cornmeal, degermed White flour Pearl barley White rice Raw pasta	Boiled pasta Boiled white rice White flour products Pastries

Appendix B: Common Foods Classified by Magnesium Content

MEAT AND POULTRY		
	Liver	Roast pork (lean)
	Beef heart	Grilled lamb
	Bacon	Beef tongue
	Corned beef	Ham
	Roast beef (lean)	Roast beef (with the fat)
	Steak	Beef kidney
	Veal	Beef brain
	Chicken	Halibut
	Turkey	Cod
MISCELLANEOUS		
Cocoa		Sugar
Bitter chocolate		
NUTS		
Cashews	Chestnuts	
Almonds		
Brazil nuts		
Peanuts		
Pecans		
Hazelnuts		
Walnuts		
VEGETABLES AND LEGUMES		
Soybeans	Parsley	Boiled potatoes
Butter beans	Sweet corn	Boiled peas
Soy flour	Okra	Boiled broccoli
Legumes (dried beans and peas, most types)	Kale	Beets
Beet greens	Kohlrabi	Boiled cauliflower
Dried seaweed (most types)	Horseradish	Carrots
Chard	Dandelion	Mushrooms
Spinach	Raw cabbage	Onions
Collards	Brussels sprouts	Eggplant
	Artichokes	Lettuce
	Potatoes (baked with skin)	Tomatoes
		Cucumber
		Asparagus

Adapted from Seelig (1964) and Pennington (1989)

If you cannot find a food you are looking for on this list, you can add it to the proper column in the table after looking up the food in the National Agriculture Library Database, which you can consult for free on the Internet. This database contains analyses of foods for many nutrients on per 100-gram serving, or per tablespoon or cup. Look up your food on the "per-100-grams" basis. The foods in Column One of the above table—the high-magnesium foods—contain more than 50 milligrams of magnesium per 100-gram serving. Column Two foods—medium-magnesium foods—have between 25 and 50 milligrams of magnesium per 100 grams. Column Three foods—low-magnesium foods—contain less than 25 milligrams magnesium per 100 grams.

To look up the magnesium content of foods in the National Agriculture Library Database, do the following:

1. Log onto the Internet and go to *www.nal.usda.gov.*
2. Click on *Publications/Databases* in the column of boxes on the left-hand side of your screen.
3. Click on *Databases,* underlined and in pink, in the center of the screen, toward the top.
4. Scroll down to the next-to-last database, *USDA Nutrient Database for Standard Reference,* and click on it.
5. Type the name of food you want to know about in the search window. You will probably get a list of foods in response. Scan the list for the one you are interested in.*
6. Select the food you want. Then select the option 100 grams of edible portion = 100 grams (a little checkmark will appear in the box at the left-hand side of that line) and click *Report*.
7. Scroll down the list of nutrients to minerals and, under that, to Magnesium. The number that appears in the center column represents the number of milligrams of magnesium in 100 grams of that food.

*If you do not get the exact food you are looking for, you can go back to the previous screen and try a slightly different version of the food name. For instance, if you type the word "blueberry" in the search screen, you may get a list of many processed food products that contain blueberry flavoring, but no listing for fresh blueberries. However, if you try again with the word "blueberries," you will find listings for fresh (raw) berries.

If the number is greater than 50, the food is a high-magnesium food and goes in Column One.

If the number is between 25 and 49, the food is a medium-magnesium food and goes in Column Two.

If the number is below 25, the food is a low-magnesium food and goes in Column Three.

Note that this database also gives you the calcium content of each food (found two rows above the magnesium content), also in milligrams per 100 grams. From this and the magnesium content you can calculate the magnesium-to-calcium ratio of the food. To do this, simply divide the magnesium value by the calcium value. If the result is greater than 1, the food has more magnesium than calcium, and so has a good magnesium-to-calcium ratio. If the result is less than 0.5, then there is at least twice as much calcium as magnesium in that food, and the ratio is beginning to be unbalanced. Remember, however, that what is important is the ratio of calcium to magnesium in your total diet, including supplements and water, not necessarily the ratio in any single food. We recommend an overall, total dietary magnesium-to-calcium ratio of 1-to-2 as a goal.

Appendix C: Magnesium in Drinking Water

As we saw in chapters 1, 9, and 11, drinking water can be a source of dietary magnesium. Both tap water and bottled water may contain magnesium. However, when it comes to mineral content, not all water is created equal.

Municipal Water Sources

Tap water can be a significant source of both magnesium and calcium. One recent study found that 2 liters of tap water from some municipal water supplies could provide up to 30 percent of the daily recommended intake (DRI) of magnesium for adults. However, tap water in many other areas is quite low in magnesium, providing no significant amounts of this mineral at all. How can you tell which category your water falls into?

We had a geologist, Dennis Hibbert, compile recent values for the magnesium and calcium levels in tap water from twenty U.S. cities. These are listed in the table that follows.

City	Magnesium (parts per million)	Calcium (parts per million)	Hardness (parts per million)
Atlanta, GA	0.3	7.3	30.0
Seattle, WA	0.5	20.0	23.0
Portland, OR	0.6	1.8	6.6
Oakland, CA	2.8	9.0	35.0
San Francisco, CA	3.4	8.9	37.0
Dallas, TX	3.8	51.0	134.0
Memphis, TN	4.5	7.9	45.4
Denver, CO	6.2	25.0	80.0
New York, NY	6.4	16.0	67.4
Washington, DC	8.0	40.0	135.0
Cleveland, OH	8.8	32.5	116.0
Chicago, IL	11.1	35.2	143.7
Los Angeles, CA	12.2	16.3	137.3
St. Louis, MO	12.6	26.4	124.5
Austin, TX	15.0	15.0	104.0
San Diego, CA	17.7	44.9	202.3
Lincoln, NE	19.0	64.0	220.0
Honolulu, HI	6.0–23.0	9.0–26.0	Not known
Salt Lake City, UT	30.2	78.9	311.9
New Orleans, LA	41.0	109.0	150.0

The above figures must be considered imprecise and of variable accuracy. They depend upon averages and then averages of averages, and there is no uniformity in methods of either analysis or calculation. Beyond this, there is a story for each of these numbers. For example, in Honolulu, municipal water is drawn from several different wells. In general, the wells closer to the mountains have more magnesium than calcium, while those closer to the ocean have slightly more calcium than magnesium. Yet all of these well sources are interconnected in Honolulu's municipal water system, so that any given resident might get mountain-source water one day and seacoast-source water the next. Your own city or town undoubtedly has its own water story. To get any real idea of the magnesium content of your local water supply, you should call the water company and interview someone in the chemistry or analytical laboratory.

That said, there are some general trends. For the most part, the recent values Dennis compiled fall into the same order, generally, as values from a large survey of U.S. cities' water that was conducted in 1962 and published in the U.S. Geologic Survey Water-Supply Paper No. 1812. This lends credibility to both sets of numbers. The other pertinent fact is that in both 1962 and 2000, in all cities except Honolulu, the level of calcium is much higher than that of magnesium. It is interesting to note that Hawaii has traditionally had one of the lowest rates of heart disease death of all fifty of the United States.

The values in the preceding table represent part per million (ppm), or the number of milligrams per liter (a little more than one quart) of water. Most people drink two to two and a half liters of tap water per day, and you can use that figure to calculate the milligrams of magnesium your tap water supplies each day. You can also calculate the amount of calcium your tap water provides you daily.

If your city is not on this list—or even if it is—you can call your local water department and ask for the latest values for magnesium and calcium. They may be able to tell you only the water's hardness. This is a combination of both the calcium and magnesium. If they cannot give you a value for magnesium but do have a value for both calcium and hardness, you can use the following calculation to estimate the magnesium content:

1. Multiply the calcium concentration in ppm by 2.5.
2. Subtract the result of step 1 from the hardness in ppm.
3. Divide the result of step 2 by 4.1. This should give you a rough estimate of the magnesium in that water.

This calculation works sometimes, but not always. It assumes a lot of chemistry that may not hold true for your situation, so do not be too surprised if you come up with a seemingly strange number, such as a negative magnesium value.

Some municipalities soften their water, and some people have household systems that soften the water at point of use (POU), as it flows into the home. The water-softening process yields water in which soap can form suds. This is accomplished by removing calcium and magnesium and adding sodium (calcium and magnesium bind with soap so that it does not make suds, but instead produces a scum that can stay on clothes, dishes, and in drainage pipes, whereas sodium does not impede suds formation). No matter what the magnesium content of your municipal water supply is, if you use softened water, your water is not a significant source of magnesium.

Bottled Water Sources

The range of magnesium, calcium, and sodium levels in bottled waters is enormous. To determine the magnesium, calcium, and sodium content of bottled water, whether a European or North American brand, consult the following websites:

- *www.pmgeiser.ch/cgi-bin/mineral?sort=mg*
- *www.mgwater.com/waters.shtml*

You can also get this information from *The Good Water Guide*, by Maureen and Timothy Green (Rosendale Press, 1985). Although currently out of print, you may be able to get a copy from an online bookseller such as *Amazon.com* or find one in your local public library. This book details magnesium, calcium, and sodium levels for seventy-three European bottled waters. Another source of information is *The Pocket Guide to Bottled Water,* by Arthur von Wiesenberger (NTC/Contemporary Publishing, 1991).

Many bottled waters in North America are distilled or deionized water, and as such they have almost zero magnesium. Often a bit of sodium is added for taste. There is at least one product designed to fortify such deionized or distilled water with magnesium. ConcenTrace trace mineral drops, produced by Trace Mineral Research of Roy, Utah, is said to contain magnesium and other elements in proportions found in the Salt Lake. It is available in health-food stores.

Appendix D: Magnesium in Salt Substitutes

The average consumption of table salt in the United States is 11 grams per day per person. Substituting all or some of this salt with a magnesium-containing salt, used during cooking or sprinkled on food, is a good way to add magnesium to the diet without major changes in the foods one eats. A few of these salts and how to obtain them are discussed in this appendix.

Salt Substitutes Containing Magnesium

There are three table salt products we know of that contain magnesium: Cardia Salt, SmartSalt, and Celtic sea salt. Using any one of them in cooking and at the table can give you a significant, simple source of magnesium. Two of them, Cardia Salt and SmartSalt, are commercial salts that are specifically formulated to add magnesium and potassium to table salt.

Cardia Salt

This product is specifically formulated to add magnesium and potassium to table salt. It contains ordinary salt (sodium chloride), potassium chloride, and magnesium sulfate. If you were to consume 11 grams of Cardia Salt in a day, you would take in about 120 milligrams of magnesium. This would take care of the magnesium gap for many people. It also would mean reducing your sodium intake by more than half and increasing your potassium intake by 1,600 milligrams per day.

In Finland, where the product originated, Cardia Salt is sold under the brand name Pansuola and is widely used in home kitchens and by some sausage makers and bakers in the food industry. Since it has been used in Finland (at the same time that a major education program has been undertaken to increase vegetable intake and reduce the amount of fat consumed), there has been a documented reduction in blood pressure among Finnish people, as well as reductions in the incidence of stroke and coronary artery disease between 1972 and 1992.

Cardia Salt can be purchased at many drugstores and other retail outlets. You can also contact the manufacturer directly as follows:

Nutrition 21
4 Manhattanville Road
Purchase, NY 10577-2197
888-422-7342 or 800-699-3533

SmartSalt

SmartSalt is produced by means of evaporation from water from Utah's Great Salt Lake, which is essentially an inland sea that contains higher concentrations of minerals than oceanic seawater. Salt harvested from this source has more magnesium, less calcium, less sodium, and fewer heavy metals than Celtic sea salt (see under "Whole Sea Salt."). The producers of SmartSalt add an FDA-permissible amount of potassium. Eleven grams of SmartSalt contain 626 milligrams of magnesium and 865 milligrams of potassium, with only 1,596 milligrams of sodium—

about one-third the amount of sodium in an equal weight of ordinary table salt. If someone were to consume half the RDA of sodium from SmartSalt, he would also consume over 100 percent of the RDA of magnesium and 20 percent of the RDA of potassium. SmartSalt also provides naturally occurring trace elements such as boron and selenium with very low levels of heavy metals.

SmartSalt can be obtained from the manufacturer, who can be contacted as follows:

Mineral Resources International
1990 West and 3300 South
Ogden, UT 84401
800-731-7866

Whole Sea Salt

Sea salt is becoming more and more popular as a healthy alternative to traditional table salt. However, caution is to be used in choosing sea salt products. There are two old processes of gathering salt, with two different results:

1. When sea water is evaporated down to just less than 10 percent moisture, sodium chloride crystallizes out first. Solid salt crystals removed from such a source are almost 99 percent sodium chloride, just the same nutritionally as the ordinary table salt of the modern world. Most sea salt sold in grocery and health-food stores is this type of salt. It is essentially sodium chloride and contains no magnesium.
2. When sea water is evaporated to less than 10 percent moisture, the salt crystals contain more than just sodium chloride. Present are all the salts of the sea, and magnesium is a good part of that. Hawaiians call this *whole salt*.

If we assume that a person uses 11 grams of sodium chloride in the form of whole salt each day, he or she would also take in 50 milligrams of magnesium (more than the RDA) and 14 milligrams of calcium, for a magnesium-to-calcium ratio greater than 3 to 1. This is *very* healthy salt in terms of magnesium-to-calcium ratio, and it also contains other trace minerals.

Where does one get such salt? There is a company that sells Celtic sea salt over the Internet. It is expensive, averaging about ten dollars a pound, although some suppliers have membership programs that cut this price in half. And this is not your usual salt. Switching to Celtic sea salt is *not* as simple a lifestyle change as switching to Cardia Salt or SmartSalt.

Celtic sea salt is made from seawater of the Celtic Sea, a region of the North Atlantic located roughly between the southern coast of Ireland and extending somewhat past the coast of Brittany in northwestern France. Celtic sea salt is not sold over the counter, but is available from several suppliers via the Internet. If you perform a search for "Celtic sea salt," you will locate a number of different suppliers. One source of Celtic sea salt is the Grain and Salt Society, which can be reached at 800-867-7258.

All of the salts discussed above tend to retain moisture and can be hard to pour from a shaker. If you decide to use one of them, adding a couple of grains of uncooked rice to the salt shaker can sometimes help (the rice absorbs moisture).

Other magnesium- and potassium-salt substitute products also are available. But stop thinking of them as salt substitutes; think of them instead as magnesium and/or potassium supplements that are easy to use and well absorbed—in addition to being safer and less expensive than supplements taken in pill form. Be aware, however, that if you have kidney disease, you must not use any salt supplements containing substantial amounts of either magnesium or potassium.

Other Salt Substitutes

There are other sodium-salt reducing products available for purchase that contain potassium without magnesium. Two of these lower the sodium chloride content by replacing half (LiteSalt) or all (NoSalt) with potassium chloride. While these obviously cannot help address your magnesium status, they can help you reduce your intake of sodium while increasing that of potassium.

Appendix E: Problems Associated with Low Magnesium Levels

This book has focused extensively on some of the most serious long-term health consequences of magnesium deficiency, namely cardiovascular disease and type II diabetes. Because magnesium is vital for the functioning of organs and systems throughout the body, deficiency can also have myriad other effects. A more complete list of some of the most prominent effects are outlined on the following page:

Body System	Effect of Magnesium Deficiency
Cardiovascular	Arrhythmias (irregular heartbeats) Cardiac arrest, sudden death Heart palpitations Hypertension (high blood pressure) Mitral valve prolapse Vasospastic angina (chest pain due to spasms, rather than blockage, of coronary arteries)
Digestive	Constipation Difficulty swallowing
Genitourinary	Kidney stones Urinary spasms
Gynecological/ reproductive	Menstrual cramps Pregnancy-induced hypertension (pre-eclampsia) progressing to convulsions (eclampsia) Premenstrual syndrome (PMS) Spontaneous abortion, miscarriage, low birth weight
Metabolic	Carbohydrate intolerance Insulin resistance Low serum calcium that cannot be corrected with calcium supplements Low serum potassium that cannot be corrected with potassium supplements Elevated serum phosphorus Vitamin D resistance
Musculoskeletal	Muscle cramps Muscle soreness, including backache, neck pain, tension headache, temporomandibular joint dysfunction Muscle tension Muscle tetany (painful spasms and tremors) Muscle twitches
Neurological	Convulsions of severe deficiency Migraine, other headaches Hearing loss, ringing in ear Hyperactivity, restlessness, constant movement Insomnia Numbness Tingling Tinnitus (persistent buzzing or ringing noise in the ears)
Mental	Agoraphobia Anxiety Depression Irritability Panic attacks

Other	Chest tightness, often expressed as "I can't seem to take a deep breath" or seen as sighing in children Chronic fatigue Cravings for carbohydrates Cravings for salt Sensitivity to bright lights in the absence of eye disease Sensitivity to loud noise

Appendix F: Guidelines for Magnesium Injections

Some people—fortunately very few—require very large amounts of magnesium that must be provided by injection, continuous infusions, or sustained slow tube feeding. These procedures require skilled medical care. Such needs are mostly found in people with a genetic inability to absorb or retain magnesium (see chapter 7). If you should require this type of treatment, the following are some things you should know about it.

Should your physician advise you to self-administer intramuscular injections, (s)he will have to provide a prescription for both injectable magnesium (usually in the form of magnesium sulfate) and the syringes to administer it. These are intramuscular (IM), not intravenous (IV), injections. You can inject the magnesium into the upper thigh or obtain assistance for injections deep into the muscle of the buttocks. The shot can cause pain *after* the injection for anywhere from ten minutes to a half hour (or more). Some people have reported that the injections hurt more when their magnesium status is low, and when the magnesium status of the body has been built up, the injections cause less pain, hurt for a shorter time, or do not hurt at all.

For people who need to take injections regularly over the long-term, lumps can form in the muscle. This can be minimized by using extra-long needles.

Appendix G: Soft Drinks Made with and without Phosphoric Acid

Too much phosphorus intake during a sub-optimal or deficient magnesium state can worsen the magnesium inadequacy (see appendix A). While phosphorus-containing food additives, mostly in baked goods and processed meats, can contribute substantial amounts of phosphorus to the diet, sodas with phosphoric acid can also be a substantial source.

The adult daily reference intake (DRI) for phosphorus is 700 milligrams per day.

All colas and Dr Pepper–type drinks—with or without caffeine, with or without sugar—have phosphoric acid in them. Here's how much:

Size of Drink	Phosphorus content
Standard aluminum can (12 ounces)	39–44 milligrams
Small fountain drink (16 ounces)	52–59 milligrams
Medium fountain drink (22 ounces)	71–81 milligrams
Large fountain drink (32 ounces)	104–118 milligrams
Extra-large fountain drink (44 ounces)	143–162 milligrams

Other types of soda have no phosphorus, including the following:

- All lemon-lime drinks (7UP, Fresca, Sprite, Squirt, and others)
- Ginger ale
- Root beer
- Orange sodas (Fanta and others)
- Mountain Dew
- Cream sodas
- Fruit-flavored sodas (black cherry, grape, and others)

Source: U.S. Department of Agriculture, Agricultural Research Service. 2001. USDA Nutrient Database for Standard Reference, Release 14. Nutrient Data Laboratory Home Page, *www.nal.usda.gov/fnic/foodcomp*

Appendix H: Common Medications That Affect Magnesium Status

There are several medications, both over-the-counter and physician prescribed that can affect magnesium status. Some increase magnesium intake, a few increase the retention of magnesium, while others cause magnesium loss. These need to be considered when assessing magnesium status and/or magnesium need.

Medications That Can Increase Magnesium

Milk of magnesia, taken as a laxative or antacid, can increase magnesium intake as follows:

- Used as a laxative, the recommended dose is 2 to 4 tablespoons. This provides 990 to 1,950 milligrams of magnesium.

- Used as an antacid, the recommended dose is 1 to 3 teaspoons. This provides 165 to 500 milligrams of magnesium.

Drugs used in the treatment of heart attack (myocardial infarction) and other conditions can cause magnesium retention, somewhat, and can result in sustained increase in a person's magnesium levels (see chapter 1). These include:

- aspirin
- beta-blockers
- ACE inhibitors

Medications That Deplete Magnesium

There are numerous medications used for a wide variety of purposes that decrease body magnesium levels by increasing its excretion in the urine.

DRUGS USED TO TREAT HEART DISEASE

Magnesium-depleting drugs in this category include:

- Some drugs used to treat irregular heartbeat, among them amiodarone (also sold under the brand name Cordarone), bretylium, quinidine (Cardioquin, Quinaglute, Quinidex, Quin-Release), and sotalol (Betapace).
- Some drugs used in the treatment of heart failure and/or irregular heartbeat, among them digoxin (Lanoxicaps, Lanoxin), Quinidex, and Cordarone.
- Diuretics, which may be used in the treatment of high blood pressure and/or congestive heart failure, among them ethacrynic acid (Edecrin), furosemide (Lasix), osmotic agents such as mannitol, and thiazides, a class of drugs that usually have both generic and brand names ending in *-zide*.

DRUGS USED TO TREAT ALLERGIES AND ASTHMA

- Some antiasthmatic drugs, among them epinephrine (Adrenalin, AsthmaNefrin, EpiPen, microNefrin, Nephron, Vaponefrin, and other brand names) and agents that mimic its effects, such as isoproterenol (Isuprel, Medihaler-Iso, and other brand names), as well as aminophylline (Phyllocontin; Truphylline)

DRUGS USED TO TREAT PSYCHIATRIC AND NEUROLOGICAL DISORDERS

- Some antipsychotic and antischizophrenic drugs, among them pimozide (Orap, also used to treat Tourette's syndrome), thioridazine (Mellaril, also used as a sedative and to treat Huntington's chorea), and trifluoperazine (Stelazine, also sometimes used to treat severe nausea and vomiting)

DRUGS USED TO TREAT INFECTION

- Aminoglycoside antibiotics, among them gentamicin (Garamycin, G-Mycin, Jenamicin) and tobramycin (Nebcin)
- Some penicillin-class antibiotics, among them carbenicillin (Geocillin, Geopen) and ticarcillin (Ticar)
- Broad-spectrum antibiotics of the tetracycline class
- The antifungal and antiparasitic drug amphotericin B.

OTHER MEDICATIONS

- Antineoplastic (cancer chemotherapy) drugs and radiation
- Immunosuppressant drugs, among them cisplatin (Platinol) and cyclosporine (Neoral, Sandimmune)
- Corticosteroid drugs, among them hydrocortisone (A-hydroCort, Hydrocortone)
- Pentamidine (Nebupent, Pentam), which is used to prevent and treat fungal pneumonia.

In addition, antacids can affect the absorption of other drugs. Many of these contain magnesium, however. Taking high doses of calcium and/or vitamin D, and consuming large quantities of caffeine can also lead to magnesium depletion.

Appendix I: Alternative Names for Sugar

Large amounts of highly refined sugar in the diet can cause increased excretion of magnesium in the urine. This is because sugar initiates the secretion of insulin, and insulin acts on the kidneys in a way that allows more magnesium to pass in the urine.

If you decide to limit or eliminate sugar from your diet, you need to watch the ingredient lists for sugar in all its forms. Following are some of the many terms that indicate the presence of sugar:

- All-natural sweetener (remember, sugar is a natural substance that has been highly refined)
- Au miel
- Barbados molasses
- Barbados sugar
- Barley malt
- Beet juice
- Beet sugar
- Blackstrap molasses (this is high in calcium)
- Brown rice sweetener
- Brown rice syrup

- Brown sugar
- Cane sugar
- Cane syrup
- Caramel
- Caramel color
- Clarified grape juice
- Concentrated fruit juices
- Confectioner's sugar
- Cooked honey
- Corn sugar
- Corn sweetener
- Corn syrup
- Dark brown sugar
- Date paste
- Date sugar
- Date syrup
- Dehydrated cane juice
- Dextrin
- Dextrose
- Disaccharides
- Dried fruits such as dates, raisins, figs, apricots
- Evaporated cane juice
- Fig syrup
- Filtered honey
- Fructooligo saccharides (FOS)
- Fructose
- Fruit juice concentrate (any kind)
- Fruit sugar
- Fruit sweetener
- Galactose
- Glucose
- Granulated sugar
- Heavy syrup
- High-fructose corn syrup
- Honey
- Hydrogenated glucose syrup
- -ides, any additive with this suffix: monosodium glycerides, saccharides, trisaccharides, disaccharides, etc.
- Invert sugar
- Invert sugar syrup
- Jaggery
- Lactose
- Levulose
- Light brown sugar
- Light sugar
- Light syrup
- Lite sugar
- Lite syrup
- Lo-sugar
- Low sugar
- Malt (any kind)
- Malt syrup
- Malted
- Malted grains (corn, barley, rice)
- Malto-anything
- Maltodextrin
- Maltodextrose
- Maltose
- Mannitol
- Maple sugar
- Maple syrup
- Miel
- Molasses (though molasses is high in magnesium)
- Mono- and disaccharides
- Monosaccharides

- Natural cane sweetener
- Natural fruit concentrates: raspberry, strawberry, blueberry, blackberry, grape
- Natural honey
- Natural sucrose
- Natural syrup
- Naturally malted organic corn and barley extract
- Naturally sweetened
- Nectar (any kind)
- 100% natural sweetener
- -ol, any additive with this suffix: mannitol, sorbitol, inversol, hexitol, etc.
- Organic brown rice syrup
- Organic malted cereal syrup: barley, corn, oat, rice
- Organic sugar
- -ose, any additive with this suffix: manose, polydextrose, polytose, ribose, zylose, etc.
- Pineapple juice
- Pineapple powder
- Polysaccharides
- Powdered sugar
- Pure honey
- Pure natural sweetener
- Pure sweetener
- Raisin juice concentrate
- Raisin juice
- Raisin paste
- Raisin syrup
- Raw honey
- Raw sugar
- Ribbon cane syrup
- Ribose
- Rice malt
- Rice syrup
- Sorbitol
- Sorghum molasses
- Sorghum syrup
- Stevia
- Succanat
- Sucralose
- Sucrose
- Sugar (any type)
- Sugar cubes
- Sugar packets
- Sweetener
- Turbinado sugar
- Unbleached water-filtered beet sugar
- Uncooked honey
- Unfiltered honey
- White grape juice
- White sugar

Adapted from "The 99 Names of Sugar," Food Addicts Anonymous, Inc. © 1993 and "Names of Sugar, Flour, and Wheat," Food Addicts Anonymous, Inc. © 2003. Used with permission.

Appendix J: The Essential Nutrients

Magnesium is only one of more than forty essential nutrients for humans. We all need an adequate amount of each nutrient daily as well as an overall balance of these essential nutrients for optimal health and to optimize the healing capabilities of the body. These forty-plus essential nutrients are listed below by the categories of essential nutrients: vitamins, minerals, essential fatty acids, and essential amino acids (found in protein foods).

The Vitamins	The Minerals
WATER-SOLUBLE VITAMINS	BULK MINERALS
B vitamins:	Calcium
• Vitamin B_1 (thiamin)	Magnesium
• Vitamin B_2 (riboflavin)	Phosophorus
• Vitamin B_3 (niacin)	Potassium
• Vitamin B_6 (pyridoxine)	Sodium
• Vitamin B_{12} (cobalamin)	Iodine
• Biotin	TRACE MINEARLS
• Folic acid	Arsenic
• Pantothenic acid	Boron
Vitamin C	Chromium
FAT-SOLUBLE VITAMINS	Cobalt
Vitamin A	Copper
Vitamin D	Iron
Vitamin E	Manganese
Vitamin K	Molybdenum
	Nickel
Essential Fatty Acids	Selenium
Arachidonic acid	Silicon
Linoleic acid	Vanadium
Linolenic acid	Zinc
	STILL IN QUESTION
Essential Amino Acids	Bromine
Histidine (for infants)	Fluorine
Isoleucine	Lead
Leucine	Tin
Lysine	
Methionine—Cystine	
Phenylalanine—Tyrosine	
Threonine	
Tryptophan	
Valine	

Resources

American Dietetics Association
216 West Jackson Boulevard
Chicago, IL 50505-0995
800-366-1655 or 312-899-0400
www.eatright.org

Compulsive Eaters Anonymous—HOW program
5500 East Atherton Street, Suite 227-B
Long Beach, CA 90815-4017
562–342–9344
www.cea.org

Food Addicts Anonymous
4623 Forest Hill Boulevard
Suite 109-4

West Palm Beach, FL 33415-9120
561–967–3871
www.foodaddictsanonymous.org

Overeaters Anonymous
World Services Office
P.O. Box 44020
Rio Rancho, New Mexico 87174-4020
505–891–2664
www.overeatersanonymous.org

Also consult your local telephone directory to find meetings in your area.

References

Chapter One

Magnesium: The Mineral That Combats Heart Disease and Keeps Blood Vessels Healthy

Introduction

American Heart Association. *2000 Heart and Stroke Statistical Update*. Dallas, TX: American Heart Association, 1999.

A Typical Story

Pierce, James B. *Heart Healthy Magnesium: Your Nutritional Key to Cardiovascular Wellness*. Garden City Park, NY: Avery Publishing Group, 1994.

Heart Disease—A Twentieth-Century Epidemic (Epidemiology)

Aleksandrowicz, J., *Natural Environment and Health Protection of Man's Natural Environment* (Cracow, Poland: Polish Scientific Publications, 1973), pp. 518–528.

Anderson, T.W., Leriche, W.H., Hewitt, D., Neri, L.C. "Magnesium, Water Hardness, and Heart Disease," in *Magnesium in Health and Disease,* ed. M. Cantin and M.S. Seelig (New York: Spectrum, 1980), pp. 565–571.

Azoicai, D., Ivan, A., Alexa, L., et al., "[Multidisciplinary Epidemiological Observations on the Role of Mineral Elements and Other Environmental Factors in Inducing Essential Arterial Hypertension]," *Revista Medico-Chirurgicala a Societatii de Medici si Naturalisti din Iasi* (Romanian) 100 (1996): 88–93.

Dawson, E.B., Frey, M.J., Moore, T.D., et al., "Relationship of Metal Metabolism to Vascular Disease Mortality Rates in Texas," *American Journal of Clinical Nutrition* 31 (1978):1188–1197.

Elwood, P.C., Sweetnam, P.M., Beasley, W.H., et al., "Magnesium and Calcium in the Myocardium: Cause of Death and Area Differences," *Lancet* 2 (1980): 720–722.

Ford, E.S., "Serum Magnesium and Ischaemic Heart Disease: Findings from a National Sample of U.S. Adults," *International Journal of Epidemiology* 28 (1999): 645–651.

Karppanen, H., "Ischaemic Heart Disease. An Epidemiological Perspective with Special Reference to Electrolytes," *Drugs* 28 (1984) (Supplement 1): 1:17–27.

Ma, J., Folsom, A.R., Melnick, S.L., et al., "Associations of Serum and Dietary Magnesium with Cardiovascular Disease, Hypertension, Diabetes, Insulin, and Carotid Arterial Wall Thickness: The ARIC Study. Atherosclerosis Risk in Communities Study," *Journal of Clinical Epidemiology* 48 (1995): 927–940.

Marier, J.R., "Quantitative Factors Regarding Magnesium Status in the Modern-Day World," *Magnesium* 1 (1982): 3–15.

Marier, J.R., "The Importance of Dietary Magnesium with Particular Reference to Humans," *Zeitschrift Vitalstoffe Zivilisationskrankh* 13 (1968): 144–149.

Masironi, R., "Geochemistry, Soils and Cardiovascular Diseases," *Experientia* 43 (1987): 68–74.

Meyers, D.H., and Williams, G. "Mortality from All Causes, and from Ischaemic Heart Disease, in the Australian Capital Cities," *Medical Journal of Australia* 2 (1977): 504–505.

Neri, L.C., Johansen, H.L., Hewitt, D., et al., "Magnesium and Certain Other Elements and Cardiovascular Disease," *The Science of the Total Environment* 42 (1985): 49–75.

Saphir, O., Ohringer, L., and Silverstone, H., "Coronary Arteriosclerotic Heart Disease in the Younger Age Group: Its Greater Frequency in This Group among an Increasingly Older Necropsy Population," *The American Journal of the Medical Sciences* 231 (1956): 494–501.

Seelig, M.S. *Magnesium Deficiency in the Pathogenesis of Disease, Early Roots of Cardiovascular, Skeletal, and Renal Abnormalities.* New York and London: Plenum Medical Book Co., 1980.

DIET AND MAGNESIUM DEFICIENCY

Dawson, E.B., Frey, M.J., Moore, T.D., et al., "Relationship of Metal Metabolism to Vascular Disease Mortality Rates in Texas," *American Journal of Clinical Nutrition* 31 (1978): 1188–1197.

Kruse, H.D., Orent, E.R., and McCollum, E.V., "Studies on Magnesium Deficiency in Animals," *The Journal of Biological Chemistry* 96 (1932): 519–539.

Marier, J.R., "Dietary Magnesium and Drinking Water: Effects on Human Health Status. Compendium on Magnesium and Its Role in Biology," *Nutrition and Physiology* 26 (1990): 85–104.

Pennington, J.A.T., Young, B.E., and Wilson, D.B., "Nutritional Elements in U.S. Diets: Results from the Total Diet Study, 1982–1986," *Journal of the American Dietetic Association* 89 (1989): 659–664.

Seelig, Mildred S., "Epidemiologic Data on Magnesium Deficiency–Associated Cardiovascular Disease and Osteoporosis; Consideration of Risks of Current Recommendations for High Calcium Intake," in *Advances in Magnesium Research: Nutrition and Health: Proceedings of the Ninth International Symposium on Magnesium (Vichy, France)*, ed. Yves Rayssiguier, André Mazur, and Jean Durlach, (London, England: John Libbey & Company, 2001), pp. 177–190.

Seelig, Mildred S., "The Requirement of Magnesium by the Normal Adult," *American Journal of Clinical Nutrition* 14 (1964): 342–390.

Sjollema, B., "Nutritional and Metabolic Disorders in Cattle," *Nutrition Abstracts and Reviews* 1 (1932): 621–632.

Syme, S.L., Hyman, M.M., and Enterline, P.E., "Some Social and Cultural Factors Associated with the Occurrence of Coronary Heart Disease," *Journal of Chronic Disorders* 17 (1964): 277–289.

CARDIOVASCULAR DISEASE (CVD) AND MAGNESIUM DEFICIENCY AND TREATMENT

Altura, B.M., and Altura B.T., "Cardiovascular Risk Factors and Magnesium: Relationships to Atherosclerosis, Ischemic Heart Disease and Hypertension," *Magnesium and Trace Elements* 10 (1991): 182–192.

Burch, G.E., and Giles, T.D., "The Importance of Magnesium Deficiency in Cardiovascular Disease," *American Heart Journal* 94 (1977): 649–657.

Chipperfield, B., and Chipperfield, J.R., "Magnesium and the Heart," *American Heart Journal* 93 (1977): 679–682.

Heggtveit, H.A., "The Cardiomyopathy of Magnesium Deficiency," in *Electrolytes and Cardiovascular Disease,* ed. E. Bajusz (Basel, Switzerland: S. Karger AG, 1965), pp. 204–220.

CARDIOVASCULAR DISEASE, MAGNESIUM, AND BLOOD CLOTTING IN VESSELS

Cazenave, J.P., Packham, M.A., Guccione, M.A., et al., "Inhibition of Platelet Adherence to Damaged Surface of Rabbit Aorta," *The Journal of Laboratory and Clinical Medicine* 86 (1975): 551–563.

Gawaz, M., Ott, I., Reininger, A.J., et al., "Effects of Magnesium on Platelet Aggregation and Adhesion. Magnesium Modulates Surface Expression of Glycoproteins on Platelets In Vitro And Ex Vivo." *Thrombosis and Haemostasis* 72 (1994): 912–918.

Gawaz, M., "[Antithrombocytic Effectiveness of Magnesium]," *Fortschritte der Medizin* 114 (1996): 329–332.

Herrmann, R.G., Lacefield, W.B., and Crowe, V.G., "Effect of Ionic Calcium and Magnesium on Human Platelet Aggregation," *Proceedings of the Society for Experimental Biology and Medicine* 135 (1970): 100–103.

Herzog, W.R., Atar, D., Gurbel, P.A., et al., "Effect of Magnesium Sulphate Infusion on Ex Vivo Platelet Aggregation in Swine," *Magnesium Research* 6 (1993): 349–353.

Ravn, H.B., Kristensen, S.D., Vissinger, H., et al., "Magnesium Inhibits Human Platelets," *Blood Coagulation and Fibrinolysis* 7 (1996): 241–244.

Serebruany, V.L., Herzog, W.R., Schlossberg, M.L., et al., "Bolus Magnesium Infusion in Humans Is Associated with Predominantly Unfavourable Changes in Platelet Aggregation and Certain Haemostatic Factors," *Pharmacological Research* 36 (1997): 17–22.

Shechter, M., Merz, C.N., Paul-Labrador, M., et al., "Oral Magnesium Supplementation Inhibits Platelet-Dependent Thrombosis in Patients with Coronary Artery Disease," *The American Journal of Cardiology* 84 (1999): 152–156.

Stevenson, M.M., and Yoder, I.I., "Studies of Platelet Aggregation, Plasma Adenosine Diphosphate Breakdown and Blood Coagulation in Magnesium Deficient Calves and Rats," *Thrombosis et Diathesis Haemorrhagica* 23 (1970): 299–305.

CARDIOVASCULAR DISEASE AND MAGNESIUM: BLOOD VESSEL CONSTRICTION

Altura, B.M., and Altura B.T., "New Perspectives on the Role of Magnesium in the Pathophysiology of the Cardiovascular System. I. Clinical Aspects," *Magnesium* 4 (1985): 226–244.

Altura, B.M., and Altura B.T., "New Perspectives on the Role of Magnesium in the Pathophysiology of the Cardiovascular System. I. Experimental Aspects," *Magnesium* 4 (1985): 245–271.

Yang, Z.W., Wang, J., Zheng, T., et al., "Low [Mg(2+)](o) Induces Contraction of Cerebral Arteries: Roles of Tyrosine and Mitogen-Activated Protein Kinases," *The American Journal of Physiology. Heart and Circulatory Physiology* 279 (2000): H185–H194.

Yang, Z.W., Gebrewold, A., Nowakowski, M., et al., "Mg(2+)–Induced Endothelium-Dependent Relaxation of Blood Vessels and Blood Pressure Lowering: Role of NO," *The American Journal of Physiology. Regulatory, Integrative, and Comparative Physiology* 278 (2000): R628–R639.

Yang, Z., Wang, J., Altura, B.T., et al., "Extracellular Magnesium Deficiency Induces Contraction of Arterial Muscle: Role of PI3–Kinases and MAPK Signaling Pathways," *Pflugers Archiv* 439 (2000): 240–247.

Zhang, A., Carella, A., Altura, B.T., et al., "Interactions of Magnesium and Chloride Ions on Tone and Contractility of Vascular Muscle," *European Journal of Pharmacology* 203 (1991): 223–235.

Zhang, A., Cheng, T.P., and Altura, B.M., "Magnesium Regulates Intracellular Free Ionized Calcium Concentration and Cell Geometry in Vascular Smooth Muscle Cells," *Biochimica et Biophysica Acta* 1134 (1992): 25–29.

CARDIOVASCULAR DISEASE AND MAGNESIUM: ARRHYTHMIAS

Bigg, R.P.C., and Chia, R., "Magnesium Deficiency—Role in Arrhythmias Complicating Acute Myocardial Infarction," *Medical Journal of Australia* ii (1981): 346–348.

Bogdan, M., Nartowicz, E., Ukleja-Adamowicz, M., et al., "[Congestive Heart Failure and Ventricular Arrhythmia in Relation to Magnesium, Potassium and Sodium in Serum and Erythrocytes]," *Kardiologia Polska* (Polish) 38 (1993): 417–420; discussion, 421.

Bolognesi, R., Tsialtas, D., Cortesi, G., et al., "[Anti–Arrhythmic Action of Magnesium Sulfate in "Torsade de Pointes" Ventricular Arrhythmia]," *Giornale Italiano di Cardiologia* (Italian) 14 (1984): 1077–1080.

Borrello, G., Montagnani, M., Francini, G., et al., "[Behavior of Blood and Urinary Magnesium in Digitalis-Induced Arrhythmia. Therapeutic Role of Magnesium Sulfate]," *Minerva Cardioangiologica* (Italian) 27 (1979): 187–195.

Bradding, P., and Withers, N., "Acute Magnesium Administration and Frequency of Ventricular Arrhythmia in Heart Failure," *Circulation* 90 (1994): 2566.

Chadda, K.D., Gupta, P.K., and Lichtenstein, E., "Magnesium in Cardiac Arrhythmia," *The New England Journal of Medicine* 287 (1972): 1102.

Colquhoun, I.W., Berg, G.A., el-Fiky, M., et al., "Arrhythmia Prophylaxis after Coronary Artery Surgery. A Randomised Controlled Trial of Intravenous Magnesium Chloride," *European Journal of Cardiothoracic Surgery* 7 (1993): 520–523.

Ferone, A., De Meo, F., De Meo, M., et al., "[Prevention and treatment of arrhythmia with magnesium sulfate in resuscitation]. *Minerva Anestesiologica* (Italian) 57 (1991): 924–925.

Foucher, A., Davy, J.M., Le Feuvre, C., et al., "[Clinical Electrophysiologic Properties of Magnesium and Correlations with Its Anti-Arrhythmia Efficacy in Acquired Torsade de Pointes]," *Annales de Cardiologil et d'Angeiologie (Paris)* (French) 38 (1989): 645–650.

Golden, J.S., and Brams, W.A., "Mechanism of Toxic Effects from Combined Use of Calcium and Digitalis," *Annals of Internal Medicine* 11 (1938): 1084–1088.

Gulker, H., Haverkamp, W., and Hindricks, G., "[Ion Regulation Disorders and Cardiac Arrhythmia. The Relevance of Sodium, Potassium, Calcium, and Magnesium]," *Arzneimittelforschung* (German) 39 (1989): 130–134.

Holzgartner, H., Maier, E., and Vierling, W., "[High-Dosage Oral Magnesium Therapy in Arrhythmias. Results of an Observational Study in 1.160 Patients with Arrhythmia]," *Fortschritte der Medizin* (German) 108 (1990): 539–542.

Horner, S., "Magnesium and Arrhythmias in Acute Myocardial Infarction," *Coronary Artery Disease* 7 (1996): 359–363.

Iseri, L.T., Ginkel, M.L., Allen, B.J., et al., "Magnesium-Potassium Interactions in Cardiac Arrhythmia. Examples of Ionic Medicine," *Magnesium and Trace Elements* 10 (1991): 193–204.

Kuhn, P., Oberthaler, G., and Oswald, J., "[Anti-Arrhythmia Effectiveness of Potassium-Magnesium-Aspartate Infusion]," *Wiener Medizinische Wochenschrift* (German) 141 (1991): 64–65.

Lewandowicz, J., "[Action of Potassium and Magnesium Salts in the Treatment of Arrhythmia]," *Polski Tygodnik Lekarski* (Polish) 25 (1970): 1700–1703.

Longobardi, G., Ferrara, N., Abete, P., et al., "[Protective Effects of Magnesium Sulfate against Reperfusion-Induced Arrhythmia in Isolated and Perfused Rat Hearts]," *Cardiologia* 32 (1987): 359–362.

Papaceit, J., Moral, V., Recio, J., et al., "[Severe Heart Arrhythmia Secondary to Magnesium Depletion. Torsade de Pointes]," *Revista Espanola de Anestesiologia y Reanimacion* 37 (1990): 28–31.

Parikka, H., Toivonen, L., Verkkala, K., et al., "Ventricular Arrhythmia Suppression by Magnesium Treatment after Coronary Artery Bypass Surgery," *International Journal of Angiology* 8 (1999): 165–170.

Speziale, G., Ruvolo, G., Fattouch, K., et al., "Arrhythmia Prophylaxis after Coronary Artery Bypass Grafting: Regimens of Magnesium Sulfate Administration," *Thoracic and Cardiovascular Surgery* 48 (2000): 22–26.

Woods, K.L., "Possible Pharmacological Actions of Magnesium in Acute Myocardial Infarction," *British Journal of Clinical Pharmacology* 32 (1991): 3–10.

Worthley, L.I., "Lithium Toxicity and Refractory Cardiac Arrhythmia Treated with

Intravenous Magnesium," *Anaesthesia and Intensive Care* 2 (1974): 357–360.

Xiang, S., and Zhao, H., "Interrelationship Between Magnesium and Potassium in Preventing Myocardial Ischemia-Reperfusion Arrhythmia," *Chinese Medical Journal* (English) 109 (1996): 282–285.

CARDIOVASCULAR DISEASE AND MAGNESIUM: CARDIAC ARREST, SUDDEN DEATH, MAGNESIUM IN HEART

Anderson, T.W., Le Riche, W.H., MacKay, J.S., "Sudden Death and Ischemic Heart Disease. Correlation with Hardness of Local Water Supply," *The New England Journal of Medicine* 280 (1969): 805–807.

Bernardi, D., Dini, F.L., Azzarelli, A., et al., "Sudden Cardiac Death Rate in an Area Characterized by High Incidence of Coronary Artery Disease and Low Hardness of Drinking Water," *Angiology* 46 (1995): 145–149.

Chipperfield, B., and Chipperfield, J.R., "Heart-Muscle Magnesium, Potassium, and Zinc Concentrations after Sudden Death from Heart-Disease," *Lancet* 2 (1973): 293–296.

Eisenberg, M.J., "Magnesium Deficiency and Sudden Death," *American Heart Journal* 124 (1992): 544–549.

CARDIOVASCULAR DISEASE AND MAGNESIUM: ISCHEMIC-CORONARY HEART DISEASE, MAGNESIUM IN HEART

Altura, B.M., "Ischemic Heart Disease and Magnesium," *Magnesium* 7 (1988): 57–67.

Anderson, T.W., Neri, L.C., Schreiber G, et al., "Ischemic Heart Disease, Water Hardness, and Myocardial Magnesium," *Canadian Medical Association Journal* 113 (1975): 199–203.

Chipperfield, B., and Chipperfield, J.R., "Differences in Metal Content of the Heart Muscle in Death from Ischemic Heart Disease," *American Heart Journal* 95 (1978): 732–737.

Heggtveit, H.A., Tanser, P., and Hunt, B., "Magnesium Content of Normal and Ischemic Human Hearts," *Proceedings of the Seventh International Congress of Clinical Pathology* (1969): 53.

Johnson, C.J., Peterson, D.R., and Smith, E.K., "Myocardial Tissue Concentrations of Magnesium and Potassium in Men Dying Suddenly from Ischemic Heart Disease," *American Journal of Clinical Nutrition* 32 (1979): 967–970.

Seelig, M.S., and Heggtveit, H.A., "Magnesium Interrelationships in Ischemic Heart Disease: A Review," *American Journal of Clinical Nutrition* 27 (1974): 59–79.

CARDIOVASCULAR DISEASE AND MAGNESIUM: HEART ATTACKS, MYOCARDIAL INFARCTION

Studies of Table 1.3

Rasmussen, H. S., Gronbaek, M., Cintin, C., Balslov, S., Norregard, P., McNair, P., "One-Year Death Rate in 270 Patients with Suspected Acute Myocardial Infarction Initially Treated with Intravenous Magnesium or Placebo," *Clinical Cardiology* 11 (1988): 377–381.

Shechter, M., Hod, H., "Magnesium Therapy in Aged Patients with Acute Myocardial Infarction," *Magnesium Bulletin* 13 (1991): 7–9.

Woods, K. L., Fletcher, S., Roffe, C., Haider, Y., "Intravenous Magnesium Sulphate in Suspected Acute Myocardial Infarction: Results of the Second Leicester Intravenous Magnesium Intervention Trial (LIMIT-2)," *Lancet* 339 (1992): 1553–1558.

MEGA-TRIALS

1515-4 Collaborative Group, "Fourth International Study of Infarct Survival: Protocol for a Large Simple Study of the Effects of Oral Mononitrate, of Oral Captopril, and of Intravenous Magnesium, *The American Journal of Cardiology* 68 (1991): 87D–100D. See Table 1.3.

Antman, E.M., "Magnesium in Coronaries. The MAGIC Study," in XXIVth Congress of the European Society of Cardiology: In-Depth Late-Breaking Clinical Trials I: GRACIA, PRAGUE-2, MAGIC, GIPS, RITA-3: www.medscape.com/viewarticle/441094, 2002. See Table 1.3.

Studies of Magnesium Treatment for Acute Myocardial Infarction (by Year of Report). Studies used in Table 1.3 are so marked.

Malkiel-Shapiro, B., Bershon, I., et al., "Parenteral Magnesium Sulphate Therapy in Coronary Heart Disease. A Preliminary Report on its Clinical and Laboratory Aspects," *Medical Procedure* 2 (1956): 455–462.

Parsons, R.S., Butler, T.C., and Sellars, E.P., "The Treatment of Coronary Artery Disease," *Medical Procedure* 5 (1959): 487–498.

Chadda, K.D., Lichstein, E., and Gupta, P.K., "Magnesium and Cardiac Arrhythmia in Patients with Acute Infarction—Preliminary Observations," in *Magnesium in Health and Disease,* ed. M. Cantin and M.S. Seelig, eds. (New York: Spectrum, 1980), pp 545–549.

Speich, M., Bosquet, B., Nicolas, G., et al., "[Incidence of Myocardial Infarction; Magnesium Plasma, Erythrocyte and Cardiac Levels]," *Revue Francaise d'Endocrinologie Clinique Nutrition et Metabolisme* (French) 20 (1979): 159–163.

Smith, L.F., Heagerty, A.M., Bing, R.F., et al., "Intravenous Infusion of Magnesium Sulphate after Acute Myocardial Infarction: Effects on Arrhythmias and Mortality," *International Journal of Cardiology* 12 (1986): 175–183.

Abraham, A.S., Rosenmann, D., Kramer, M., et al., "Magnesium in the Prevention of Lethal Arrhythmias in Acute Myocardial Infarction," *Archives of Internal Medicine* 147 (1987): 753–755.

Abraham, A.S., "Magnesium Therapy for Acute Myocardial Infarction," *Comprehensive Therapy* 14 (1988): 64–68.

Ceremuzynski, L., Jurgiel, R., Kulakowski, P., et al., "Threatening Arrhythmias in Acute Myocardial Infarction Are Prevented by Intravenous Magnesium Sulfate," *American Heart Journal* 118 (1989): 1333–1334.

Abraham, A.S., "Treatment of Patients with Acute Myocardial Infarction with Intravenous Magnesium," *Magnesium and Trace Elements* 9 (1990): 177–185.

Shechter, M., "Beneficial Effect of Magnesium in Acute Myocardial Infarction. A Review of the Literature," *Magnesium Bulletin* 12 (1990): 1–6.

Shechter, M., and Hod, H., "Magnesium Therapy in Aged Patients with Acute Myocardial Infarction," *Magnesium Bulletin* 13 (1991): 7–9. Table 1.3.

Horner, S.M., "Efficacy of Intravenous Magnesium in Acute Myocardial Infarction in Reducing Arrhythmias and Mortality. Meta-Analysis of Magnesium in Acute Myocardial Infarction," *Circulation* 86 (1992): 774–779.

Pohl, W., Mory, P., Nurnberg, M., et al., "[Serum Magnesium, Serum Potassium and Arrhythmia Profile in Patients with Acute Myocardial Infarct]," *Wiener Klinische Wochenschrift* (German) 105 (1993): 163–166.

Teo, K.K., and Yusuf, S., "Role of Magnesium in Reducing Mortality in Acute Myocardial Infarction. A Review of the Evidence," *Drugs* 46 (1993): 347–359.

Thogersen, A.M., Johnson, O., and Wester, P.O., "Effects of Magnesium Infusion on Thrombolytic and Non-Thrombolytic Treated Patients with Acute Myocardial Infarction," *International Journal of Cardiology* 39 (1993): 13–22.

Heesch, C.M., and Eichhorn, E.J., "Magnesium in Acute Myocardial Infarction," *Annals of Emergency Medicine* 24 (1994): 1154–1160.

Orlov, M.V., Brodsky, M.A., and Douban, S., "A Review of Magnesium, Acute Myocardial Infarction and Arrhythmia," *Journal of the American College of Nutrition* 13 (1994): 127–132.

Thogersen, A.M., Johnson, O., and Wester, P.O., "Effects of Intravenous Magnesium Sulfate in Suspected Acute Myocardial Infarction on Arrhythmia and Long-Term Outcome," *International Journal of Cardiology* 49 (1995): 143–151.

Horner, S., "Magnesium and Arrhythmias in Acute Myocardial Infarction," *Coronary Artery Disease* 7 (1996): 359–363.

Thiele, R., Protze, F., Winnefeld, K., et al., "Application of Magnesium (Intravenously and Per Os) in Patients with Acute Myocardial Infarction and the Effect on Tachycardiac Ventricular Arrhythmias," *Magnesium Bulletin* 19 (1997): 69–73.

Raghu, C., Peddeswara Rao, P., and Seshagiri Rao, D., "Protective Effect of Intravenous Magnesium in Acute Myocardial

Infarction Following Thrombolytic Therapy," *International Journal of Cardiology* 71 (1999): 209–215.

Thiele, R., Protze, F., Winnefeld, K., et al., "Effect of Intravenous Magnesium on Ventricular Tachyarrhythmias Associated with Acute Myocardial Infarction," *Magnesium Research* 13 (2000): 111–122.

Need for Timely Magnesium Treatment

Antman, E.M., "Magnesium in Acute MI. Timing Is Critical," *Circulation* 92 (1995): 2367–2372.

Antman, E.M., "Randomized Trials of Magnesium in Acute Myocardial Infarction: Big Numbers Do Not Tell the Whole Story," *American Journal of Cardiology* 75 (1995): 391–393.

Antman, E.M., Seelig, M.S., Fleischmann, K., et al., "Magnesium in Acute Myocardial Infarction: Scientific, Statistical, and Economic Rationale for Its Use," editorial, *Cardiovascular Drugs and Therapy* 10 (1996): 297–301.

Antman, E.M., Yang, P., and Smetana, R., "Magnesium in Acute Myocardial Infarction: Clinical Benefits of Intravenous Magnesium Therapy," *Magnesium Bulletin* 18 (1996): 74–76.

Baxter, G.F., Sumeray, M.S., and Walker, J.M., "Infarct Size and Magnesium: Insights into LIMIT–2 and ISIS–4 from Experimental Studies," *Lancet* 348 (1996): 1424–1426.

Casscells, W., "Magnesium and Myocardial Infarction," commentary, *Lancet* 343 (1994): 807–809.

Fernandes, J.S., "Early Intravenous Magnesium Administration in Acute Myocardial Infarction," *Magnesium Research* 7 (1994): 341–343.

Gyamlani, G., Parikh, C., and Kulkarni, A.G., "Clinical Benefits of Magnesium in Acute Myocardial Infarction: Timing Is Crucial," 139 *American Heart Journal* (2000): 703.

Herzog, W.R., and Serebruany, V.L., "How Magnesium Therapy May Influence Clinical Outcome in Acute Myocardial Infarction: Review of Potential Mechanisms," *Coronary Artery Disease* 7 (1996): 364–371.

Rasmussen, H.S., et al., "Substituting Magnesium in Acute Myocardial Infarction: A Life-Saver?" *Magnesium Bulletin* 8 (1986): 257.

Rasmussen, H.S., Gronbaek, M., Cintin, C., et al., "One-Year Death Rate in 270 Patients with Suspected Acute Myocardial Infarction Initially Treated with Intravenous Magnesium or Placebo," *Clinical Cardiology* 11 (1988): 377–381. Table 1.3.

Rasmussen, H.S., "Justification for Intravenous Magnesium Therapy in Acute Myocardial Infarction," *Magnesium Research* 1 (1988): 59–73.

Rasmussen, H.S., "Clinical Intervention Studies on Magnesium in Myocardial Infarction," *Magnesium* 8 (1989): 316–325.

Rasmussen, H.S., "Justification for Intravenous Magnesium Therapy in Acute Ischaemic Heart Disease," *Danish Medical Bulletin* 40 (1993): 84–99.

Shechter, M., Hod, H., Couraqui, P., et al., "Magnesium Therapy in Acute Myocardial Infarction When Patients Are Not Candidates for Thrombolytic Therapy," *The American Journal of Cardiology* 75 (1995): 321–323.

Shechter, M., Hod, H., Chouraqui, P., et al., "Acute Myocardial Infarction without Thrombolytic Therapy: Beneficial Effects of Magnesium Sulfate," *Herz* 22 (1997): (Supplement 1): 73–76.

Shechter, M., Hod, H., Marks, N., et al., "Beneficial Effect of Magnesium Sulfate in Acute Myocardial Infarction," *The American Journal of Cardiology* 66 (1990): 271–274.

Shechter, M., Hod, H., Kaplinsky, E., et al., "The Rationale of Magnesium as Alternative Therapy for Patients with Acute Myocardial Infarction without Thrombolytic Therapy," *American Heart Journal* 132 (1996): 483–486; discussion 496–502.

Shechter, M., Hod, H., Rabinowitz, B., et al., "Long-Term Outcome in Patients with Acute Myocardial Infarction Ineligible for Thrombolysis Treated with Intravenous Magnesium," American Heart Association Conference, 1999.

Shechter, M., Kaplinsky, E., and Rabinowitz, B., "The Rationale of Magnesium Supplementation in Acute Myocardial Infarction. A Review of the Literature,"

Archives of Internal Medicine 152 (1992): 2189–2196.

Shechter, M., Kaplinsky, E., and Rabinowitz, B., "Review of Clinical Evidence—Is There a Role for Supplemental Magnesium in Acute Myocardial Infarction in High-Risk Populations (Patients Ineligible for Thrombolysis and the Elderly)?" *Coronary Artery Disease* 7 (1996): 352–358.

Woods, K.L., "Possible Pharmacological Actions of Magnesium in Acute Myocardial Infarction," *British Journal of Clinical Pharmacology* 32 (1991): 3–10.

Woods, K.L., "Review of Research Methodology Used in Clinical Trials of Magnesium and Myocardial Infarction—Why Does Controversy Persist Despite ISIS–4?" *Coronary Artery Disease* 7 (1996): 348–351.

Woods, K.L., and Fletcher, S., "Long-Term Outcome after Intravenous Magnesium Sulphate in Suspected Acute Myocardial Infarction: The Second Leicester Intravenous Magnesium Intervention Trial (LIMIT–2)," *Lancet* 343 (1994): 816–819.

Woods, K.L., Fletcher, S., Roffe, C., et al., "Intravenous Magnesium Sulphate in Suspected Acute Myocardial Infarction: Results of the Second Leicester Intravenous Magnesium Intervention Trial (LIMIT–2). *Lancet* 339 (1992): 1553–1558. Table 1.3.

MEGA-TRIALS

ISIS–4 Collaborative Group, "Fourth International Study of Infarct Survival: Protocol for a Large Simple Study of the Effects of Oral Mononitrate, of Oral Captopril, and of Intravenous Magnesium," *The American Journal of Cardiology* 68 (1991): 87D–100D. Table 1.3.

The MAGIC Steering Committee, "Rationale and Design of the Magnesium in Coronaries (MAGIC) Study: A Clinical Trial to Reevaluate the Efficacy of Early Administration of Magnesium in Acute Myocardial Infarction," *American Heart Journal* 139 (2000): 10–14.

Antman, E.M., "Magnesium in Coronaries. The MAGIC Study," in XXIVth Congress of the European Society of Cardiology: In-Depth Late-Breaking Clinical Trials I: GRACIA, PRAGUE–2, MAGIC, GIPS, RITA–3, at www.medscape.com/viewarticle/441094, 2002. Table 1.3.

CARDIOVASCULAR DISEASE AND MAGNESIUM—EFFECTS OF DRUGS USED IN TREATMENT OF CARDIOVASCULAR DISEASE AND HEART ATTACKS

Aspirin

Elliott, H.C., and Murdaugh, H.V., "Effect of Aspirin in Cation Excretion," *Clinical Research* 13 (1965): 305.

Ramsay, A.G., and Elliott, H.C., "Effect of Acetylsalicylic Acid on Ionic Reabsorption in the Renal Tubule," *The American Journal of Physiology* 213 (1967): 323–327.

Shechter, M., Merz, C.N., Paul-Labrador, M., et al., "Beneficial Antithrombotic Effects of the Association of Pharmacological Oral Magnesium Therapy with Aspirin in Coronary Heart Disease Patients," *Magnesium Research* 13 (2000): 275–284.

Winter, J.E., and Richey, C.H., "Human Absorption of Magnesium with and without Aspirin and Other Adjuvants," *Journal of Pharmacology and Experimental Therapeutics* 42 (1931): 179–183.

Beta-Blockers

Green, M., Guideri, G., and Lehr, D., "Effectiveness of Antiarrhythmic Agents in Preventing Death in Ventricular Fibrillation Induced by Isoprenaline in Desoxycorticosterone-Pretreated Rats," *Cardiovascular Research* 17 (1983): 562–567.

Leary, W.P., "Renal Excretory Actions of Antihypertensive Agents. Effects of Rilmenidine," *American Journal of Medicine* 87 (1989): 63S–66S.

Landmark, K., and Urdal, P., "Serum Magnesium and Potassium in Acute Myocardial Infarction: Relationship to Existing Beta-Blockade and Infarct Size," *Angiology* 44 (1993): 347–352.

Pastori, C., Delva, P., Degan, M., et al., "Preliminary Communication on Intralymphocyte Ionized Magnesium in Hypertensive Patients under Treatment with Beta-Blockers," *Magnesium Research* 12 (1999): 49–55.

Maslow, A.D., Regan, M.M., Heindle, S., et al., "Postoperative Atrial Tachyarrhythmias in Patients Undergoing Coronary Artery Bypass Graft Surgery without Cardiopulmonary Bypass: A Role for Intraoperative Magnesium Supplementation," *Journal of Cardiothoracic and Vascular Anesthesia* 14 (2000): 524–530.

Lehr, D., "Studies on the Cardiotoxicity of Alpha- and Beta-Andrenergic amines," in *Cardiac Toxicology,* ed. T. Balazs (Boca Raton, FL: CRC Press, Inc., 1981) pp. 75–112.

Reyes, A.J., "Mechanisms and Extent of the Decrease in Magnesiuresis Induced by Antikaliuretic Diuretics in Man," in *Magnesium in Health and Disease,* ed. Y. Itokawa and J. Durlach (London, England: John Libbey & Company, 1989) pp. 415–422.

ACE Inhibitors

Barbagallo, M., Dominguez, L.J., and Resnick, L.M., "Protective Effects of Captopril against Ischemic Stress: Role of Cellular Mg," *Hypertension* 34 (1999): 958–963.

Haenni, A., Berglund, L., Reneland, R., et al., "The Alterations in Insulin Sensitivity during Angiotensin Converting Enzyme Inhibitor Treatment Are Related to Changes in the Calcium/Magnesium Balance," *American Journal of Hypertension* 10 (1997): 145–51.

Di Bianco, R., "Captopril in the Treatment of Congestive Heart Failure," *Herz* 12 (1987) (Supplement 1): 27–37.

Dietz, R., and Osterziel, K.J., "[Effects of Angiotensin-Converting Enzyme Inhibitors in Heart Failure]," *Zeitschrift für Kardiologie* 77 (1988) (Supplement 3): 89–93.

Freedman, A.M., Cassidy, M.M., and Weglicki, W.B., "Captopril Protects against Myocardial Injury Induced by Magnesium Deficiency," *Hypertension* 18 (1991): 142–147.

Leary, W.P., "Interactions between Magnesium and Drugs in the Treatment of Hypertension," *Magnesium Bulletin* 9 (1987): 62–73.

O'Keeffe, S., Grimes, H., Finn, J., et al., "Effect of Captopril Therapy on Lymphocyte Potassium and Magnesium Concentrations in Patients with Congestive Heart Failure," *Cardiology* 80 (1992): 100–105.

Oladapo, O.O., and Falase, A.O., "Serum and Urinary Magnesium during Treatment of Patients with Chronic Congestive Heart Failure," *African Journal of Medicine and Medical Sciences* 29 (2000): 301–303.

Reyes, A.J., "Mechanisms and Extent of the Decrease in Magnesiuresis Induced by Antikaliuretic Diuretics in Man," in *Magnesium in Health and Disease,* ed. Y. Itokawa and J. Durlach (London, England: J., eds., London: John Libbey & Company, 1989) pp. 415–422.

Riegger, A.J., "ACE Inhibitors in Congestive Heart Failure," *Cardiology* 76 (1989) (Supplement 2): 42–49.

Stevenson, R.N., Keywood, C., Amadi, A.A., et al., "Angiotensin Converting Enzyme Inhibitors and Magnesium Conservation in Patients with Congestive Cardiac Failure," *British Heart Journal* 66 (1991): 19–21.

Weglicki, W.B., Bloom, S., Cassidy, M.M., et al., "Antioxidants and the Cardiomyopathy of Mg-Deficiency," *American Journal of Cardiovascular Pathology* 4 (1992): 210–215.

CARDIOVASCULAR DISEASE AND MAGNESIUM: HEART FAILURE

Altura, B.M., and Altura, B.T., "Biochemistry and Pathophysiology of Congestive Heart Failure: Is There a Role for Magnesium?" *Magnesium* 5 (1986): 134–43.

Smetana, R., Pacher, R., Baumgartner, W., et al., "Moderate Magnesium-Sparing Effect of High Dosage ACE-Inhibitor Therapy in Chronic Heart Failure," *Magnesium Bulletin* 16 (1994): 98–100.

Sueta, C.A., Clarke, S.W., Dunlap, S.H., et al., "Effect of Acute Magnesium Administration on the Frequency of Ventricular Arrhythmia in Patients with Heart Failure," *Circulation* 89 (1994): 660–666.

Wu, F., Zou, L., Altura, B.T., et al., "Low Extracellular Magnesium Results in Cardiac Failure in Isolated Perfused Rat Hearts," *Magnesium and Trace Elements* 10 (1991): 364–73.

Wu, F., Altura, B.T., Gao, J., et al., "Ferrylmyoglobin Formation Induced by Acute Magnesium Deficiency in Perfused Rat

Heart Causes Cardiac Failure," *Biochimica et Biophysica Acta* 1225 (1994): 158–164.

CARDIOVASCULAR DISEASE AND MAGNESIUM: HIGH BLOOD PRESSURE

Altura, B.M., and Altura B.T., "Interactions of Mg and K on Blood Vessels—Aspects in View of Hypertension. Review of Present Status and New Findings," *Magnesium* 3 (1984): 175–194.

Altura, B.M., and Altura B.T., "Cardiovascular Risk Factors and Magnesium: Relationships to Atherosclerosis, Ischemic Heart Disease and Hypertension," *Schriftenreihe des Vereins für Wasser-, Boden- und Lufthygiene* 88 (1993): 451–473.

Durlach, J., Durlach, V., Rayssiguier, Y., et al., "Magnesium and Blood Pressure. II. Clinical Studies," *Magnesium Research* 5 (1992): 147–153.

CARDIOVASCULAR DISEASE AND MAGNESIUM: STROKE

Altura, B.T., and Altura, B.M., "Interactions of Mg and K on Cerebral Vessels—Aspects in View of Stroke. Review of Present Status and New Findings," *Magnesium* 3 (1984): 195–211.

Altura, B.T., Memon, Z.I., Zhang, A., et al., "Low Levels of Serum Ionized Magnesium Are Found in Patients Early after Stroke Which Result in Rapid Elevation in Cytosolic Free Calcium and Spasm in Cerebral Vascular Muscle Cells," *Neuroscience Letters* 230 (1997): 37–40.

CARDIOVASCULAR DISEASE AND MAGNESIUM: WATER HARDNESS

Abu-Zeid, H.A., "The Water Factor and Mortality from Ischemic Heart Disease: A Review and Possible Explanations for Inconsistent Findings with Additional Data from Manitoba," *Archives of Environmental Health* 34 (1979): 328–336.

Andelman, J.B., *Water Chemistry and Analysis of Trace Elements in Relation to Hardness and Cardiovascular Mortality* (Geneva, Switzerland: Joint WHO/IAEA Research Project, 1971).

Anderson, T.W., Neri, L.C., Schreiber, G., et al., "Ischemic Heart Disease, Water Hardness, and Myocardial Magnesium," *Canadian Medical Association Journal* 113 (1975): 199–203.

Anderson, T.W., "Water Hardness and Heart Disease," *Counterpoint* (1976): 21–22.

Anderson, T.W., Leriche, W.H., Hewitt, D., et al., "Magnesium, Water Hardness, and Heart Disease," in: *Magnesium in Health and Disease,* ed. M. Cantin and M.S. Seelig (New York: Spectrum, 1980): 565–571.

Bernardi, D., Dini, F.L., Azzarelli, A., et al., "Sudden Cardiac Death Rate in an Area Characterized by High Incidence of Coronary Artery Disease and Low Hardness of Drinking Water," *Angiology* 46 (1995): 145–149.

Chipperfield, B., Chipperfield, J.R., Behr, G., et al., "Magnesium and Potassium Content of Normal Heart Muscle in Areas of Hard and Soft Water," *Lancet* 1 (1976): 121–122.

Chipperfield, B., and Chipperfield, J.R., "Magnesium and the Heart," *American Heart Journal* 93(1977): 679–682.

Chipperfield, B., and Chipperfield, J.R., "Relation of Myocardial Metal Concentrations to Water Hardness and Death Rates from Ischaemic Heart Disease," *Lancet* 2 (1979): 709–712.

Chorazy, W., "[Coal Mine Waters Containing Magnesium as Natural Source of That Element.]," *Magnesium Bulletin* (German) 8 (1986): 114–116.

Comstock, G.W., "The Epidemiologic Perspective: Water Hardness and Cardiovascular Disease," *Journal of Environmental Pathology and Toxicology* 4 (1980): 9–25.

Comstock, G.W., Cauthen, G.M., and Helsing, K.J., "Water Hardness at Home and Deaths from Arteriosclerotic Heart Disease in Washington County, Maryland," *American Journal of Epidemiology* 112 (1980): 209–216.

Crawford, M.D., "Hardness of Drinking Water and Cardiovascular Disease," *The Proceedings of the Nutrition Society* 31 (1972): 347–353.

Crawford, T., and Crawford, M.D., "Prevalence and Pathological Changes of Ischaemic Heart Disease in a Hard-Water and in a Soft-Water Area," *Lancet* 1 (1967): 229–232.

Crawford, M.D., Gardner, M.J., and Morris, J.N., "Mortality and Hardness of Local Water Supplies," *Lancet* 1 (1968): 827–831.

Crawford, M.D., Gardner, M.J., and Morris, J.N., "Mortality and Hardness of Water," *Lancet* 1 (1968): 1092.

Crawford, M.D., Gardner, M.J., and Morris, J.N., "Cardiovascular Disease and the Mineral Content of Drinking Water," *British Medical Bulletin* 27 (1971): 21–24.

Crawford, M.D., Gardner, M.J., and Morris, J.N., "Changes in Water Hardness and Local Death Rates," *Lancet* 2 (1971): 327–329.

Crawford, M.D., Gardner, M.J., and Morris, J.N., "Water Hardness, Rainfall, and Cardiovascular Mortality," *Lancet* 1 (1972): 1396–1397.

Duran, J., "Hardness of Local Water Supplies and Mortality from Cardiovascular Disease," *Lancet* 1 (1961): 1171.

Durlach, J., Bara, M., and Guiet-Bara, A., "Magnesium Level in Drinking Water and Cardiovascular Risk Factor: A Hypothesis," *Magnesium* 4 (1985): 5–15.

Durlach, J., Bara, M., and Guiet-Bara, A, "Magnesium Level in Drinking Water; Its Importance in Cardiovascular Risk," in *Magnesium in Health and Disease,* ed. Y. Itokawa and J. Durlach (London, England: John Libbey & Company, 1989), pp. 173–182.

Dzik, A.J., "Cerebrovascular Disease Mortality Rates and Water Hardness in North Dakota," *South Dakota Journal of Medicine* 42 (1989): 5–7.

Feder, G.L., and Hopps, H.C., "Variations in Drinking Water Quality and the Possible Effects on Human Health," *Trace Substances and Environmental Health* 15 (1981): 96–103.

Fodor, J.G., Pfeiffer, C.J., and Papezik, V.S., "Relationship of Drinking Water Quality (Hardness-Softness) to Cardiovascular Mortality in Newfoundland," *Canadian Medical Association Journal* 108 (1973): 1369–1373.

Folsom, A.R., and Prineas, R.J., "Drinking Water Composition and Blood Pressure: A Review of the Epidemiology," *American Journal of Epidemiology* 115 (1982): 818–832.

Gimeno, O.A., Jimenez, R.R., Blanco, A.M., et al., "[Relationship of Several Physico-Chemical Components in Drinking Water, Hypertension and Cardiovascular Disease Mortality]," *Revista de Sanidad y Higiene Publica (Madrid)* (Spanish) 64 (7–) (July–August 1990): 377–385.

Glattre, E., Askevold, R., and Bay, I.G., "Norwegian Water Story," *Lancet* 2 (1977): 1038.

Gyllerup, S., Lanke, J., Lindholm, L.H., et al., "Water Hardness Does Not Contribute Substantially to the High Coronary Mortality in Cold Regions of Sweden," *Journal of Internal Medicine* 230 (1991): 487–492.

Hewitt, D., and Neri, L.C., "Development of the 'Water Story': Some Recent Canadian Studies," *Journal of Environmental Pathology and Toxicology* 4 (1980): 51–63.

Heyden, S., "The Hard Facts Behind the Hard-Water Theory and Ischemic Heart Disease," *Journal of Chronic Disorders* 29 (1976): 149–157.

Hopps, H.C., "A Report of Some Studies Relating Geochemical Environment to Health and Disease," *The Science of the Total Environment* 4 (1975): 316–319.

Hopps, H.C., and Feder, G.L., "Chemical Qualities of Water That Contribute to Human Health in a Positive Way," *The Science of the Total Environment* 54 (1986): 207–216.

Jeppesen, B.B., "Greenland, a Soft-Water Area with a Low Incidence of Ischemic Heart Death," *Magnesium* 6 (1987): 307–313.

Kobayashi, J., "On Geographical Relationship Between the Chemical Nature of River Water and Death Rate from Apoplexy," *Berichte des Ohara Instituts für Landwirtshaftliche Biologie* 11 (1957): 12–21.

Leary, W.P., "Content of Magnesium in Drinking Water and Deaths from Ischaemic Heart Disease in White South Africans," *Magnesium* 5 (1986): 150–153.

Loseva, M.I., and Krasnikova, L.B., "[The Prevalence of Arterial Hypertension and Stenocardia of Effort among the Rural Population Living in Geochemically Contrasted Regions of the Novosibirsk Province]," *Kardiologiia* (Russian) 28 (1988): 31–34.

Luoma, H., Aromaa, A., Helminen, S., et al., "Risk of Myocardial Infarction in Finnish Men in Relation to Fluoride, Magnesium and Calcium Concentration in

Drinking Water," *Acta Medica Scandinavica* 213 (1983): 171–176.

Luoma, H., "Risk of Myocardial Infarction in Relation to Magnesium and Calcium Concentrations in Drinking Water, with Some Aspects on the Magnesium vs. Fluoride Interactions," in *Magnesium in Health and Disease,* ed. Y. Itokawa and J. Durlach (London, England: John Libbey & Company, 1989), pp. 183–190.

Mackinnon, A.U., and Taylor, S.H., "Relationship Between 'Sudden' Coronary Deaths and Drinking Water Hardness in Five Yorkshire Cities and Towns," International Journal of Epidemiology 9 (1980): 247–249.

Maheswaran, R., Morris, S., Falconer, S., et al., "Magnesium in Drinking Water Supplies and Mortality from Acute Myocardial Infarction in North West England," *Heart* 82 (1999): 455–460.

Maksimovic, Z.J., Jovanovic, T., Rsumovic, M., et al., *Magnesium and Calcium in Drinking Water and Cardiovascular Mortality in Serbia* (Belgrade, Yugoslavia: Serbian Academy of Sciences and Art, 1998) pp. 2–3.

Marier, J.R., "Cardioprotective Contribution of Hard Waters to Magnesium Intake," *Revue Canadienne de Biologie* 37 (1978): 115–125.

Marier, J.R., Neri, L.C., and Anderson, T.W., "Water Hardness, Human Health, and the Importance of Magnesium," National Research Council of Canada Report NRCC 17581 (1979): 1–119.

Marier, J.R., "Comments on Magnesium Intake and Fluoride Intake in the Modern-Day World," *Proceedings of the Finnish Dental Society* 76 (1980): 82–92.

Marier, J.R., "Water Hardness and Heart Disease," *Journal of the American Medical Association* 245 (1981): 1315–1316.

Marier, J.R., "Nutritional and Myocardial Aspects of Magnesium in Drinking Water," *Magnesium Bulletin* 1a (1981): 48–54.

Marier, J.R., and Neri, L.C., "Quantifying the Role of Magnesium in the Interrelationship between Human Mortality/Morbidity and Water Hardness," *Magnesium* 4 (1985): 53–59.

Marier, J.R., "Role of Magnesium in the "Hard-Water Story," *Magnesium Bulletin* 8 (1986): 194–198.

Marier, J.R., "Dietary Magnesium and Drinking Water: Effects on Human Health Status. Compendium on Mg and Its Role in Biology," *Nutrition and Physiology* 26 (1990): 85–104.

Marx, A., and Neutra, R.R., "Magnesium in Drinking Water and Ischemic Heart Disease," *Epidemiologic Reviews* 19 (1997): 258–272.

Masironi, R., "Cardiovascular Mortality in Relation to Radioactivity and Hardness of Local Water Supplies in the USA," *Bulletin of the World Health Organization* 43 (1970): 687–697.

Masironi, R., Pisa, Z., and Clayton, D., "Myocardial Infarction and Water Hardness in the WHO Myocardial Infarction Registry Network," *Bulletin of the World Health Organization* 57 (1979): 291–299.

Masironi, R., "Geochemistry and Cardiovascular Diseases," *Philosophical Transactions of the Royal Society of London. Series B: Biological Sciences* 288 (1979): 193–203.

Masironi, R., Pisa, Z., and Clayton, D., "Myocardial Infarction and Water Hardness in European Towns," *Journal of Environmental Pathology and Toxicology* 4 (1980): 77–87.

Masironi, R., and Shaper, A.G., "Epidemiological Studies of Health Effects of Water from Different Sources," *Annual Review of Nutrition* 1 (1981): 375–400.

Menaker, W., "Cardiovascular Disease and Hardness of Water," correspondence, *Journal of the American Medical Association* 174 (1960): 1346–1347.

Menotti, A., and Signoretti, P., "[Characteristics of Drinking Water and Coronary Heart Disease. An Epidemiological Experience]," *Giornale Italiano di Cardiologia* (Italian) 9 (1979): 674–677.

Morris, J.N., Crawford, M.D., and Heady, J.A., "Hardness of Local Water Supplies and Mortality from Cardiovascular Disease in the County Boroughs of England and Wales," *Lancet* 1 (1961): 860–862.

Morris, J.N., Crawford, M.D., and Heady, J.A., "Hardness of Local Water Supplies and Mortality from Cardiovascular Disease," *Lancet* 2 (1962): 506–507.

Morton, W.E., "Hypertension and Drinking Water. A Pilot Statewide Ecological Study in Colorado," *Journal of Chronic Disorders* 23 (1971): 537–545.

Neri, L.C., Hewitt, D., and Mandel, J.S., "Risk of Sudden Death in Soft Water Areas," *American Journal of Epidemiology* 94 (1971): 101–104.

Neutra, RR., "Epidemiology vs. Physiology? Drinking Water Magnesium and Cardiac Mortality," *Epidemiology* 10 (1999): 4–6.

Peterson, D.R., Thompson, D.J., and Nam, J.M., "Water Hardness, Arteriosclerotic Heart Disease and Sudden Death," *American Journal of Epidemiology* 92 (1970): 90–93.

Punsar, S., Erametsa, O., Karvonen, M.J., et al., "Coronary Heart Disease and Drinking Water. A Search in Two Finnish Male Cohorts for Epidemiologic Evidence of a Water Factor," *Journal of Chronic Disorders* 28 (1975): 259–287.

Punsar, S., and Karvonen, M.J., "Drinking Water Quality and Sudden Death: Observations from West and East Finland," *Cardiology* 64 (1979): 24–34.

Rubenowitz, E., Axelsson, G., and Rylander, R., "Magnesium in Drinking Water and Death from Acute Myocardial Infarction," *American Journal of Epidemiology* 143 (1996): 456–462.

Rubenowitz, E., Axelsson, G., and Rylander, R., "Magnesium in Drinking Water and Body Magnesium Status Measured Using an Oral Loading Test," *Scandinavian Journal of Clinical and Laboratory Investigation* 58 (1998): 423–428.

Rubenowitz, E., Axelsson, G., and Rylander, R., "Magnesium and Calcium in Drinking Water and Death from Acute Myocardial Infarction in Women," *Epidemiology* 10 (1999): 31–36.

Rylander, R., Bonevik, H., and Rubenowitz, E., "Magnesium and Calcium in Drinking Water and Cardiovascular Mortality," *Scandinavian Journal of Work, Environment, and Health* 17 (1991): 91–94.

Schroeder, H.A., "Relation between Mortality from Cardiovascular Disease and Treated Water Supplies," *Journal of the American Medical Association* 172 (1960): 1902–1908.

Schroeder, H.A., "Relations between Hardness of Water and Death Rates from Certain Chronic and Degenerative Diseases in the United States," *Journal of Chronic Disorders* 12 (1960): 586–591.

Schroeder, H.A., "Municipal Drinking Water and Cardiovascular Death Rates," *Journal of the American Medical Association* 195 (1966): 81–85.

Schroeder, H.A., "The Water Factor," *The New England Journal of Medicine* 280 (1969): 836–838.

Schroeder, H.A., and Kraemer, L.A., "Cardiovascular Mortality, Municipal Water, and Corrosion," *Archives of Environmental Health* 28 (1974): 303–311.

Seelig, M.S., "Epidemiology of Water Magnesium; Evidence of Contributions to Health," in *Advances in Magnesium Research: Nutrition and Health: Proceedings of the Ninth International Symposium on Magnesium (Vichy, France)*, ed. Yves Rayssiguier, André Mazur, and Jean Durlach, (London, England: John Libbey & Company, 2001), pp. 211–218.

Shaper, A.G., "Soft Water, Heart Attacks, and Stroke," *Journal of the American Medical Association* 230 (1974): 130–131.

Sharrett, A.R., "The Role of Chemical Constituents of Drinking Water in Cardiovascular Diseases," *American Journal of Epidemiology* 110 (1979): 401–419.

Sharrett, A.R., "Water Hardness and Cardiovascular Disease," *Circulation* 63 (1981): 247A–250A.

Singh, A., Uppal, A.K., and Singh, K., "Serum Magnesium and Consumed Water Magnesium Levels in Cases of Acute Myocardial Infarction and in Controls," *Indian Journal of Medical Sciences* 37 (1983): 81–84.

Sonneborn, M., and Mandelkow, J., "German Studies on Health Effects of Inorganic Drinking Water Constituents," *The Science of the Total Environment* 18 (1981): 47–60.

Stitt, F.W., Clayton, D.G., Crawford, M.D., et al., "Clinical and Biochemical Indicators of Cardiovascular Disease among Men Living in Hard and Soft Water Areas," *Lancet* 1 (1973): 122–126.

Teitge, J.E., "[Incidence in Myocardial Infarct and Mineral Content of the Drinking Water]," *Zeitschrift für die Gesamte Innere Medizin und Ihre Grenzgebiete* 45 (1990): 478–485.

"Water Quality, Trace Elements, and Cardiovascular Disease," *WHO Chronicles* 27 (1973): 534–538.

Yang, C.Y., and Chiu, H.F., "Calcium and

Magnesium in Drinking Water and the Risk of Death from Hypertension," *American Journal of Hypertension* 12 (1999): 894–899.

MAGNESIUM IN THE HEART AND BLOOD VESSELS

Abraham, A.S., Bar-On, E., and Eylath, U., "Changes in the Magnesium Content of Tissues Following Myocardial Damage in Rats," *Medical Biology* 59 (1981): 99–102.

Anderson, T.W., Neri, L.C., Schreiber, G., et al., "Ischemic Heart Disease, Water Hardness, and Myocardial Magnesium," *Canadian Medical Association Journal* 113 (1975): 199–203.

Barbour, R.L., Altura, B.M., Reiner, S.D., et al., "Influence of Mg2+ on Cardiac Performance, Intracellular Free Mg2+ and pH in Perfused Hearts as Assessed with 31P Nuclear Magnetic Resonance Spectroscopy," *Magnesium and Trace Elements* 10 (1991): 99–116.

Behr, G., and Burton, P., "Heart-Muscle Magnesium, *Lancet* 2 (1973): 450.

Hearse, D.J., Stewart, D.A., and Braimbridge, M.V., "Myocardial Protection during Oschemic Cardiac Arrest. The Importance of Magnesium in Cardioplegic Infusates," *Journal of Thoracic and Cardiovascular Surgery* 75 (1978): 877–885.

Krasner, B.S., Girdwood, R., and Smith, H., "The Effect of Slow Releasing Oral Magnesium Chloride on the QTc Interval of the Electrocardiogram during Open Heart Surgery," *Canadian Anaesthetists' Society Journal* 28 (1981): 329–333.

Wu, F., Altura, B.T., Gao, J., et al., "Ferrylmyoglobin Formation Induced by Acute Magnesium Deficiency in Perfused Rat Heart Causes Cardiac Failure," *Biochimica et Biophysica Acta* 1225 (1994): 158–164.

MAGNESIUM IN ENZYMES

Altura, B.T., and Altura, B.M., "Interactions of Mg and K on Cerebral Vessels—Aspects in View of Stroke. Review of Present Status and New Findings," *Magnesium* 3 (1984): 195–211.

Altura, B.M., "Basic Biochemistry and Physiology of Magnesium: A Brief Review," *Magnesium and Trace Elements* 10 (1991): 167–171.

Altura, B.M., "Introduction: Importance of Mg in Physiology and Medicine and the Need for Ion Selective Electrodes," *Scandinavian Journal of Clinical and Laboratory Investigation* 217 (1994) (Supplement): 5–9.

Altura, B.M., and Altura, B.T., "Role of Magnesium and Calcium in Alcohol-Induced Hypertension and Strokes as Probed by In Vivo Television Microscopy, Digital Image Microscopy, Optical Spectroscopy, 31P–NMR, Spectroscopy and a Unique Magnesium Ion-Selective Electrode," *Alcoholism, Clinical and Experimental Research* 18 (1994): 1057–1068.

Altura, B.M., and Altura B.T., "Role of Magnesium in Patho-Physiological Processes and the Clinical Utility of Magnesium Ion Selective Electrodes," *Scandinavian Journal of Clinical and Laboratory Investigation* 224 (1996) (Supplement): 211–234.

Herzog, W.R., and Serebruany, V.L., "How Magnesium Therapy May Influence Clinical Outcome in Acute Myocardial Infarction: Review of Potential Mechanisms," *Coronary Artery Disease* 7 (1996): 364–371.

Rude, R.K., and Singer, F.R., "Magnesium Deficiency and Excess," *Annual Review of Medicine* 32 (1981): 245–259.

Shechter, M., Kaplinsky, E., and Rabinowitz, B., "The Rationale of Magnesium Supplementation in Acute Myocardial Infarction. A Review of the Literature," *Archives of Internal Medicine* 152 (1992): 2189–2196.

Turnland, J.R., "Copper," in *Modern Nutrition in Health and Disease,* ed. Maurice E. Shils, James A. Olson, Moshe Shike, and Catherine A. Ross (Philadelphia: Lippincott Williams & Wilkins, 1999): p. 235.

MAGNESIUM IN CELLS

Altura, B.M., "Sudden-Death Ischemic Heart Disease and Dietary Magnesium Intake: Is the Target Site Coronary Vascular Smooth Muscle?" *Medical Hypotheses* 5 (1979): 843–848.

Lehr, D., "Magnesium and Cardiac Necrosis," *Magnesium Bulletin* 1a (1981): 178–191.

Shechter, M., Paul-Labrador, M.J., Rude, R.K., et al., "Intracellular Magnesium Predicts Functional Capacity in Patients with Coronary Artery Disease," *Cardiology* 90 (1998): 168–172.

MAGNESIUM AND CALCIUM: A DELICATE BALANCE

Altura, B.M., Altura, B.T., Carella, A., et al., "Hypomagnesemia and Vasoconstriction: Possible Relationship to Etiology of Sudden Death Ischemic Heart Disease and Hypertensive Vascular Diseases," *Artery* 9 (1981): 212–231.

Bloom, S., and Peric-Golia, L., "Geographic Variation in the Incidence of Myocardial Calcification Associated with Acute Myocardial Infarction," *Human Pathology* 20 (1989): 726–731.

Herrmann, R.G., Lacefield, W.B., and Crowe, V.G., "Effect of Ionic Calcium and Magnesium on Human Platelet Aggregation," *Proceedings of the Society for Experimental Biology and Medicine* 135 (1970): 100–103.

Herzog, W.R., and Serebruany, V.L., "How Magnesium Therapy May Influence Clinical Outcome in Acute Myocardial Infarction: Review of Potential Mechanisms," *Coronary Artery Disease* 7 (1996): 364–371.

Horner, S., "Magnesium and Arrhythmias in Acute Myocardial Infarction," *Coronary Artery Disease* 7 (1996): 359–363.

Karppanen, H., Pennanen, R., and Passinen, L., "Minerals, Coronary Heart Disease and Sudden Coronary Death," *Advances in Cardiology* 25 (1978): 9–24.

WHY ARE THE HEALTH BENEFITS OF MAGNESIUM NOT COMMONLY KNOWN?

Avery, O.T., MacLeod, C.M., and McCarty, M., "Studies on the Chemical Nature of the Substance Inducing Transformation of Pneumococcal Types. Induction of Transformation by a Desoxyribonucleic Acid Fraction Isolated from Pneumococcus Type III. 1944," *Molecular Medicine* 1 (1995): 344–365.

Hammer, D.I., and Heyden, S., "Water Hardness and Cardiovascular Mortality. An Idea That Has Served Its Purpose," *Journal of the American Medical Association* 243 (1980): 2399–2400.

Hershey, A.D., and Chase, M., "Independent Functions of Viral Protein and Nucleic Acid in Growth of Bacteriophage," *The Journal of General Physiology* 36 (1952): 39–56.

Johnson, S., "The Multifaceted and Widespread Pathology of Magnesium Deficiency," *Medical Hypotheses* 56 (2001): 163–170.

ARRHYTHMIA, SUDDEN CARDIAC DEATH, AND MAGNESIUM

Boyd, L.J., and Scherf, D., "Magnesium Sulfate in Paroxysmal Tachycardia," *The American Journal of the Medical Sciencess* 206 (1943): 43–48.

Dorup, I., Skajaa, K., and Thybo, N.K., "Oral Magnesium Supplementation Restores the Concentrations of Magnesium, Potassium and Sodium-Potassium Pumps in Skeletal Muscle of Patients Receiving Diuretic Treatment," *Journal of Internal Medicine* 233 (1993): 117–123.

Douban, S., Brodsky, M.A., Whang, D.D., et al., "Significance of Magnesium in Congestive Heart Failure," *American Heart Journal* 132 (1996): 664–671.

Dyckner, T., and Wester, P.O., "Ventricular Extrasystoles and Intracellular Electrolytes before and after Potassium and Magnesium Infusions in Patients on Diuretic Treatment," *American Heart Journal* 97 (1979): 12–18.

Dyckner, T., and Wester, P.O., "Extra– and Intracellular Potassium and Magnesium, Diuretics and Arrhythmias," in *Potassium: Its Biologic Significance,* ed. R. Whang (Boca Raton, FL: CRC Press, 1983), pp. 137–154.

Dyckner, T., and Wester, P.O., "Potassium/Magnesium Depletion in Patients with Cardiovascular Disease," *The American Journal of Medicine* 82 (1987): 11–17.

Fazekas, T., Scherlag, B.J., Vos, M., et al., "Magnesium and the Heart: Antiarrhythmic Therapy with Magnesium," *Clinical Cardiology* 16 (1993): 768–774.

Gottlieb, S.S., Fisher, M.L., Pressel, M.D., et al., "Effects of Intravenous Magnesium Sulfate on Arrhythmias in Patients with Congestive Heart Failure," *American Heart Journal* 125 (1993): 1645–1650.

Hollifield, J.W., "Thiazide Treatment of Systemic Hypertension: Effects on Serum Magnesium and Ventricular Ectopic Activity," *The American Journal of Cardiology* 63 (1989): 22G–25G.

Iseri, L.T., Allen, B.J., and Brodsky, M.A., "Magnesium Therapy of Cardiac Arrhythmias in Critical-Care Medicine," *Magnesium* 8 (1989): 299–306.

Iseri, L.T., Freed, J., and Bures, A.R., "Magnesium Deficiency and Cardiac Disorders," *The American Journal of Medicine* 58 (1975): 837–846.

Iseri, L.T., and French, J.H., "Magnesium: Nature's Physiologic Calcium Blocker" (editorial), *American Heart Journal* 108 (1984): 188–193.

Iseri, L.T., Ginkel, M.L., Allen, B.J., et al., "Magnesium-Potassium Interactions in Cardiac Arrhythmia. Examples of Ionic Medicine," *Magnesium and Trace Elements* 10 (1991): 193–204.

Keren, A., and Tzivoni, D., "Magnesium Therapy in Ventricular Arrhythmias," *Pacing and Clinical Electrophysiology* 13 (1990): 937–945.

Kurita, T. "Antiarrhythmic Effect of Parenteral Magnesium on Ventricular Tachycardia Associated with Long QT Syndrome," *Magnesium Research* 7 (1994): 155–157.

Lewis, R., Durnin, C., McLay, J., et al., "Magnesium Deficiency May Be an Important Determinant of Ventricular Ectopy in Digitalised Patients with Chronic Atrial Fibrillation," *British Journal of Clinical Pharmacology* 31 (1991): 200–203.

Lim P., Jacob E. Magnesium deficiency in patients on long-term diuretic therapy for heart failure. *British Medical Journal* 1972; 3:620–2.

Nayler W.G. The heart cell: some metabolic aspects of cardiac arrhythmias. *Acta Medica Scandinavica* 647 (1981) (Supplement): 17–31.

Raehl, C.L., Patel, A.K., and LeRoy, M., "Drug-Induced Torsade de Pointes," *Clinical Pharmacy* 4 (1985): 675–690.

Reyes, A.J., and Leary, W.P., "Cardiovascular Toxicity of Diuretics Related to Magnesium Depletion," *Human Toxicology* 3 (1984): 351–371.

Roden, D.M., "Magnesium Treatment of Ventricular Arrhythmias," *The American Journal of Cardiology* 63 (1989): 43G–46G.

Ryan, M.P., "Magnesium and Potassium-Sparing Diuretics," *Magnesium* 5 (1986): 282–292.

Tzivoni, D., Keren, A., Cohen, A.M., et al., "Magnesium Therapy for Torsade de Pointes," *The American Journal of Cardiology* 53 (1984): 528–530.

Whang, R., Hampton, E.M., and Whang, D.D., "Magnesium Homeostasis and Clinical Disorders of Magnesium Deficiency," *The Annals of Pharmacotherapy* 28 (1994): 220–226.

Chapter Two

METABOLIC SYNDROME X, DIABETES, AND MAGNESIUM

INTRODUCTION AND METABOLIC SYNDROME X

Resnick, L.M., "Cellular Ions in Hypertension, Insulin Resistance, Obesity, and Diabetes: A Unifying Theme," *Journal of the American Society of Nephrology* 3 (1992): S78–S85.

A LOOK AT THE RESEARCH THAT DISCOVERED METABOLIC SYNDROME X

Diabetes Line of Research

Baillie, G.M., Sherer, J.T., and Weart, C.W., "Insulin and Coronary Artery Disease: Is Syndrome X the Unifying Hypothesis?" *The Annals of Pharmacotherapy* 32 (1998): 233–247.

Chisholm, D.J., Campbell, L.V., and Kraegen, E.W., "Pathogenesis of the Insulin Resistance Syndrome (Syndrome X)," *Clinical and Experimental Pharmacology and Physiology* 24 (1997): 782–784.

DeFronzo, R.A., and Ferrannini, E., "Insulin Resistance. A Multifaceted Syndrome Responsible for NIDDM, Obesity, Hypertension, Dyslipidemia, and Atherosclerotic Cardiovascular Disease," *Diabetes Care* 14 (1991): 173–194.

DeFronzo, R.A., "Insulin Resistance: A Multifaceted Syndrome Responsible for NIDDM, Obesity, Hypertension, Dyslipidaemia and Atherosclerosis," *The Netherlands Journal of Medicine* (1997): 50:191–7.

Ferrannini E. Syndrome X. *Hormone Research* (1993): 39 (Supplement 3:107–11.

Hjermann I. "The Metabolic Cardiovascular Syndrome: Syndrome X, Reaven's Syndrome, Insulin Resistance Syndrome, Atherothrombogenic Syndrome." *The Jour-*

nal of Cardiovascular Pharmacology 20 (Supplement 8) (1992): S5–S10.

Karam, J.H., "Type II Diabetes and Syndrome X. Pathogenesis and Glycemic Management," *Endocrinology and Metabolism Clinics of North America* 21 (1992): 329–350.

Kotake, H., and Oikawa, S., "[Syndrome X]," *Nippon Rinsho* (Japanese) 57 (1999): 622–626.

Matsuzawa, Y., Funahashi, T., and Nakamura, T., "Molecular Mechanism of Metabolic Syndrome X: Contribution of Adipocytokines Adipocyte-Derived Bioactive Substances," *Annals of the New York Academy of Sciences* 892 (1999): 146–154.

McCarty, M.F., "Hemostatic Concomitants of Syndrome X," *Medical Hypotheses* 44 (1995): 179–193.

Reaven, G.M., "Role of Insulin Resistance in Human Disease (Syndrome X): An Expanded Definition," *Annual Review of Medicine* 44 (1993): 121–131.

Reaven, G.M., "Syndrome X: 6 Years Later," *Journal of Internal Medicine* (Supplement 736 (Supplement) (1994): 13–22.

Reaven, G., Strom, T. K., and Fox, B., *Syndrome X: The Silent Killer* (New York: Simon & Schuster, 2000).

Reaven G.M. Banting lecture 1988. Role of insulin resistance in human disease. *Diabetes* (1988): 37:1595–607.

Reddy, S.S., "Reducing the Incidence of Coronary Heart Disease by Managing Hypertension: Implications Of Syndrome X," *Canadian Journal of Public Health* 85 (Supplement 2) (1994): S51–S53.

Roberts, K., Dunn, K., Jean, S.K., et al., "Syndrome X: Medical Nutrition Therapy," *Nutrition Reviews* 58 (2000): 154–160.

Sakkinen, P.A., Wahl, P., Cushman, M., et al., "Clustering of Procoagulation, Inflammation, and Fibrinolysis Variables with Metabolic Factors in Insulin Resistance Syndrome," *American Journal of Epidemiology* 152 (2000): 897–907.

Shen, D.C., Shieh, S.M., Fuh, M.M., et al., "Resistance to Insulin-Stimulated-Glucose Uptake in Patients with Hypertension," *The Journal of Clinical Endocrinology and Metabolism* 66 (1988): 580–583.

Stern, M.P., "'Syndrome X': Is It a Significant Cause of Hypertension? Affirmative," *Hospital Practice* (Office Edition) 27 (Supplement 1) (1992): 37–40, discussion 44–45.

Timar, O., Sestier, F., and Levy, E., "Metabolic Syndrome X: A Review," *Canadian Journal of Cardiology* 16 (2000): 779–789.

Wajchenberg, B.L., Malerbi, D.A., Rocha, M.S., et al., "Syndrome X: A Syndrome of Insulin Resistance. Epidemiological and Clinical evidence," *Diabetes/Metabolism Reviews* 10 (1994): 19–29.

Cardiovascular Line of Research

Bory, M., "[Does Syndrome X Exist?]" *Archives des Maladies du Coeur et des Vaisseaux* (French) 87 (1994): 1739–1743.

Chauhan, A., "Syndrome X—Angina and Normal Coronary Angiography," *Postgraduate Medical Journal* 71 (1995): 341–345.

Chen, J.W., Lin, S.J., and Ting, C.T., "Syndrome X: Pathophysiology and Clinical Management," *Zhonghua Yi Xue Za Zhi (Taipei)* 60 (1997): 177–183.

Favaro, L., Masini, F., Maffei, M.L., et al., "[Syndrome X]," *Recenti Progressi in Medicina* (Italian) 80 (1989): 281–285.

Ferrara, L., Tagliamonte, E., Cice, G., et al., "[Syndrome X and Microvascular Angina]," *Minerva Cardioangiologica* (Italian) 46 (1998): 181–193.

Friedberg, C.K., and Horn, H., "Acute Myocardial Infarction Not Due to Coronary Artery Occlusion," *Journal of the American Medical Association* 112 (1939): 1673–1679.

Henderson, A.H., "Syndrome X," *Cardiovascular Drugs and Therapy* 3 (1989) (Supplement 1): 271–274.

Holdright, D.R., Rosano, G.M., Sarrel, P.M., et al., "The ST Segment—The Herald of Ischaemia, the Siren of Misdiagnosis, or Syndrome X?" *International Journal of Cardiology* 35 (1992): 293–301.

Iglesias, I., Velasco, S., Alegria, E., et al., "[Update on Coronary Syndrome X]," *Revista de Medicina de la Universidad de Navarra* (Spanish) 34 (1990): 203–207.

Kaski, J.C., and Russo, G., "Cardiac Syndrome X: An Overview," *Hospital Practice (Office Edition)* 35 (2000): 75–76, 79–82, 85–88.

Kaski, J.C., and Russo, G., "Microvascular Angina in Patients with Syndrome X,"

Zeitschrift für Kardiologie 89 (2000) (Supplement 9): 121–125.

Kern, M.J., "Syndrome X: Understanding and Evaluating the Patient with Chest Pain and Normal Coronary Arteriograms," *Heart Disease and Stroke* 1 (1992): 299–302.

Lanza, G.A., "Abnormal Cardiac Nerve Function in Syndrome X," *Herz* 24 (1999): 97–106.

Poole-Wilson, P.A., and Crake, T., "The Enigma of Syndrome X," *International Journal of Microcirculation, Clinical and Experimental* 8 (1989): 423–432.

Rosano, G.M., Lindsay, D.C., and Poole-Wilson, P.A., "Syndrome X: An Hypothesis for Cardiac Pain without Ischaemia," *Cardiologia* 36 (1991): 885–895.

Hypertension Line of Research

Barbagallo, M., Novo, S., Licata, G., et al., "Diabetes, Hypertension and Atherosclerosis: Pathophysiological Role of Intracellular Ions," *International Angiology* 12 (1993): 365–370.

Resnick, L.M., "Cellular Ions in Hypertension, Insulin Resistance, Obesity, and Diabetes: A Unifying Theme," *Journal of the American Society of Nephrology* 3 (1992): S78–S85.

Resnick, L.M., "Ionic Basis of Hypertension, Insulin Resistance, Vascular Disease, and Related Disorders. The Mechanism of 'Syndrome X,'" *American Journal of Hypertension* 6 (1993): 123S–134S.

Resnick, L.M., Altura, B.T., Gupta, R.K., et al., "Intracellular and Extracellular Magnesium Depletion in Type 2 (Non-Insulin-Dependent) Diabetes Mellitus," *Diabetologia* 36 (1993): 767–770.

Resnick, L.M., Militianu, D., Cunnings, A.J., et al., "Direct Magnetic Resonance Determination of Aortic Distensibility in Essential Hypertension: Relation to Age, Abdominal Visceral Fat, and In Situ Intracellular Free Magnesium," *Hypertension* 30 (1997): 654–659.

Resnick, L.M., "The Cellular Ionic Basis of Hypertension and Allied Clinical Conditions," *Progress in Cardiovascular Diseases* 42 (1999): 1–22.

Sowers, J.R., and Draznin, B., "Insulin, Cation Metabolism and Insulin Resistance," *Journal of Basic and Clinical Physiology and Pharmacology* 9 (1998): 223–233.

Low Cellular Magnesium and Metabolic Syndrome X

de Valk, H.W., "Magnesium in Diabetes Mellitus," *The Netherlands Journal of Medicine* 54 (1999): 139–146.

Garland, H.O., "New Experimental Data on the Relationship Between Diabetes Mellitus and Magnesium," *Magnesium Research* 5 (1992): 193–202.

Kao, W.H., Folsom, A.R., Nieto, F.J., et al., "Serum and Dietary Magnesium and the Risk for Type 2 Diabetes Mellitus: The Atherosclerosis Risk in Communities Study," *Archives of Internal Medicine* 159 (1999): 2151–2159.

Matsuda, M., Mandarino, L., and DeFronzo, R.A., "Synergistic Interaction of Magnesium and Vanadate on Glucose Metabolism in Diabetic Rats," *Metabolism* 48 (1999): 725–731.

Nagase, N., "Hypertension and Serum Mg in the Patients with Diabetes and Coronary Heart Disease," *Hypertension Research* 19 (1996) (Supplement 1): S65–S68.

Paolisso, G., and Barbagallo, M., "Hypertension, Diabetes Mellitus, and Insulin Resistance: The Role of Intracellular Magnesium," *American Journal of Hypertension* 10 (1997): 346–355.

Piia, P., Simonen, P.P., Gylling, H.K., et al, "Diabetes Contributes to Cholesterol Metabolism Regardless of Obesity," *Diabetes Care* 25 (2002): 1511–1515.

Resnick, L.M., "Ionic Basis of Hypertension, Insulin Resistance, Vascular Disease, and Related Disorders. The Mechanism of 'Syndrome X,'" *American Journal of Hypertension* 6 (1993): 123S–134S.

Rosolova, H., Mayer, O., Jr., and Reaven, G., "Effect of Variations in Plasma Magnesium Concentration on Resistance to Insulin-Mediated Glucose Disposal in Nondiabetic Subjects," *The Journal of Clinical Endocrinology and Metabolism* 82 (1997): 3783–3785.

Rosolova, H., Mayer, O., Jr., and Reaven, G.M., "Insulin-Mediated Glucose Disposal Is Decreased in Normal Subjects with Relatively Low Plasma Magnesium Concentrations," *Metabolism* 49 (2000): 418–420.

Rude, R.K., "Magnesium Deficiency and

Diabetes Mellitus. Causes and Effects," *Postgraduate Medicine* 92 (1992): 217–219, 222–224.

Srivastava, V.K., Chauhan, A.K., and Lahiri, V.L., "The Significance of Serum Magnesium in Diabetes Mellitus," *Indian Journal of Medical Sciences* 47 (1993): 119–123.

Uriu–Hare, J.Y., Stern, J.S., Reaven, G.M., et al., "The Effect of Maternal Diabetes on Trace Element Status and Fetal Development in the Rat," *Diabetes* 34 (1985): 1031–1040.

White, J.R., Jr., and Campbell, R.K., "Magnesium and Diabetes: A Review," *The Annals of Pharmacotherapy* 27 (1993): 775–780.

Yang, C.Y., Chiu, H.F., Cheng, M.F., et al., "Magnesium in Drinking Water and the Risk of Death from Diabetes Mellitus," *Magnesium Research* 12 (1999): 131–137.

Table: Specific Cellular Reactions to Low Cellular Magnesium/High Calcium

Hwang, D.L., Yen, C.F., and Nadler, J.L., "Effect of Extracellular Magnesium on Platelet Activation and Intracellular Calcium Mobilization," *American Journal of Hypertension* 5 (1992): 700–706.

Nadler, J.L., Malayan, S., Luong, H., et al., "Intracellular Free Magnesium Deficiency Plays a Key Role in Increased Platelet Reactivity in Type II Diabetes Mellitus," *Diabetes Care* 15 (1992): 835–841.

Nadler, J.L., Buchanan, T., Natarajan, R., et al., "Magnesium Deficiency Produces Insulin Resistance and Increased Thromboxane Synthesis," *Hypertension* 21 (1993): 1024–1029.

Resnick, L.M., "Ionic Basis of Hypertension, Insulin Resistance, Vascular Disease, and Related Disorders. The Mechanism of 'Syndrome X,'" *American Journal of Hypertension* 6 (1993): 123S–134S.

Resnick, L., "The Cellular Ionic Basis of Hypertension and Allied Clinical Conditions," *Progress in Cardiovascular Diseases* 42 (1999): 1–22.

Resnick, L.M., "Cellular Calcium and Magnesium Metabolism in the Pathophysiology and Treatment of Hypertension and Related Metabolic Disorders," *The American Journal of Medicine* 93 (1992): 11S–20S.

Resnick, L.M., "Calcium Metabolism in Hypertension and Allied Metabolic Disorders," *Diabetes Care* 14 (1991): 505–520.

Rosolova, H., Mayer, O., Jr., and Reaven, G.M., "Insulin-Mediated Glucose Disposal Is Decreased in Normal Subjects with Relatively Low Plasma Magnesium Concentrations," *Metabolism* 49 (2000) 418–420.

How Certain Conditions Affect Cellular Magnesium Ion

Barbagallo, M., Novo, S., Licata, G., et al., "Diabetes, Hypertension and Atherosclerosis: Pathophysiological Role of Intracellular Ions," *International Angiology* 12 (1993): 365–370.

Barbagallo, M., Dominguez, L.J., and Resnick, L.M., "Protective Effects of Captopril against Ischemic Stress: Role of Cellular Mg," *Hypertension* 34 (1999): 958–963.

Barbagallo, M., Dominguez, L.J., Tagliamonte, M.R., et al., "Effects of Glutathione on Red Blood Cell Intracellular Magnesium: Relation to Glucose Metabolism," *Hypertension* 34 (1999): 76–82.

Komers, R., and Vrana, A., "Thiazolidinediones—Tools for the Research of Metabolic Syndrome X," *Physiological Research* 47 (1998): 215–225.

Resnick, L.M., Barbagallo, M., Gupta, R.K., et al., "Ionic Basis of Hypertension in Diabetes Mellitus. Role of Hyperglycemia," *American Journal of Hypertension* 6 (1993): 413–417.

DIABETES, HEART DISEASE, AND MAGNESIUM

Acton, R.T., Roseman, J.M., Bell, D.S., et al., Genes within the Major Histocompatibility Complex Predict NIDDM in African–American Women in Alabama," *Diabetes Care* 17 (1994): 1491–1494.

Aitman, T.J., and Todd, J.A., "Molecular Genetics of Diabetes Mellitus," *Baillieres Clinical Endocrinology and Metabolism* 9 (1995): 631–656.

Baillie, G.M., Sherer, J.T., and Weart, C.W., "Insulin and Coronary Artery Disease: Is Syndrome X the Unifying Hypothesis?" *The Annals of Pharmacotherapy* 32 (1998): 233–247.

Chisholm, D.J., Campbell, L.V., and Kraegen, E.W., "Pathogenesis of the Insulin

Resistance Syndrome (Syndrome X)," *Clinical and Experimental Pharmacology and Physiology* 24 (1997): 782–784.

DeFronzo, R.A., and Ferrannini, E., "Insulin Resistance. A Multifaceted Syndrome Responsible for NIDDM, Obesity, Hypertension, Dyslipidemia, and Atherosclerotic Cardiovascular Disease," *Diabetes Care* 14 (1991): 173–194.

DeFronzo, R.A., "Insulin Resistance: A Multifaceted Syndrome Responsible for NIDDM, Obesity, Hypertension, Dyslipidaemia and Atherosclerosis," *The Netherlands Journal of Medicine* 50 (1997): 191–197.

Dittmer, I., Woodfield, G., and Simpson, I., "Non-Insulin-Dependent Diabetes Mellitus in New Zealand Maori: A relationship with Class I but Not Class II Histocompatibility Locus Antigens," *The New Zealand Medical Journal* 111 (1998): 294–296.

Djurhuus, M.S., "New Data on the Mechanisms of Hypermagnesuria in Type I Diabetes Mellitus," *Magnesium Research* 14 (2001): 217–223.

Ferrannini, E., "Syndrome X," *Hormone Research* 39 (1993) (Supplement 3): 107–111.

Garland, H.O., "New Experimental Data on the Relationship Between Diabetes Mellitus and Magnesium," *Magnesium Research* 5 (1992): 193–202.

Ghabanbasani, M.Z., Spaepen, M., Buyse, I., et al., "Increased and Decreased Relative Risk for Non-Insulin-Dependent Diabetes Mellitus Conferred by HLA Class II and by CD4 Alleles," *Clinical Genetics* 47 (1995): 225–230.

Hjermann, I., "The Metabolic Cardiovascular Syndrome: Syndrome X, Reaven's Syndrome, Insulin Resistance Syndrome, Atherothrombogenic Syndrome," *The Journal of Cardiovascular Pharmacology* 20 (1992) (Supplement 8): S5–S10.

Karam, J.H., "Type II Diabetes and Syndrome X. Pathogenesis and Glycemic Management," *Endocrinology and Metabolism Clinics of North America* 21 (1992): 329–350.

Kotake, H., and Oikawa, S., "[Syndrome X]," *Nippon Rinsho. Japanese Journal of Medicine* 57 (1999): 622–626.

Lavric, J., and Zaversnik, H., "Drinking of Mineral Water Donat Mg and Its Influence on the Serum Magnesium Concentration in Diabetics," *Magnesium Bulletin* 8 (1986): 275.

Lindeman, R.D., "Influence of Various Nutrients and Hormones on Urinary Divalent Cation Excretion," *Annals of the New York Academy of Sciences* 162 (1969): 802–809.

Lostroh, A.J., and Krahl, M.E., "Magnesium, a Second Messenger for Insulin: Ion Translocation Coupled to Transport Activity," *Advances in Enzyme Regulation* 12 (1974): 73–81.

Martin, H.E., and Wertman, M., "Serum Potassium, Magnesium and Calcium Levels in Diabetic Acidosis," *The Journal of Clinical Investigations* 26 (1947): 217–228.

Martin, H.E., Mehl, J., and Wertman, M., "Clinical Studies of Magnesium Metabolism," *The Medical Clinics of North America* 36 1952): 1157–1171.

Matsuzawa, Y., Funahashi, T., and Nakamura, T., "Molecular Mechanism of Metabolic Syndrome X: Contribution of Adipocytokines Adipocyte-Derived Bioactive Substances," *Annals of the New York Academy of Sciences* 892 (1999): 146–154.

McCarty, M.F., "Hemostatic Concomitants of Syndrome X," *Medical Hypotheses* 44 (1995): 179–193.

Pandey, J.P., Zamani, M., and Cassiman, J.J., "Epistatic Effects of Genes Encoding Tumor Necrosis Factor-Alpha, Immunoglobulin Allotypes, and HLA Antigens on Susceptibility to Non-Insulin-Dependent (Type 2) Diabetes Mellitus," *Immunogenetics* 49 (1999): 860–864.

Piia, P., Simonen, P.P., Gylling, H.K., et al., "Diabetes Contributes to Cholesterol Metabolism Regardless of Obesity," *Diabetes Care* 25 (2002): 1511–1515.

Rajala, U., Laakso, M., Paivansalo, M., et al., "Low Insulin Sensitivity Measured by Both Quantitative Insulin Sensitivity Check Index and Homeostasis Model Assessment Method as a Risk Factor of Increased Intima-Media Thickness of the Carotid Artery," *The Journal of Clinical Endocrinology and Metabolism* 87 (2002): 5092–5097.

Reaven, G.M. "Banting lecture 1988. Role of Insulin Resistance in Human Disease," *Diabetes* 37 (1988): 1595–1607.

Reaven, G.M., "Role of Insulin Resistance in Human Disease (Syndrome X): An Expanded Definition," *Annual Review of Medicine* 44 (1993): 121–131.

Reaven, G.M., "Syndrome X: 6 Years Later," *Journal of Internal Medicine* 736 (1994) (Supplement): 13–22.

Reaven, Gerald, Strom, Terry Kristen, and Fox, Barry, *Syndrome X: The Silent Killer* (New York: Simon & Schuster, 2000).

Reddy, S.S., "Reducing the Incidence of Coronary Heart Disease by Managing Hypertension: Implications of Syndrome X," *Canadian Journal of Public Health* 85 (1994) (Supplement 2): S51–S53.

Rich, S.S., French, L.R., Sprafka, J.M., et al., "HLA-Associated Susceptibility to Type 2 (Non-Insulin-Dependent) Diabetes Mellitus: The Wadena City Health Study," *Diabetologia* 36 (1993): 234–238.

Roberts, K., Dunn, K., Jean, S.K., et al., "Syndrome X: Medical Nutrition Therapy," *Nutrition Reviews* 58 (2000): 154–160.

Rude, R.K., "Magnesium Deficiency and Diabetes Mellitus. Causes and Effects," *Postgraduate Medicine* 92 (1992): 217–219, 222–224.

Sakkinen, P.A., Wahl, P., Cushman, M., et al., "Clustering of Procoagulation, Inflammation, and Fibrinolysis Variables with Metabolic Factors in Insulin Resistance Syndrome," *American Journal of Epidemiology* 152 (2000): 897–907.

Shen, D.C., Shieh, S.M., Fuh, M.M., et al., "Resistance to Insulin-Stimulated Glucose Uptake in Patients with Hypertension," *The Journal of Clinical Endocrinology and Metabolism* 66 (1988): 580–583.

Sjogren, A., Floren, C.H., and Nilsson, A., "Oral Administration of Magnesium Hydroxide to Subjects with Insulin-Dependent Diabetes Mellitus: Effects on Magnesium and Potassium Levels and on Insulin Requirements," *Magnesium* 7 (1988): 117–122.

Srivastava, V.K., Chauhan, A.K., and Lahiri, V.L., "The Significance of Serum Magnesium in Diabetes Mellitus," *Indian Journal of Medical Sciences* 47 (1993): 119–123.

Stern, M.P., "'Syndrome X': Is It a Significant Cause of Hypertension? Affirmative," *Hospital Practice (Office Ed.)* 27 (1992) (Supplement 1): 37–40; discussion 44–5.

Thorsby, P., Undlien, D.E., Berg, J.P., et al., "[Diabetes Mellitus—A Complex Interaction Between Heredity and Environment]," *Tidsskrift for den Norske Laegeforening* 118 (1998): 2519–2524.

Timar, O., Sestier, F., and Levy, E., "Metabolic Syndrome X: A Review," *Canadian Journal of Cardiology* 16 (2000): 779–789.

Tuomi, T., Carlsson, A., Li, H., et al., "Clinical and Genetic Characteristics of Type 2 Diabetes with and without GAD Antibodies," *Diabetes* 48 (1999): 150–157.

Tuomilehto-Wolf, E., Tuomilehto, J., Hitman, G.A., et al., "Genetic Susceptibility to Non-Insulin-Dependent Diabetes Mellitus and Glucose Intolerance Are Located in HLA Region," *British Medical Journal* 307 (1993): 155–159.

Wajchenberg, B.L., Malerbi, D.A., Rocha, M.S., et al., "Syndrome X: A Syndrome of Insulin Resistance. Epidemiological and Clinical EvidenceM" *Diabetes/Metabolism Reviews* 10 (1994): 19–29.

Yang, C.Y., Chiu, H.F., Cheng, M.F., et al., "Magnesium in Drinking Water and the Risk of Death from Diabetes Mellitus," *Magnesium Research* 12 (1999): 131–137.

CURRENT MEDICAL THOUGHT ON METABOLIC SYNDROME X

Chabot, V., "[Syndrome 'X']," *Schweizerische Rundschau für Medizin Praxis* 82 (1993): 858–863.

Ford, E.S., Giles, W.H., and Dietz, W.H., "Prevalence of the Metabolic Syndrome among U.S. Adults: Findings from the Third National Health and Nutrition Examination Survey," *Journal of the American Medical Association* (2002): 287:356–9.

Hjermann, I., "The Metabolic Cardiovascular Syndrome: Syndrome X, Reaven's Syndrome, Insulin Resistance Syndrome, Atherothrombogenic Syndrome," *The Journal of Cardiovascular Pharmacology* 20 (1992) (Supplement 8): S5–S10.

Karam, J.H., "Type II Diabetes and Syndrome X. Pathogenesis and Glycemic Management," *Endocrinology and Metabolism Clinics of North America* 21 (1992): 329–350.

Minchoff, L.E., and Grandin, J.A., "Syndrome X. Recognition and Management of this Metabolic Disorder in Primary Care," *The Nurse Practitioner* 21 (1996): 74–75, 79–80, 83–86.

Nilsson, P., "Diabetes and Syndrome X in Hypertension—Population Aspects," *Journal of Human Hypertension* 10 (1996) (Supplement 1): S81–S84.

Timar, O., Sestier, F., Levy, E., "Metabolic Syndrome X: A Review," *Canadian Journal of Cardiology* 16 (2000): 779–789.

Weight-Loss Diets for Metabolic Syndrome X

Daubresse, J.C., "[The Importance of Syndrome X in Daily Practice]," *Revue Medicale de Bruxelles* (French) 21 (2000): 473–477.

Parillo, M., Coulston, A., Hollenbeck, C., et al., "Effect of a Low Fat Diet on Carbohydrate Metabolism in Patients with Hypertension," *Hypertension* 11 (1988): 244–248.

Reaven, G.M., "Do High Carbohydrate Diets Prevent the Development or Attenuate the Manifestations (or Both) of Syndrome X? A Viewpoint Strongly Against," *Current Opinion in Lipidology* 8 (1997): 23–27.

Reaven, G.M., "Diet and Syndrome X," *Current Atherosclerosis Reports* 2 (2000): 503–507.

Reaven, Gerald, Strom, Terry Kristen, and Fox, Barry, *Syndrome X: The Silent Killer* (New York: Simon & Schuster, 2000).

Roberts, K., Dunn, K., Jean, S.K., et al., "Syndrome X: Medical Nutrition Therapy," *Nutrition Reviews* 58 (2000): 154–160.

Singh, R.B., Rastogi, V., Rastogi, S.S., et al., "Effect of Diet and Moderate Exercise on Central Obesity and Associated Disturbances, Myocardial Infarction and Mortality in Patients with and without Coronary Artery Disease," *Journal of the American College of Nutrition* 15 (1996): 592–601.

Drugs for Metabolic Syndrome X

Chisholm, D.J., Campbell, L.V., and Kraegen, E.W., "Pathogenesis of the Insulin Resistance Syndrome (Syndrome X)," *Clinical and Experimental Pharmacology and Physiology* 24 (1997): 782–784.

Feldman, R., "ACE Inhibitors Versus AT1 Blockers in the Treatment of Hypertension and Syndrome X," *Canadian Journal of Cardiology* 16 (2000) (Supplement E): 41E–44E.

Ferrara, L., Tagliamonte, E., Cice, G., et al., "[Syndrome X and Microvascular Angina]," *Minerva Cardioangiologica* (Italian) 46 (1998): 181–193.

Komers, R., and Vrana, A., "Thiazolidinediones—Tools for the Research of Metabolic Syndrome X," *Physiological Research* 47 (1998): 215–225.

Reaven, Gerald, Strom, Terry Kristen, and Fox, Barry, *Syndrome X: The Silent Killer* (New York: Simon & Schuster, 2000).

Napoli, Kaiser, Bern & Associates, LLP, "Diabetes Drug on Trial: At Issue Is When Drugmaker Knew Of Rezulin's Risks," http://www.rezulin-eresource.com/pfizer4.cfm, 2002.

COMPREHENSIVE TREATMENT FOR METABOLIC SYNDROME X

Baillie, G.M., Sherer, J.T., and Weart, C.W., "Insulin and Coronary Artery Disease: Is Syndrome X the Unifying Hypothesis?" *The Annals of Pharmacotherapy* 32 (1998): 233–247.

Halmos, T., and Jermendy, G., "[Metabolic Syndrome X at the Turn of the Millennium (Theoretical Aspects with Practical Consequences)]," *Orvosi Hetilap* 141 (2000): 2701–2709.

Kotake, H., and Oikawa, S., "[Syndrome X]," *Nippon Rinsho. Japanese Journal of Medicine* 57 (1999): 622–626.

Reddy, S.S., "Reducing the Incidence of Coronary Heart Disease by Managing Hypertension: Implications of Syndrome X," *Canadian Journal of Public Health* 85 (1994) (Supplement 2): S51–S53.

Chapter Three

HIGH BLOOD PRESSURE, SALT, AND MAGNESIUM

INTRODUCTION—HISTORY

Altura, B.M., and Altura, B.T., "Cardiovascular Risk Factors and Magnesium: Relationships to Atherosclerosis, Ischemic Heart Disease, and Hypertension," *Magnesium and Trace Elements* 10 (1991): 182–192.

Postel-Vinay, N., *A Century of Arterial Hypertension 1896–1996* (New York: John Wiley & Sons/IMOTHEP, 1996).

Riesman, D., "High Blood Pressure and Longevity," *Journal of the American Medical Association* 96 (1931): 1105–1111.

Cook, N.R., Cohen, J., Hebert, P.R., et al., "Implications of Small Reductions in Diastolic Blood Pressure for Primary Prevention," *Archives of Internal Medicine* 155 (1995): 701–709.

Fang, J., Madhavan, S., Cohen, H., et al., "Measures of Blood Pressure and Myocardial Infarction in Treated Hypertensive Patients," *Journal of Hypertension* 13 (1995): 413–419.

Isles, C.G., Walker, L.M., Beevers, G.D., et al., "Mortality in Patients of the Glasgow Blood Pressure Clinic," *Journal of Hypertension* 4 (1986): 141–156.

Alderman, M.H., "Quantifying Cardiovascular Risk in Hypertension," *Cardiology Clinics* 13 (1995): 519–527.

THE EFFECT OF MAGNESIUM ON HIGH BLOOD PRESSURE

Altura, B.M., and Altura, B.T., "Role of Magnesium Ions in Contractility of Blood Vessels and Skeletal Muscles, *Magnesium Bulletin* 3 (1981): 102–114.

Altura, B.M., Altura, B.T., and Carella, A., "Magnesium Deficiency–Induced Spasms of Umbilical Vessels: Relation to Preeclampsia, Hypertension, Growth Retardation," *Science* 221 (1983): 376–378.

Altura, B.M., Altura, B.T., Carella, A, et al., "Hypomagnesemia and Vasoconstriction: Possible Relationship to Etiology of Sudden Death Ischemic Heart Disease and Hypertensive Vascular Diseases," *Artery* 9 1981): 212–231.

Altura, B.M., Altura, B.T., Gebrewold, A., et al., "Magnesium Deficiency and Hypertension: Correlation between Magnesium-Deficient Diets and Microcirculatory Changes In Situ," *Science* 223 (1984): 1315–1317.

Altura, B.T., and Altura, B.M., "Cardiovascular Actions of Magnesium: Importance in Etiology and Treatment of High Blood Pressure," *Magnesium Bulletin* 9 (1987): 6–21.

Delhumeau, A., Granry, J.C., Cottineau, C., et al., "[Comparison of Vascular Effects of Magnesium Sulfate and Nicardipine during Extracorporeal Circulation]," *Annales Francaises d'Anesthesie et de Reanimation* 14 (1995): 149–153.

Nastou, H., Sarros, G., Nastos, A., et al., "Prophylactic Effects of Intravenous Magnesium on Hypertensive Emergencies after Cataract Surgery. A New Contribution to the Pharmacological Use of Magnesium in Anaesthesiology," *Magnesium Research* 8 (1995): 271–276.

Ryan, M.P., and Brady, H.R., "The Role of Magnesium in the Prevention and Control of Hypertension," *Annals of Clinical Research* 16 (1984) (Supplement 43): 81–88.

Seelig, M.S., and Heggtveit, H.A., "Magnesium Interrelationships in Ischemic Heart Disease: A Review," *American Journal of Clinical Nutrition* 27 (1974): 59–79.

Shils, M.E., "Experimental Human Magnesium Depletion," *Medicine (Baltimore)* 48 (1969): 61–85.

Singh, R.B., Rastogi, S.S., Mehta, P.J., et al., "Magnesium Metabolism in Essential Hypertension," *Acta Cardiologica* 44 (1989): 313–322.

Witteman, J.C., Willett, W.C., Stampfer, M.J., et al., "A Prospective Study of Nutritional Factors and Hypertension among U.S. Women," *Circulation* 80 (1989): 1320–1327.

Magnesium and Hypertension Research

The following studies are those numbered in Table 3.1:

1. Nowson, C.A., and Morgan, T.O., "Magnesium Supplementation in Mild Hypertensive Patients on a Moderately Low Sodium Diet," *Clinical and Experimental Pharmacology and Physiology* 16 (1989): 299–302.
2. Dyckner, T., and Wester, P.O., "Effect of Magnesium on Blood Pressure," *British Medical Journal (Clinical Research Edition)* 286 (1983): 1847–1849.
3. Cappuccio, F.P., Markandu, N.D., Beynon, G.W., et al., "Lack of Effect of Oral Magnesium on High Blood Pressure: A Double Blind Study," *British Medical Journal (Clinical Research Edition)* 291 (1985): 235–238.
4. Lind, L., Lithell, H., Pollare, T., et al., "Blood Pressure Response during Long-Term Treatment with Magnesium Is Dependent on Magnesium Status. A Double-Blind, Placebo-Controlled Study in Essential Hypertension and in

Subjects with High-Normal Blood Pressure," *American Journal of Hypertension* 4 (1991): 674–679.

5. "The Effects of Nonpharmacologic Interventions on Blood Pressure of Persons with High Normal Levels. Results of the Trials of Hypertension Prevention, Phase I," *Journal of the American Medical Association* 267 (1992): 1213–1220.
6. Ferrara, L.A., Iannuzzi, R., Castaldo, A., et al., "Long-Term Magnesium Supplementation in Essential Hypertension," *Cardiology* 81 (1992): 25–33.
7. Plum-Wirell, M., Stegmayr, B.G., and Wester, P.O., "Nutritional Magnesium Supplementation Does Not Change Blood Pressure nor Serum or Muscle Potassium and Magnesium in Untreated Hypertension. A Double-Blind Crossover Study," *Magnesium Research* 7 (1994): 277–283.
8. Wirell, M.P., Wester, P.O., and Stegmayr, B.G., "Nutritional Dose of Magnesium in Hypertensive Patients on Beta-Blockers Lowers Systolic Blood Pressure: A Double-Blind, Crossover Study," *Journal of Internal Medicine* 236 (1994): 189–195.
9. Yamamoto, M.E., Applegate, W.B., Klag, M.J., et al., "Lack of Blood Pressure Effect with Calcium and Magnesium Supplementation in Adults with High-Normal Blood Pressure. Results from Phase I of the Trials of Hypertension Prevention (TOHP). Trials of Hypertension Prevention (TOHP) Collaborative Research Group," *Annals of Epidemiology* 5 (1995): 96–107.
10. Sacks, F.M., Brown, L.E., Appel, L., et al., "Combinations of Potassium, Calcium, and Magnesium Supplements in Hypertension," *Hypertension* 26 (1995): 950–956.
11. Whelton, P.K., Kumanyika, S.K., Cook, N.R., et al., "Efficacy of Nonpharmacologic Interventions in Adults with High-Normal Blood Pressure: Results from Phase 1 of the Trials of Hypertension Prevention. Trials of Hypertension Prevention Collaborative Research Group," *American Journal of Clinical Nutrition* 65 (1997): 652S–660S.
12. Witteman, J.C., Grobbee, D.E., Derkx, F.H., et al., "Reduction of Blood Pressure with Oral Magnesium Supplementation in Women with Mild to Moderate Hypertension," *American Journal of Clinical Nutrition* 60 (1994): 129–135.
13. Kawano, Y., Matsuoka, H., Takishita, S., et al., "Effects of Magnesium Supplementation in Hypertensive Patients: Assessment by Office, Home, and Ambulatory Blood Pressures," *Hypertension* 32 (1998): 260–265.
14. Sanjuliani, A.F., de Abreu Fagundes, V.G., and Francischetti, E.A., "Effects of Magnesium on Blood Pressure and Intracellular Ion Levels of Brazilian Hypertensive Patients," *International Journal of Cardiology* 56 (1996): 177–183.
15. Widman, L., Wester, P.O., Stegmayr, B.K., et al., "The Dose-Dependent Reduction in Blood Pressure through Administration of Magnesium. A Double Blind Placebo Controlled Crossover Study," *American Journal of Hypertension* 6 (1993): 41–45.
16. Zemel, P.C., Zemel, M.B., Urberg, M., et al., "Metabolic and Hemodynamic Effects of Magnesium Supplementation in Patients with Essential Hypertension," *American Journal of Clinical Nutrition* 51 (1990): 665–669.

The Role of Potassium

Addison, W.L., "The Use of Sodium Chloride, Potassium Chloride, Sodium Bromide, and Potassium Bromide in Cases of Arterial Hypertension Which Are Amenable to Potassium Chloride," *The Canadian Medical Association Journal* XVIII (1928): 281–285.

Barden, A.E., Vandongen, R., Beilin, L.J., et al., "Potassium Supplementation Does Not Lower Blood Pressure in Normotensive Women," *Journal of Hypertension* 4 (1986): 339–343.

Cooper, G.M., *Dietary Potassium and Health: Potential Benefits of Supplemental Addition in Reducing the Incidence or Severity of Cardiovascular Diseases, Osteoporosis and Kidney Stones* (Woodstock, IL: Morton Salt, 1996).

Karen, B., *Everything You Always Wanted to Know About Potassium but Were Too Tired to Ask* (Novato, CA: Nutrition Encounter, Inc., 1992).

Moore, Richard, and Webb, George, *The K Factor, Reversing and Preventing High Blood Pressure without Drugs* (New York: MacMillan Publishing Company, 1986).

"Pressure Drop, (Intake of Potassium Improves Blood Pressure)," *FDA Consumer* 32 (1998): 4.

Priddle, W.W., "Observations on the Management of Hypertension," *Canadian Medical Association Journal* 25 (1931): 5–8.

The Effect of Potassium Supplements on High Blood Pressure

Arzilli, F., Taddei, S., Graziadei, L., et al., "A. Potassium-Rich and Sodium-Poor Salt Reduces Blood Pressure in Hospitalized Patients," *Journal of Hypertension* 4 (1986) (Supplement): S347–S350.

Brancati, F.L., Appel, L.J., Seidler, A.J., et al., "Effect of Potassium Supplementation on Blood Pressure in African Americans on a Low-Potassium Diet. A Randomized, Double-Blind, Placebo-Controlled Trial," *Archives of Internal Medicine* 156 (1996): 61–67.

Cappuccio, F.P., and MacGregor, G.A., "Does Potassium Supplementation Lower Blood Pressure? A Meta-Analysis of Published Trials," *Journal of Hypertension* 9 (1991): 465–473.

Patki, P.S., Singh, J., Gokhale, S.V., et al., "Efficacy of Potassium and Magnesium in Essential Hypertension: A Double-Blind, Placebo-Controlled, Crossover Study," *British Medical Journal* 301 (1990): 521–523.

"Potassium Supplementation for High Blood Pressure," *Executive Health's Good Health Report* 35 (1999): 6.

Siani, A., Strazzullo, P., Giacco, A., et al., "Increasing the Dietary Potassium Intake Reduces the Need for Antihypertensive Medication," *Annals of Internal Medicine* 115 (1991): 753–759.

Smith, S.R., Klotman, P.E., and Svetkey, L.P., "Potassium Chloride Lowers Blood Pressure and Causes Natriuresis in Older Patients with Hypertension," *Journal of the American Society of Nephrology* 2 (1992): 1302–1309.

Svetkey, L.P., Yarger, W.E., Feussner, J.R., et al., "Double-Blind, Placebo-Controlled Trial of Potassium Chloride in the Treatment of Mild Hypertension," *Hypertension* 9 (1987): 444–450.

Valdes, G., Vio, C.P., Montero, J., et al., "Potassium Supplementation Lowers Blood Pressure and Increases Urinary Kallikrein in Essential Hypertensives," *Journal of Human Hypertension* 5 (1991): 91–96.

Whelton, P.K., He, J., Cutler, J.A., et al., "Effects of Oral Potassium on Blood Pressure. Meta-Analysis of Randomized Controlled Clinical Trials," *Journal of the American Medical Association* 277 (1997): 1624–1632.

Wilson, D.K., Sica, D.A., Devens, M., et al., "The Influence of Potassium Intake on Dipper and Nondipper Blood Pressure Status in an African-American Adolescent Population," *Blood Pressure Monitoring* 1 (1996): 447–455.

Wilson, D.K., Sica, D.A., and Miller, S.B., "Effects of Potassium on Blood Pressure in Salt-Sensitive and Salt-Resistant Black Adolescents," *Hypertension* 34 (1999): 181–186.

Magnesium and Potassium in the Regulation of Blood Pressure

Dyckner, T., and Wester, P.O., "Intracellular Potassium after Magnesium Infusion," *British Medical Journal* 1 (1978): 822–823.

Kamen, B., *Everything You Always Wanted to Know About Potassium but Were Too Tired to Ask* (Novato, CA: Nutrition Encounter, Inc., 1992).

Karppanen, H., "Ischaemic Heart Disease. An Epidemiological Perspective with Special Reference to Electrolytes," *Drugs* 28 (1984) (Supplement 1): 17–27.

Rubenowitz, E., Landin, K., and Wilhelmsen, L., "Skeletal Muscle Magnesium and Potassium by Gender and Hypertensive Status," *Scandinavian Journal of Clinical and Laboratory Investigation* 58 (1998): 47–54.

Rude, R.K., "Physiology of Magnesium Metabolism and the Important Role of Magnesium in Potassium Deficiency," *The American Journal of Cardiology* 63 (1989): 31G–34G.

Sanjuliani, A.F., de Abreu Fagundes, V.G., and Francischetti, E.A., "Effects of Magnesium on Blood Pressure and Intracellular Ion Levels of Brazilian Hypertensive Patients," *International Journal of Cardiology* 56 (1996): 177–183.

Suter, P.M., "The Effects of Potassium, Magnesium, Calcium, and Fiber on Risk of Stroke," *Nutrition Reviews* 57 (1999): 84–88.

Whang, R., and Aikawa, J.K., "Magnesium Deficiency and Refractoriness to Potassium Repletion," *Journal of Chronic Disorders* 30 (1977): 65–68.

CURRENT TREATMENTS FOR HYPERTENSION

Lindholm, L.H., "Cardiovascular Risk Factors and Their Interactions in Hypertensives," *Journal of Hypertension* 9 (1991) (Supplement): S3–S6.

Madhavan, S., Cohen, H., and Alderman, M.H., "Angina Pectoris by Rose Questionnaire Does Not Predict Cardiovascular Disease in Treated Hypertensive Patients," *Journal of Hypertension* 13 (1995): 1307–1312.

Multiple Risk Factor Intervention Trial Research Group, "Multiple Risk Factor Intervention Trial. Risk Factor Changes and Mortality Results," *Journal of the American Medical Association* 248 (1982): 1465–1477.

Wong, Z.Y., Stebbing, M., Ellis, J.A., et al., "Genetic Linkage of Beta and Gamma Subunits of Epithelial Sodium Channel to Systolic Blood Pressure," *Lancet* 353 (1999): 1222–1225.

Medications for Hypertension

American Heart Association, *Guide to Heart Attack. Treatment, Recovery, Prevention* (New York: Times Books-Random House, 1996).

Basile, J.N., "ACE Inhibitor-Associated Cough Lessened with Iron Supplementation," *Journal of Clinical Hypertension (Greenwich)* 4 (2002): 49–50.

Goldberg, E.L., Comstock, G.W., and Graves, C.G., "Psychosocial Factors and Blood Pressure," *Psychological Medicine* 10 (1980): 243–255.

Kuller, L., Farrier, N., Caggiula, A., et al., "Relationship of Diuretic Therapy and Serum Magnesium Levels among Participants in the Multiple Risk Factor Intervention Trial," *American Journal of Epidemiology* 122 (1985): 1045–1059.

Moore, Richard, and Webb, George, *The K Factor: Reversing and Preventing High Blood Pressure without Drugs* (New York: Macmillan Publishing Company, 1986).

Multiple Risk Factor Intervention Trial Research Group, "Multiple Risk Factor Intervention Trial. Risk Factor Changes and Mortality Results," *Journal of the American Medical Association* 248 (1982): 1465–1477.

Pickering, Thomas, *Good News About High Blood Pressure. How to Take Control of Hypertension and Your Life* (New York: Simon & Schuster, 1996).

Prisant, L.M., and Herman, W., "Calcium Channel Blocker Induced Gingival Overgrowth," *Journal of Clinical Hypertension (Greenwich)* 4 (2002): 310–311.

Rangarajan U., Kochar M.S. Hypertension in women. *Wmj* (2000): 99:65–70.

Whitaker, Julian, *Reversing Hypertension. A Vital New Program to Prevent, Treat, and Reduce High Blood Pressure* (New York: Warner Books, 2000).

Diuretics

Dyckner, T., and Wester, P.O., "Intracellular Magnesium Loss after Diuretic Administration," *Drugs* 28 (1984) (Supplement 1):161–166.

Dyckner, T., Wester, P.O., and Widman, L. "Effects of Peroral Magnesium on Plasma and Skeletal Muscle Electrolytes in Patients on Long-Term Diuretic Therapy," *International Journal of Cardiology* 19 (1988): 81–87.

Dyckner T.H., Wester P.O. Magnesium-electrophysiological effects. *Magnesium Bulletin* (1986): 8:219–222.

Field, M.J., and Lawrence, J.R., "Complications of Thiazide Diuretic Therapy: An Update," *Medical Journal of Australia* 144 (1986): 641–644.

Karppanen, H., "Ischaemic Heart Disease. An Epidemiological Perspective with Special Reference to Electrolytes," *Drugs* 28 (1984) (Supplement 1):17–27.

Kuller, L., Farrier, N., Caggiula, A., et al., "Relationship of Diuretic Therapy and Serum Magnesium Levels among Participants in the Multiple Risk Factor Intervention Trial,"

American Journal of Epidemiology 122 (1985): 1045–1059.

Moser, M., "Why Are Physicians Not Prescribing Diuretics More Frequently in the Management of Hypertension?" *Journal of the American Medical Association* 279 (1998): 1813–1816.

ACE Inhibitors

Basile, J.N., "ACE Inhibitor-Associated Cough Lessened with Iron Supplementation," *Journal of Clinical Hypertension (Greenwich)* 4 (2002): 49–50.

Haenni, A., Berglund, L., Reneland, R., et al., "The Alterations in Insulin Sensitivity during Angiotensin Converting Enzyme Inhibitor Treatment Are Related to Changes in the Calcium/Magnesium Balance," *American Journal of Hypertension* 10 (1997): 145–151.

Calcium Channel Blockers

Agus, Z.S., Kelepouris, E., Dukes, I., et al., "Cytosolic Magnesium Modulates Calcium Channel Activity in Mammalian Ventricular Cells," *The American Journal of Physiology* 256 (1989): C452–C455.

Altura, B.M., and Altura, B.T., "Magnesium, Electrolyte Transport and Coronary Vascular Tone," *Drugs* 28 (1984) (Supplement 1): 120–142.

Bara, M, and Guiet-Bara, A., "Magnesium Regulation of Ca2+ Channels in Smooth Muscle and Endothelial Cells of Human Allantochorial Placental Vessels," *Magnesium Research* 14 (2001): 11–18.

Heaton, F.W., Rayssiguier, Y., "Magnesium Deficiency and Membrane Properties," in: *Magnesium in Cellular Processes and Medicine,* ed. B.M. Altura, J. Durlach, and M.S. Seelig (Basel, Switzerland: S. Karger AG, 1987), pp. 121–130.

Kelepouris, E., Kasama, R., and Agus, Z.S., "Effects of Intracellular Magnesium on Calcium, Potassium and Chloride Channels," *Mineral and Electrolyte Metabolism* 19 (1993): 277–281.

Prisant, L.M., and Herman, W., "Calcium Channel Blocker Induced Gingival Overgrowth," *Journal of Clinical Hypertension (Greenwich)* 4 (2002): 310–311.

Diet and Lifestyle Changes for Hypertension

Chalmers, J., Morgan, T., Doyle, A., et al. "Australian National Health and Medical Research Council Dietary Salt Study in Mild Hypertension," *Journal of Hypertension* 4 (1986) (Supplement): S629–S637.

Goldfarb, S., and Henrich, W.L., "Update in Nephrology," *Annals of Internal Medicine* 129 (1998): 636–642.

Midgley, J.P., Matthew, A.G., Greenwood, C.M., et al., "Effect of Reduced Dietary Sodium on Blood Pressure: A Meta-Analysis of Randomized Controlled Trials," *Journal of the American Medical Association* 275 (1996): 1590–1597.

Suter, P.M., "The Effects of Potassium, Magnesium, Calcium, and Fiber on Risk of Stroke," *Nutrition Reviews* 57 (1999): 84–88.

Svetkey, L.P., Simons-Morton, D., Vollmer, W.M., et al., "Effects of Dietary Patterns on Blood Pressure: Subgroup Analysis of the Dietary Approaches to Stop Hypertension (DASH) Randomized Clinical Trial," *Archives of Internal Medicine* 159 (1999): 285–293.

The Trials of Hypertension Prevention Collaborative Research Group, "Effects of Weight Loss and Sodium Reduction Intervention on Blood Pressure and Hypertension Incidence in Overweight People with High-Normal Blood Pressure. The Trials of Hypertension Prevention, Phase II," *Archives of Internal Medicine* 157 (1997): 657–667.

Whelton, P.K., Appel, L.J., Espeland, M.A., et al., Sodium Reduction and Weight Loss in the Treatment of Hypertension in Older Persons: A Randomized Controlled Trial of Nonpharmacologic Interventions in the Elderly (TONE). TONE Collaborative Research Group," *Journal of the American Medical Association* 279 (1998): 839–846.

Does Weight Loss Improve Hypertension?

Resnick, L.M., Militianu, D., Cunnings, A.J., et al., "Direct Magnetic Resonance Determination of Aortic Distensibility in Essential Hypertension: Relation to Age, Abdominal Visceral Fat, and In Situ Intracellular Free Magnesium," *Hypertension* 30 (1997): 654–659.

The Trials of Hypertension Prevention Collaborative Research Group, "Effects of Weight Loss and Sodium Reduction Intervention on Blood Pressure and Hypertension Incidence in Overweight People with High-Normal Blood Pressure. The Trials of Hypertension Prevention, Phase II," *Archives of Internal Medicine* 157 (1997): 657–667.

Williamson, D.F., Serdula, M.K., Anda, R.F., et al., "Weight Loss Attempts in Adults: Goals, Duration, and Rate of Weight Loss," *The American Journal of Public Health* 82 (1992): 1251–1257.

Is Salt Restriction Safer Than Antihypertensive Medications?

American Heart Associatoin Nutrition Committee, "Low Sodium Diets: For Hypertensive Patients Only?" *Patient Care* 1 (1) (30 October 1998).

Alderman, M.H., and Lamport, B., "Moderate Sodium Restriction. Do the Benefits Justify the Hazards?" *American Journal of Hypertension* 3 (1990): 499–504.

Alderman, M.H., Madhavan, S., Cohen, H., et al., "Low Urinary Sodium Is Associated with Greater Risk of Myocardial Infarction among Treated Hypertensive Men," *Hypertension* 25 (1995): 1144–1152.

Contreras, R.J., and Frank, M., "Sodium Deprivation Alters Neural Responses to Gustatory Stimuli," *The Journal of General Physiology* 73 (1979): 569–594.

Egan, B.M., and Stepniakowski, K.T., "Adverse Effects of Short-Term, Very-Low-Salt Diets in Subjects with Risk-Factor Clustering," *American Journal of Clinical Nutrition* 65 (1997): 671S–677S.

Esslinger, K.A., and Jones, P.J., "Dietary Sodium Intake and Mortality," *Nutrition Reviews* 56 (1998): 311–313.

Graudal, N.A., Galloe, A.M., and Garred, P., "Effects of Sodium Restriction on Blood Pressure, Renin, Aldosterone, Catecholamines, Cholesterols, and Triglyceride: A Meta-Analysis," *Journal of the American Medical Association* 279 (1998): 1383–1391.

Hanneman, R.L., "The Politics of Sodium Restriction," *The United States Seventh Symposium on Salt* (1993): 231–239.

Luft, F.C., and Weinberger, M.H., "Heterogeneous Responses to Changes in Dietary Salt Intake: The Salt-Sensitivity Paradigm," *American Journal of Clinical Nutrition* 65 (1997): 612S–617S.

Midgley, J.P., Matthew, A.G., Greenwood, C.M., et al., "Effect of Reduced Dietary Sodium on Blood Pressure: A Meta-Analysis of Randomized Controlled Trials," *Journal of the American Medical Association* 275 (1996): 1590–1597.

Morris, C.D., "Effect of Dietary Sodium Restriction on Overall Nutrient Intake," *American Journal of Clinical Nutrition* 65 (1997): 687S–691S.

Pregnancy-Induced Hyptertension

Conradt, A., Weidinger, H., and Algayer, H., "On the Role of Magnesium in Fetal Hypotrophy, Pregnancy Induced Hypertension, and Pre-Eclampsia," *Magnesium Bulletin* 6 (1984): 68–76.

D'Almeida, A., Carter, J.P., Anatol, A., et al., "Effects of a Combination of Evening Primrose Oil (Gamma Linolenic Acid) and Fish Oil (Eicosapentaenoic + Docosahexaenoic Acid) versus Magnesium, and versus Placebo in Preventing Pre-Eclampsia," *Women Health* 19 (1992): 117–131.

"Do Women with Pre-Eclampsia, and Their Babies, Benefit from Magnesium Sulphate? The Magpie Trial: A Randomised Placebo-Controlled Trial," *Lancet* 359 (2002): 1877–1890.

Hutton, J.D., James, D.K., Stirrat, G.M., et al., "Management of Severe Pre-Eclampsia and Eclampsia by U.K. Consultants," *British Journal of Obstetrics and Gynaecology* 99 (1992): 554–556.

Jerie, P., "[Hypertension and its treatment in pregnancy]," *Casopis Lekaru Ceskych* (Czech) 137 (1998): 467–472.

Kontopoulos, V., Seelig, M.S., Dolan, J., et al., "Influence of Parenteral Administration of Magnesium Sulfate to Normal Pregnant and to Pre-Eclamptic Women," in *Magnesium in Health and Disease,* ed. M. Cantin and M.S. Seelig (New York: Spectrum, 1980), pp. 839–848.

Lazard, E.M., "An Analysis of 575 Cases of Eclamptic and Pre-Eclamptic Toxemias Treated by Intravenous Injections of

Magnesium Sulphate," *American Journal of Obstetrics and Gynecology* 26 (1933): 647–656.

Lazard, E.M., "A Preliminary Report on the Intravenous Use of Magnesium Sulphate in Puerperal Eclampsia, 1925," *American Journal of Obstetrics and Gynecology* 174 (1996): 1390–1391.

Li, S., and Tian, H., "[Oral Low-Dose Magnesium Gluconate Preventing Pregnancy Induced Hypertension]," *Zhonghua Fu Chan Ke Za Zhi* (Chinese) 32 (1997): 613–615.

McNeile, L.G., "Conservative Treatment of Late Toxemias of Pregnancy," *Journal of the American Medical Association* 103 (1934): 549–552.

McNeile, L.G., and Vruwink, J., "Magnesium Sulphate Intravenously in the Care and Treatment of Preeclampsia and Eclampsia," *Journal of the American Medical Association* 87 (1926): 236–240.

Pritchard, J.A., "The Use of the Magnesium Ion in the Management of Eclamptic Toxemias," *Surgery, Obstetrics, and Gynecology* 100 (1955): 131–140.

Pritchard, J.A., Cunningham, F.G., and Pritchard, S.A., "The Parkland Memorial Hospital Protocol for Treatment of Eclampsia: Evaluation of 245 Cases," *American Journal of Obstetrics and Gynecology* 148 (1984): 951–963.

Robson, S.C., "Magnesium Sulphate: The Time of Reckoning," *British Journal of Obstetrics and Gynaecology* 103 (1996): 99–102.

Rudnicki, M., Frolich, A., Rasmussen, W.F., et al., "The Effect of Magnesium on Maternal Blood Pressure in Pregnancy-Induced Hypertension. A Randomized Double-Blind Placebo-Controlled Trial," *Acta Obstetricia et Gynecolica Scandinavica* 70 (1991): 445–450.

Sheth, S.S., and Chalmers, I., "Magnesium for Preventing and Treating Eclampsia: Time for International Action," *Lancet* 359 (2002): 1872–1873.

"Which Anticonvulsant for Women with Eclampsia? Evidence from the Collaborative Eclampsia Trial," *Lancet* 345 (1995): 1455–1463.

Zuspan F. P. "Treatment of severe preeclampsia and eclampsia." *Clin Obstetrics and Gynecology* 9 (1966): 954–972.

Zuspan, F.P., and Ward, M.C., "Improved Fetal Salvage in Eclampsia," *Obstetrics and Gynecology* 26 (1965): 893–897.

Hypertension in African-Americans

Aviv, A., and Gardner, J., "Racial Differences in Ion Regulation and Their Possible Links to Hypertension in Blacks," *Hypertension* 14 (1989): 584–589.

Canto, J.G., Allison, J.J., Kiefe, C.I., et al., "Relation of Race and Sex to the Use of Reperfusion Therapy in Medicare Beneficiaries with Acute Myocardial Infarction," *The New England Journal of Medicine* 342 (2000): 1094–1100.

Cooper, R., and Rotimi, C., "Hypertension in Blacks," *American Journal of Hypertension* 10 (1997): 804–812.

Falkner, B., "Is There a Black Hypertension?" *Hypertension* 10 (1987): 551–554.

Falkner, B., Hulman, S., Tannenbaum, J., et al., "Insulin Resistance and Blood Pressure in Young Black Men," *Hypertension* 16 (1990): 706–711.

Falkner, B., and Kushner, H., "Effect of Chronic Sodium Loading on Cardiovascular Response in Young Blacks and Whites," *Hypertension* 15 (1990): 36–43.

Fang, J., Madhavan, S., Cohen, H., et al., "Differential Mortality in New York City (1988–1992). Part One: Excess Mortality among Non-Hispanic Blacks," *Bulletin of the New York Academy of Medicine* 72 (1995): 470–482.

Ford, E.S., "Race, Education, and Dietary Cations: Findings from the Third National Health and Nutrition Examination Survey," *Ethnicity and Disease* 8 (1998): 10–20.

Fumo, M.T., Teeger, S., Lang, R.M., et al., "Diurnal Blood Pressure Variation and Cardiac Mass in American Blacks and Whites and South African Blacks," *American Journal of Hypertension* 5 (1992): 111–116.

Grim, C.E., and Robinson, M., "Blood Pressure Variation in Blacks: Genetic Factors," *Seminars in Nephrology* 16 (1996): 83–93.

Hyman, D.J., Ogbonnaya, K., Pavlik, V.N., et al., "Lower Hypertension Prevalence in First-Generation African Immigrants Compared to U.S.-Born African Americans," *Ethnicity and Disease* 10 (2000): 343–349.

Liu, K., Ruth, K.J., Flack, J.M., et al., "Blood Pressure in Young Blacks and Whites: Relevance of Obesity and Lifestyle Factors in Determining Differences. The CARDIA Study. Coronary Artery Risk Development in Young Adults," *Circulation* 93 (1996): 60–66.

Powers, D.R., and Wallin, J.D., "End-Stage Renal Disease in Specific Ethnic and Racial Groups: Risk Factors and Benefits of Antihypertensive Therapy," *Archives of Internal Medicine* 158 (1998): 793–800.

Touyz, R.M., Milne, F.J., and Reinach, S.G., "Intracellular Mg2+, Ca2+, Na2+ and K+ in Platelets and Erythrocytes of Essential Hypertension Patients: Relation to Blood Pressure," *Clinical and Experimental Hypertension. Part A, Theory and Practice* 14 (1992): 1189–1209.

Wilson, T.W., and Grim, C.E., "Biohistory of Slavery and Blood Pressure Differences in Blacks Today. A Hypothesis," *Hypertension* 17 (1991): I122–I128.

TEN STEPS TO HEALTHIER BLOOD PRESSURE

Altura, B.M., Altura B.T. Role of magnesium ions in contractility of blood vessels and skeletal muscles. *Magnesium Bulletin* (1981): 3:102–114.

Altura, B.M., Altura, B.T., Carella, A., et al., "Hypomagnesemia and Vasoconstriction: Possible Relationship to Etiology of Sudden Death Ischemic Heart Disease and Hypertensive Vascular Diseases," *Artery* 9 (1981): 212–231.

Altura, B.T., and Altura, B.M., "Cardiovascular Actions of Magnesium: Importance in Etiology and Treatment of High Blood Pressure," *Magnesium Bulletin* 9 (1987): 6–21.

Barbagallo, M., Dominguez, L.J., Licata, G., et al., "Effects of Aging on Serum Ionized and Cytosolic Free Calcium: Relation to Hypertension and Diabetes," *Hypertension* 34 (1999): 902–906.

Cutler, J.A., and Brittain, E., "Calcium and Blood Pressure. An Epidemiologic Perspective," *American Journal of Hypertension* 3 (1990): 137S–146S.

Moore, Richard, and Webb, George, *The K Factor, Reversing and Preventing High Blood Pressure without Drugs* (New York: MacMillan Publishing Company, 1986).

Resnick, L.M., "The Role of Dietary Calcium in Hypertension: A Hierarchical Overview," *American Journal of Hypertension* 12 (1999): 99–112.

Whitaker, Julian, *Reversing Hypertension. A Vital New Program to Prevent, Treat, and Reduce High Blood Pressure* (New York: Warner Books, 2000).

Witteman, J.C., Willett, W.C., Stampfer, M.J., et al., "A Prospective Study of Nutritional Factors and Hypertension among U.S. Women," *Circulation* 80 (1989): 1320–1327.

The following studies are those numbered in Table 3.3:

1. Geleijnse, J.M., Witteman, J.C., Bak, A.A., et al., "Reduction in Blood Pressure with a Low Sodium, High Potassium, High Magnesium Salt in Older Subjects with Mild to Moderate Hypertension," *British Medical Journal* 309 (1994): 436–440.
2. Gilleran, G., O'Leary, M., et al., "Effects of Dietary Sodium Substitution with Potassium and Magnesium in Hypertensive Type II Diabetics: A Randomised Blind Controlled Parallel Study," *Journal of Human Hypertension* 10 (1996): 517–521.
3. Margetts, B.M., Beilin, L.J., Vandongen, R., et al., "Vegetarian Diet in Mild Hypertension: A Randomised Controlled Trial," *British Medical Journal (Clinical Research Edition)* 293 (1986): 1468–1471.

Can Magnesium Supplements Be Dangerous?

Holzgartner, H., Maier, E., and Vierling, W., "[High-Dosage Oral Magnesium Therapy in Arrhythmias. Results of an Observational Study in 1,160 Patients with Arrhythmia]," *Fortschritte der Medizin* (German) 108 (1990): 539–542.

Kurtoglu, S., Caksen, H., and Poyrazoglu, M.H., "Neonatal Poisonings in Middle Anatolia of Turkey: An Analysis of 72 Cases," *The Journal of Toxicological Sciences* 25 (2000): 115–119.

Levav, A.L., Chan, L., and Wapner, R.J., "Long-Term Magnesium Sulfate Tocolysis and Maternal Osteoporosis in a Triplet Pregnancy: A Case Report," *American Journal of Perinatology* 15 (1998): 43–46.

Standing Committee on the Scientific Evaluation of Dietary Reference Intakes, Food and Nutrition Board, Institute of Medicine, *Dietary Reference Intakes for Calcium, Phosphorus, Magnesium, Vitamin D, and Fluoride* (Washington, D.C.: National Academy of Sciences, 1997).

Chapter Four
OBESITY, PHYSICAL ACTIVITY, AND MAGNESIUM

INTRODUCTION

American Heart Association, "Lifetime Risks and Costs of Heart Disease Much Higher for Obese," American Heart Association Abstract 2519, 10 November 1998.

Grundy, S.M., "Metabolic Complications of Obesity," *Endocrine* 13 (2000): 155–165.

Henry, L., "Heart Attack at 20-Something? Investigations into the Causes of Heart Attack Among Young Athletes," *Muscle & Fitness* 58 (1997): 136.

Klug, F., "Big, Bold Body, Huge Heart, and 276 Triathlons for Dave," The Associated Press, 27 December 2000.

Resnick, L.M., "Cellular Ions in Hypertension, Insulin Resistance, Obesity, and Diabetes: A Unifying Theme," *Journal of the American Society of Nephrology* 3 (1992): S78–S85.

Singh, R.B., Beegom, R., Rastogi, S.S., et al., "Association of Low Plasma Concentrations of Antioxidant Vitamins, Magnesium and Zinc with High Body Fat Percent Measured by Bioelectrical Impedance Analysis in Indian Men," *Magnesium Research* 11 (1998): 3–10.

Wilson P.W., D'Agostino, R.B., Sullivan, L., et al., "Overweight and Obesity as Determinants of Cardiovascular Risk: The Framingham Experience," *Archives of Internal Medicine* 162 (2002): 1867–1872.

HOW PROCESSED FOODS TAKE OUT MAGNESIUM AND INCREASE CALORIES

Schroeder, H.A., "Losses of Vitamins and Trace Minerals Resulting from Processing and Preservation of Foods," *American Journal of Clinical Nutrition* 24 (1971): 562–573.

U.S. Department of Agriculture Agricultural Research Service, *USDA Nutrient Database for Standard Reference,* Release 14, Nutrient Data Laboratory Home Page, www.nal.usda.gov/fnic/foodcomp (2001).

THE CONSEQUENCE OF OVEREATING REFINED FOODS

Corica, F., Allegra, A., Ientile, R., et al., "Changes in Plasma, Erythrocyte, and Platelet Magnesium Levels in Normotensive and Hypertensive Obese Subjects during Oral Glucose Tolerance Test. *American Journal of Hypertension* 12 (1999): 128–136.

Lean, M.E., "Pathophysiology of Obesity," *The Proceedings of the Nutrition Society* 59 (2000): 331–336.

Marier, J.R., "Quantitative Factors Regarding Magnesium Status in the Modern-Day World," *Magnesium* 1 (1982): 3–15.

Maison, P., Byrne, C.D., Hales, C.N., et al., "Do Different Dimensions of the Metabolic Syndrome Change Together Over Time? Evidence Supporting Obesity As the Central Feature," *Diabetes Care* 24 (2001): 1758–1763.

Marier, J.R., "Role of Environmental Magnesium in Cardiovascular Diseases," *Magnesium* 1 (1982): 266–276.

Marier, J.R., "Magnesium Content of the Food Supply in the Modern-Day World," *Magnesium* 5 (1986): 1–8.

Morris, K.L., and Zemel, M.B., "Glycemic Index, Cardiovascular Disease, and Obesity," *Nutrition Reviews* 57 (1999): 273–276.

Oberleas, D., "A New Perspective of Trace Element Deficiencies," *Trace Elements in Medicine* 12 (2002): 3.

Pennington, J.A.T., Young, B.E., and Wilson, D.B., "Nutritional Elements in U.S. Diets: Results from the TotalDiet Study, 1982–1986," *Journal of the American Dietetic Association* 89 (1989): 659–664.

Reaven, G.M., "The Kidney: An Unwilling Accomplice in Syndrome X," *American Journal of Kidney Diseases* 30 (1997): 928–931.

Resnick, L.M., "Cellular Calcium and Magnesium Metabolism in the Pathophysiology and Treatment of Hypertension and Related Metabolic Disorders," *The American Journal of Medicine* 93 (1992): 11S–20S.

Singh, R.B., Beegom, R., Rastogi, S.S., et

al., "Association of Low Plasma Concentrations of Antioxidant Vitamins, Magnesium and Zinc with High Body Fat Percent Measured by Bioelectrical Impedance Analysis in Indian Men," *Magnesium Research* 11 (1998): 3–10.

Singh, R.B., Rastogi, V., Rastogi, S.S., et al., "Effect of Diet and Moderate Exercise on Central Obesity and Associated Disturbances, Myocardial Infarction and Mortality in Patients with and without Coronary Artery Disease," *Journal of the American College of Nutrition* 15 (1996): 592–601.

ABDOMINAL OBESITY, HEART DISEASE, AND MAGNESIUM

Barzilai, N., and Gupta, G., "Interaction between Aging and Syndrome X: New Insights on the Pathophysiology of Fat Distribution," *Annals of the New York Academy of Sciences* 892 (1999): 58–72.

Bengtsson, C., Bjorkelund, C., Lapidus, L., et al., "Associations of Serum Lipid Concentrations and Obesity with Mortality in Women: 20 Year Follow Up of Participants in Prospective Population Study in Gothenburg, Sweden," *British Medical Journal* 307 (1993): 1385–1388.

Croft, J.B., Keenan, N.L., Sheridan, D.P., et al., "Waist-to-Hip Ratio in a Biracial Population: Measurement, Implications, and Cautions for Using Guidelines to Define High Risk for Cardiovascular Disease," *Journal of the American Dietetic Association* 95 (1995): 60–64.

Daubresse, J.C., "[The Importance of Syndrome X in Daily Practice]," *Revue Medicale de Bruxelles* (French) 21 (2000): 473–477.

Despres, J.P., Pascot, A., and Lemieux, I., "[Risk Factors Associated with Obesity: A Metabolic Perspective]," *Annales d'Endocrinologie (Paris)* (French) 61 (2000) (Supplement 6): 31–38.

Hughes, K., Aw, T.C., Kuperan, P., et al., "Central Obesity, Insulin Resistance, Syndrome X, Lipoprotein(A), and Cardiovascular Risk in Indians, Malays, and Chinese in Singapore," *Journal of Epidemiology and Community Health* 51 (1997): 394–399.

Iwao, S., Iwao, N., Muller, D.C., et al., "Does Waist Circumference Add to the Predictive Power of the Body Mass Index for Coronary Risk?" *Obesity Research* 9 (2001): 685–695.

Kahn, H.S., and Williamson, D.F., "Abdominal Obesity and Mortality Risk among Men in Nineteenth-Century North America," *International Journal of Obesity and Related Metabolic Disorders* 18 (1994): 686–691.

Kotake, H., and Oikawa, S., "[Syndrome X]," *Nippon Rinsho. Japanese Journal of Medicine* 57 (1999): 622–626.

Lean, M.E., "Pathophysiology of Obesity," *The Proceedings of the Nutrition Society* 59 (2000): 331–336.

Mansfield, E., McPherson, R., and Koski, K.G., "Diet and Waist-to-Hip Ratio: Important Predictors of Lipoprotein Levels in Sedentary and Active Young Men with No Evidence of Cardiovascular Disease," *Journal of the American Dietetic Association* 99 (1999): 1373–1379.

Matsuzawa, Y., Funahashi, T., and Nakamura, T., "Molecular Mechanism of Metabolic Syndrome X: Contribution of Adipocytokines Adipocyte-Derived Bioactive Substances," *Annals of the New York Academy of Sciences* 892 (1999): 146–154.

Matsuzawa, Y., Shimomura, I., Nakamura, T., et al., "Pathophysiology and Pathogenesis of Visceral Fat Obesity," *Annals of the New York Academy of Sciences* 748 (1995): 399–406.

"The Metabolic Basis for the 'Apple' and the 'Pear' Body Habitus," *Nutrition Reviews* 49 (1991): 84–86.

Moller, R., Tafeit, T.E., Sudi, T.K., et al., "Quantifying the 'Appleness' or 'Pearness' of the Human Body by Subcutaneous Adipose Tissue Distribution," *Annals of Human Biology* 27 (2000): 47–55.

Rimm, A.A., Hartz, A.J., and Fischer, M.E., "A Weight Shape Index for Assessing Risk of Disease in 44,820 Women," *Journal of Clinical Epidemiology* 41 (1988): 459–465.

Singh, R.B., Beegom, R., Rastogi, S.S., et al., "Association of Low Plasma Concentrations of Antioxidant Vitamins, Magnesium and Zinc with High Body Fat Percent Measured by Bioelectrical Impedance Analysis in Indian Men," *Magnesium Research* 11 (1998): 3–10.

Singh, R.B., Rastogi, V., Rastogi, S.S., et

al., "Effect of Diet and Moderate Exercise on Central Obesity and Associated Disturbances, Myocardial Infarction and Mortality in Patients with and without Coronary Artery Disease," *Journal of the American College of Nutrition* 15 (1996): 592–601.

ABDOMINAL OBESITY, INSULIN RESISTANCE, AND MAGNESIUM DEFICIENCY

Resnick, L.M., "Cellular Ions in Hypertension, Insulin Resistance, Obesity, and Diabetes: A Unifying Theme," *Journal of the American Society of Nephrology* 3 (1992): S78–S85.

Resnick, L.M., Militianu, D., Cunnings, A.J., et al., "Direct Magnetic Resonance Determination of Aortic Distensibility in Essential Hypertension: Relation to Age, Abdominal Visceral Fat, and In Situ Intracellular Free Magnesium," *Hypertension* 30 (1997): 654–659.

Singh, R.B., Beegom, R., Rastogi, S.S., et al., "Association of Low Plasma Concentrations of Antioxidant Vitamins, Magnesium and Zinc with High Body Fat Percent Measured by Bioelectrical Impedance Analysis in Indian Men," *Magnesium Research* 11 (1998): 3–10.

Sowers, J.R., and Draznin, B., "Insulin, Cation Metabolism and Insulin Resistance," *Journal of Basic and Clinical Physiology and Pharmacology* 9 (1998): 223–233.

THE EFFECT OF EXERCISE ON OBESITY AND METABOLIC SYNDROME

Bjorntorp, P., "Evolution of the Understanding of the Role of Exercise in Obesity and Its Complications," *International Journal of Obesity and Related Metabolic Disorders* 19 (1995) (Supplement 4): S1–S4.

Blair, S.N., and Brodney, S., "Effects of Physical Inactivity and Obesity on Morbidity and Mortality: Current Evidence and Research Issues," *Medicine and Science in Sports and Exercise* 31 (1999): S646–S662.

Church, T.S., Kampert, J.B., Gibbons, L.W., et al., "Usefulness of Cardiorespiratory Fitness as a Predictor of All-Cause and Cardiovascular Disease Mortality in Men with Systemic Hypertension," *The American Journal of Cardiology* 88 (2001): 651–656.

Erikssen, G., "Physical Fitness and Changes in Mortality: The Survival of the Fittest," *Sports Medicine* 31 (2001): 571–576.

Haapanen-Niemi, N., Miilunpalo, S., Pasanen, M., et al., "Body Mass Index, Physical Inactivity and Low Level of Physical Fitness as Determinants of All-Cause and Cardiovascular Disease Mortality—16 Year Follow-Up of Middle-Aged and Elderly Men and Women," *International Journal of Obesity and Related Metabolic Disorders* 24 (2000): 1465–1474.

Heim, D.L., Holcomb, C.A., and Loughin, T.M., "Exercise Mitigates the Association of Abdominal Obesity with High-Density Lipoprotein Cholesterol in Premenopausal Women: Results from the Third National Health and Nutrition Examination Survey," *Journal of the American Dietetic Association* 100 (2000): 1347–1353.

Kelley, D.E., and Goodpaster, B.H., "Effects of Physical Activity on Insulin Action and Glucose Tolerance in Obesity," *Medicine and Science in Sports and Exercise* 31 (1999): S619–S623.

Kriska, A.M., Hanley, A.J., Harris, S.B., et al., "Physical Activity, Physical Fitness, and Insulin and Glucose Concentrations in an Isolated Native Canadian Population Experiencing Rapid Lifestyle Change," *Diabetes Care* 24 (2001): 1787–1792.

Laukkanen, J.A., Lakka, T.A., Rauramaa, R,. et al., "Cardiovascular Fitness as a Predictor of Mortality in Men," *Archives of Internal Medicine* 161 (2001): 825–831.

Lee, I.M., Hsieh, C.C., and Paffenbarger, R.S., Jr., "Exercise Intensity and Longevity in Men. The Harvard Alumni Health Study," *Journal of the American Medical Association* 273 (1995): 1179–1184.

Liu, S., and Manson, J.E., "Dietary Carbohydrates, Physical Inactivity, Obesity, and the 'Metabolic Syndrome' as Predictors of Coronary Heart Disease," *Current Opinion in Lipidology* 12 (2001): 395–404.

Menotti, A., and Puddu, V., "Ten-Year Mortality from Coronary Heart Disease among 172,000 Men Classified by Occupational Physical Activity," *Scandinavian Journal of Work, Environment, and Health* 5 (1979): 100–108.

Samaras, K., Kelly, P.J., Chiano, M.N., et al., "Genetic and Environmental Influences on Total-Body and Central Abdominal Fat: The Effect of Physical Activity in Female Twins," *Annals of Internal Medicine* 130 (1999): 873–882.

Stefanick, M.L., "Physical Activity for Preventing and Treating Obesity-Related Dyslipoproteinemias," *Medicine and Science in Sports and Exercise* 31 (1999): S609–S618.

Stromme, S.B., and Hostmark, A.T., "[Physical Activity, Overweight and Obesity]," *Tidsskrift for den Norske Laegeforening* (Norwegian) 120 (2000): 3578–3582.

Winett, R.A., and Carpinelli, R.N., "Examining the Validity of Exercise Guidelines for the Prevention of Morbidity and All-Cause Mortality," *Annals of Behavioral Medicine* 22 (2000): 237–245.

Yagalla, M.V., Hoerr, S.L., Song, W.O, et al., "Relationship of Diet, Abdominal Obesity, and Physical Activity to Plasma Lipoprotein Levels in Asian Indian Physicians Residing in the United States," *Journal of the American Dietetic Association* 96 (1996): 257–261.

THE EFFECT OF EXERCISE ON MAGNESIUM STATUS

Abbasciano, V., Levato, F., Reali, M.G., et al., "Reduction of Erythrocyte Magnesium Concentration in Heterozygote Beta-Thalassaemic Subjects and in Normal Subjects Submitted to Physical Stress," *Magnesium Research* 1 (1988): 213–217.

Golf, S.W., Bender, S., and Gruttner, J., "On the Significance of Magnesium in Extreme Physical Stress," *Cardiovascular Drugs and Therapy* 12 (1998) (Supplement 2): 197–202.

Konig, D., Keul, J., Northoff, H., et al., "[Rationale for a Specific Diet from the Viewpoint of Sports Medicine and Sports Orthopedics. Relation to Stress Reaction and Regeneration]," *Der Orthopade* (German) 26 (1997): 942–950.

Laires, M.J., Madeira, F., Sergio, J., et al., "Preliminary Study of the Relationship between Plasma and Erythrocyte Magnesium Variations and Some Circulating Pro-Oxidant and Antioxidant Indices in a Standardized Physical Effort," *Magnesium Research* 6 (1993): 233–238.

Monteiro, C.P., Varela, A., Pinto, M., et al., "Effect of an Aerobic Training on Magnesium, Trace Elements and Antioxidant Systems in a Down Syndrome Population," *Magnesium Research* 10 (1997): 65–71.

Resina, A., Brettoni, M., Gatteschi, L., et al., "Changes in the Concentrations of Plasma and Erythrocyte Magnesium and of 2,3-Diphosphoglycerate during a Period of Aerobic Training," *European Journal of Applied Physiology and Occupational Physiology* 68 (1994): 390–394.

When Exercise Is Bad for You

Chadda, K.D., Cohen, J., Werner, B.M., et al., "Observations on Serum and Red Blood Cell Magnesium Changes in Treadmill Exercise–Induced Cardiac Ischemia," *Journal of the American College of Nutrition* 4 (1985): 157–163.

Konig, D., Keul, J., Northoff, H., et al., "[Rationale for a Specific Diet from the Viewpoint of Sports Medicine and Sports Orthopedics. Relation to Stress Reaction and Regeneration]," *Der Orthopade* (German) 26 (1997): 942–950.

Rayssiguier, Y., Guezennec, C.Y., and Durlach, J., "New Experimental and Clinical Data on the Relationship between Magnesium and Sport," *Magnesium Research* 3 (1990): 93–102.

How Magnesium Status Affects the Response to Exercise

Clarkson, P.M., and Haymes, E.M., "Exercise and Mineral Status of Athletes: Calcium, Magnesium, Phosphorus, and Iron," *Medicine and Science in Sports and Exercise* 27 (1995): 831–843.

Konig, D., Weinstock, C., Keul, J., et al., "Zinc, Iron, and Magnesium Status in Athletes—Influence on the Regulation of Exercise-Induced Stress and Immune Function," *Exercise Immunology Review* 4 (1998): 2–21.

Rayssiguier, Y., Guezennec, C.Y., and Durlach, J., "New Experimental and Clinical Data on the Relationship between Magnesium and Sport," *Magnesium Research* 3 (1990): 93–102.

Rosenfeldt, F.L., "Metabolic Supplementation with Orotic Acid and Magnesium Orotate," *Cardiovascular Drugs and Therapy* 12 (1998) (Supplement 2): 147–152.

Ruddel, H., Werner, C., and Ising, H., "Impact of Magnesium Supplementation on Performance Data in Young Swimmers," *Magnesium Research* 3 (1990): 103–107.

Shechter, M., Sharir, M., Labrador, M.J., et al., "Oral Magnesium Therapy Improves Endothelial Function in Patients with Coronary Artery Disease," *Circulation* 102 (2000): 2353–2358.

DO YOU REALLY NEED TO LOSE WEIGHT?

Overweight and Health Risks

Alpert, M.A., "Obesity Cardiomyopathy: Pathophysiology and Evolution of the Clinical Syndrome," *The American Journal of the Medical Sciences* 321 (2001): 225–236.

Andres, R., "Effect of Obesity on Total Mortality," *International Journal of Obesity* 4 (1980): 381–386.

Andres, R., "The Obesity-Mortality Association: Where is the Nadir of the U-Shaped Curve?" *Transactions of the Association of Life Insurance Medical Directors of America* 64 (1980): 185–197.

Bender, R., Jockel, K.H., Trautner, C., et al., "Effect of Age on Excess Mortality in Obesity," *Journal of the American Medical Association* 281 (1999): 1498–1504.

Bender, R., Trautner, C., Spraul, M., et al., "Assessment of Excess Mortality in Obesity," *American Journal of Epidemiology* 147 (1998): 42–48.

Burns, C.M., Tijhuis, M.A., and Seidell, J.C., "The Relationship between Quality of Life and Perceived Body Weight and Dieting History in Dutch Men and Women," *International Journal of Obesity and Related Metabolic Disorders* 25 (2001): 1386–1392.

Carmelli, D., Zhang, H., and Swan, G.E., "Obesity and 33-Year Follow-Up for Coronary Heart Disease and Cancer Mortality," *Epidemiology* 8 (1997): 378–383.

Choban, P.S., Weireter, L.J., Jr., and Maynes, C., "Obesity and Increased Mortality in Blunt Trauma," *The Journal of Trauma* 31 (1991): 1253–1257.

Croft, J.B., Keenan, N.L., Sheridan, D.P., et al., "Waist-to-Hip Ratio in a Biracial Population: Measurement, Implications, and Cautions for Using Guidelines to Define High Risk for Cardiovascular Disease," *Journal of the American Dietetic Association* 95 (1995): 60–64.

Gunnell, D.J., Frankel, S.J., Nanchahal, K., et al., "Childhood Obesity and Adult Cardiovascular Mortality: A 57-Year Follow-Up Study Based on the Boyd Orr Cohort," *American Journal of Clinical Nutrition* 67 (1998): 1111–1118.

Haapanen-Niemi, N., Miilunpalo, S., Pasanen, M., et al., "Body Mass Index, Physical Inactivity and Low Level of Physical Fitness as Determinants of All-Cause and Cardiovascular Disease Mortality—16-Year Follow-Up of Middle-Aged and Elderly Men and Women," *International Journal of Obesity and Related Metabolic Disorders* 24 (2000): 1465–1474.

Hodge, A.M., Dowse, G.K., Collins, V.R., et al., "Mortality in Micronesian Nauruans and Melanesian and Indian Fijians Is Not Associated with Obesity," *American Journal of Epidemiology* 143 (1996): 442–455.

Hoit, B.D., Gilpin, E.A., Maisel, A.A., et al., "Influence of Obesity on Morbidity and Mortality after Acute Myocardial Infarction," *American Heart Journal* 114 (1987): 1334–1341.

Katzmarzyk, P.T., Craig, C.L., and Bouchard, C., "Original Article Underweight, Overweight and Obesity: Relationships with Mortality in the 13-Year Follow-Up of the Canada Fitness Survey," *Journal of Clinical Epidemiology* 54 (2001): 916–920.

Kielmann, R., and Herpertz, S., "[Psychological Factors in Development and Treatment of Obesity]," *Herz* (German) 26 (2001): 185–193.

Lietz, K., John, R., Burke, E.A., et al., "Pretransplant Cachexia and Morbid Obesity are Predictors of Increased Mortality after Heart Transplantation," *Transplantation* 72 (2001): 277–283.

Maffeis, C., and Tato, L., "Long-Term Effects of Childhood Obesity on Morbidity and Mortality," *Hormone Research* 55 (2001) (Supplement 1): 42–45.

Pettitt, D.J., Lisse, J.R., Knowler, W.C., et al., "Mortality as a Function of Obesity and Diabetes Mellitus," *American Journal of Epidemiology* 115 (1982): 359–366.

Schroder, T., Nolte, M., Kox, W.J., et al., "[Anesthesia in Extreme Obesity]," *Herz* (German) 26 (2001): 222–228.

Seftel, H.C., "The Rarity of Coronary

Heart Disease in South African Blacks," *South African Medical Journal* 54 (1978): 99–105.

Solomon, C.G., Manson, J.E., "Obesity and Mortality: A Review of the Epidemiologic Data," *American Journal of Clinical Nutrition* 66 (1997): 1044S–1050S.

Xavier Pi-Sunyer, F., "Obesity," in *Modern Nutrition in Health and Disease*, 9th ed., ed. Maurice E. Shils, James A. Olson, Moshe Shike, and Catherine A. Ross (Philadelphia: Lippincott Williams & Wilkins, 1999): p. 1396.

Weight Loss and Cardiovascular Risk

Fisler, J.S., "Cardiac Effects of Starvation and Semistarvation Diets: Safety and Mechanisms of Action," *American Journal of Clinical Nutrition* 56 (1992): 230S–234S.

National Task Force on the Prevention and Treatment of Obesity, "Weight Cycling," *Journal of the American Medical Association* 272 (1994): 1196–1202.

Resnick, L.M., Militianu, D., Cunnings, A.J., et al., "Direct Magnetic Resonance Determination of Aortic Distensibility in Essential Hypertension: Relation to Age, Abdominal Visceral Fat, and In Situ Intracellular Free Magnesium," *Hypertension* 30 (1997): 654–659.

Singh, R.B., Rastogi, V., Rastogi, S.S., et al., "Effect of Diet and Moderate Exercise on Central Obesity and Associated Disturbances, Myocardial Infarction and Mortality in Patients with and without Coronary Artery Disease," *Journal of the American College of Nutrition* 15 (1996): 592–601.

Weinsier, R.L., Wilson, L.J., and Lee, J., "Medically Safe Rate of Weight Loss for the Treatment of Obesity: A Guideline Based on Risk of Gallstone Formation," *The American Journal of Medicine* 98 (1995): 115–117.

Williamson, D.F., Serdula, M.K., Anda, R.F., et al., "Weight Loss Attempts in Adults: Goals, Duration, and Rate of Weight Loss," *The American Journal of Public Health* 82 (1992): 1251–1257.

Weight Loss and Life Expectancy

Alexander, J.K., "Obesity and Coronary Heart Disease," *The American Journal of the Medical Sciences* 321 (2001): 215–224.

Allison, D.B., Zannolli, R., Faith, M.S., et al., "Weight Loss Increases and Fat Loss Decreases All-Cause Mortality Rate: Results from Two Independent Cohort Studies," *International Journal of Obesity and Related Metabolic Disorders* 23 (1999): 603–611.

French, S.A., Folsom, A.R., Jeffery, R.W., et al., "Prospective Study of Intentionality of Weight Loss and Mortality in Older Women: The Iowa Women's Health Study," *American Journal of Epidemiology* 149 (1999): 504–514.

Iribarren, C., Sharp, D.S., Burchfiel, C.M., et al., "Association of Weight Loss and Weight Fluctuation with Mortality among Japanese American Men," *The New England Journal of Medicine* 333 (1995): 686–692.

Pamuk, E.R., Williamson, D.F., Madans, J., et al., "Weight Loss and Mortality in a National Cohort of Adults, 1971–1987," *American Journal of Epidemiology* 136 (1992): 686–697.

Payette, H., Coulombe, C., Boutier, V., et al., "Weight Loss and Mortality among Free-Living Frail Elders: A Prospective Study," *The Journals of Gerontology. Series A, Biological Sciences and Medical Sciences* 54 (1999): M440–M445.

Ryan, C., Bryant, E., Eleazer, P., et al., "Unintentional Weight Loss in Long-Term Care: Predictor of Mortality in the Elderly," *Southern Medical Journal* 88 (1995): 721–724.

Williamson, D.F., "Weight Cycling and Mortality: How Do the Epidemiologists Explain the Role of Intentional Weight Loss?" *Journal of the American College of Nutrition* 15 (1996): 6–13.

Williamson, D.F., "Intentional Weight Loss: Patterns in the General Population and its Association with Morbidity and Mortality," *International Journal of Obesity and Related Metabolic Disorders* 21 (1997) (Supplement 1): S14–S19; discussion S20–S21.

Williamson, D.F., Pamuk, E., Thun, M., et al., "Prospective Study of Intentional Weight Loss and Mortality in Never-Smoking Overweight U.S. White Women Aged 40–64 Years," *American Journal of Epidemiology* 141 (1995): 1128–1141.

Yaari, S., and Goldbourt, U., "Voluntary and Involuntary Weight Loss: Associations with Long Term Mortality in 9,228 Middle-Aged and Elderly Men," *American Journal of Epidemiology* 148 (1998): 546–555.

THE RISING TREND OF OBESITY—A WORLDWIDE EPIDEMIC?

Eckersley, R.M., "Losing the Battle of the Bulge: Causes and Consequences of Increasing Obesity," *Medical Journal of Australia* 174 (2001): 590–592.

Flegal, K.M., "The Obesity Epidemic in Children and Adults: Current Evidence and Research Issues," *Medicine and Science in Sports and Exercise* 31 (1999): S509–S514.

James, W.P., "The Epidemiology of Obesity," *Ciba Foundation Symposium* 201 (1996): 1–11; discussion 11–16, 32–36.

Lyznicki, J.M., Young, D.C., Riggs, J.A., et al., "Obesity: Assessment and Management in Primary Care," *American Family Physician* 63 (2001): 2185–2196.

Ulmer, H., Diem, G., Bischof, H.P., et al., "Recent Trends and Sociodemographic Distribution of Cardiovascular Risk Factors: Results from Two Population Surveys in the Austrian WHO CINDI Demonstration Area," *Wiener Klinische Wochenschrift* (German) 113 (2001): 573–579.

IF YOU DECIDE YOU WANT TO LOSE WEIGHT

American Heart Association, *Your Heart: American Heart Association's Complete Guide to Heart Health, An Owner's Manual* (Prentice Hall Trade, 1995).

American Heart Association, *American Heart Association Low-Fat, Low-Cholesterol Cook Book: Heart-Healthy, Easy-To-Make Recipes That Taste Great,* 2nd ed. (New York: Clarkson Potter, 1997).

Appleton, Nancy, *Lick the Sugar Habit* (New York: Avery/Penguin Putnam, 1996).

Atkins, Robert C., *Dr. Atkins' New Diet Revolution* (New York: Avon Books, 1992).

Bruch Hilde, *Eating Disorders: Obesity, Anorexia Nervosa, and the Person Within* (New York: Basic Books, Inc., 1973).

Bruch, Hilde, *The Golden Cage: The Enigma of Anorexia Nervosa* (Cambridge, MA: Harvard University Press, 1978).

Cooper, Kenneth H., *The Aerobics Program for Total Well-Being: Exercise, Diet, Emotional Balance* (New York: Bantam Books, 1983).

Cooper, Kenneth H., *Aerobics* (New York: Bantam Books, 1988).

Harrup, T., and Hansen, B., "Substance Dependency—Food Dependency," in *Health Promotion in the Workplace,* ed. M.P. O'Donnell and T. Ainsworth (New York: John Wiley & Sons, 1984), pp. 456–462.

Heller Richard F., and Heller, Rachael F., *The Carbohydrate Addict's Diet* (New York: Signet Penguin Books, 1993).

Monteforte, M.J., and Turkelson, C.M., "Bariatric Surgery for Morbid Obesity," *Obesity Surgery* 10 (2000): 391–401.

Ornish, Dean, *Dr. Dean Ornish's Program for Reversing Heart Disease,* reprint ed. (New York: Ivy Books, 1996).

Reaven, Gerald, Strom, Terry Kristen, and Fox, Barry, *Syndrome X: The Silent Killer* (New York: Simon & Schuster, 2000).

Sjostrom, L., "Surgical Intervention as a Strategy for Treatment of Obesity," *Endocrine* 13 (2000): 213–230.

Steward, H. L., Bethea, M. C., Andrews, S. S., et al., *Sugar Busters! Cut Sugar to Trim Fat* (New York: Ballantine Books, 1998).

Svetkey, L.P., Simons-Morton, D., Vollmer, W.M., et al., "Effects of Dietary Patterns on Blood Pressure: Subgroup Analysis of the Dietary Approaches to Stop Hypertension (DASH) Randomized Clinical Trial," *Archives of Internal Medicine* 159 (1999): 285–293.

Wangsness, M., "Pharmacological Treatment of Obesity. Past, Present, and Future," *Minnesota Medicine* 83 (2000): 21–26.

Chapter Five

FAT, CHOLESTEROL, AND MAGNESIUM

WHAT IS CHOLESTEROL?

Boden, W.E., "High-Density Lipoprotein Cholesterol as an Independent Risk Factor in Cardiovascular Disease: Assessing the Data from Framingham to the Veterans Affairs High-Density Lipoprotein Intervention Trial," *The American Journal of Cardiology* 86 (2000): 19L–22L.

Castelli, W.P., Doyle, J.T., Gordon, T., et al., "HDL Cholesterol and Other Lipids in Coronary Heart Disease. The Cooperative Lipoprotein Phenotyping Study," *Circulation* 55 (1977): 767–772.

Erasmus, Udo, *Fats That Heal, Fats That Kill* (Burnaby, BC, Canada: Alive Books, 1993).

Lehninger, Albert L., *Principles of Biochemistry* (New York: Worth Publishers, Inc., 1982).

THE EFFECT OF MAGNESIUM INTAKE ON CHOLESTEROL

Corica, F., Allegra, A., Di Benedetto, A., et al., "Effects of Oral Magnesium Supplementation on Plasma Lipid Concentrations in Patients with Non-Insulin-Dependent Diabetes Mellitus," *Magnesium Research* 7 (1994): 43–47.

De Leeuw, I., Engelen, W., Vertommen J., et al., "Effect of Intensive I.V. + Oral Magnesium Supplementation on Circulating Ion Levels, Lipid Parameters and Metabolic Control in Mg-Depleted Insulin-Dependent Diabetic Patients (IDDM)," *Magnesium Research* 10 (1997): 135–141.

Djurhuus, M.S., Henriksen, J.E., Klitgaard, N.A., et al., "Effect of Moderate Improvement in Metabolic Control on Magnesium and Lipid Concentrations in Patients with Type 1 Diabetes," *Diabetes Care* 22 (1999): 546–554.

Gupta, B.K., Glicklich, D., and Tellis, V.A., "Magnesium Repletion Therapy Improved Lipid Metabolism in Hypomagnesemic Renal Transplant Recipients: A Pilot Study," *Transplantation* 67, (1999): 1485–1487.

Hagg, E., Carlberg, B.C., Hillorn, V.S., et al., "Magnesium Therapy in Type 1 Diabetes. A Double Blind Study Concerning the Effects on Kidney Function and Serum Lipid Levels," *Magnesium Research* 12 (1999): 123–130.

Helbig, J.. "[Serum Magnesium Levels in Subjects on a Low Calorie Diet with and without Magnesium Replacement]," *Magnesium Bulletin* 1 (1979): 167–169.

Hoogerbrugge, N., Cobbaert, C., de Heide, L., et al., "Oral Physiological Magnesium Supplementation for 6 Weeks with 1 g/d Magnesium Oxide Does Not Affect Increased Lp(a) Levels in Hypercholesterolaemic Subjects," *Magnesium Research* 9 (1996): 129–132.

Kisters, K., Hausberg, M., Tokmak, F., et al., "Hypomagnesaemia, Borderline Hypertension and Hyperlipidaemia," *Magnesium Bulletin* 21 (1999): 31–34.

Knipscheer, H.C., Kindt, I., van den Ende, A., et al., "Magnesium Pyridoxal-5'-Phosphate Glutamate, 'A Vitamin B_6 Derivative,' Does Not Affect Lipoprotein Levels in Patients with Familial Hypercholesterolaemia," *European Journal of Clinical Pharmacology* 51 (1997): 499–503.

Marken, P.A., Weart, C.W., Carson, D.S., et al., "Effects of Magnesium Oxide on the Lipid Profile of Healthy Volunteers," *Atherosclerosis* 77 (1989): 37–42.

Parsons, R.S., Butler, T.C., and Sellars, E.P., "The Treatment of Coronary Artery Disease," *Medical Proceedings* 5 (1959): 487–498.

Parsons, R.S., Butler, T.C., and Sellars, E.P., "Coronary Artery Disease. Further Investigations on its Treatment with Parenteral Magnesium Sulphate and Incorporating Minimal Doses of Heparin," *Medical Proceedings* 6 (1960): 479–486.

Purvis, J.R., Cummings, D.M., Landsman, P., et al., "Effect of Oral Magnesium Supplementation on Selected Cardiovascular Risk Factors in Non-Insulin-Dependent Diabetics," *Archives of Family Medicine* 3 (1994): 503–508.

Seelig, M.S., and Vitale, J.J., "Lipids and Magnesium Deficit," in *Proceedings of the First International Symposium on Magnesium (Vittel, France)*, ed. Jean Durlach, pp. 515–522.

Singh, R.B., Rastogi, S.S., Mani, U.V., et al., "Does Dietary Magnesium Modulate Blood Lipids?" *Biological Trace Element Research* 30 (1991): 59–64.

HOW MAGNESIUM CONTROLS COMPONENTS OF BLOOD CHOLESTEROL

Magnesium and Enzyme Regulation—HMG CoA Reductase

Beg, Z.H., Stonik, J.A., and Brewer, H.B., Jr., "3-Hydroxy-3-Methylglutaryl Coenzyme A Reductase: Regulation of Enzymatic Activity by Phosphorylation and Dephosphorylation," *Proceedings of the National Academy of Sciences of the United States of America* 75 (1978): 3678–3682.

Beg, Z.H., Stonik, J.A., and Brewer, H.B.,

Jr. "In Vivo Modulation of Rat Liver 3-Hydroxy-3-Methylglutaryl-Coenzyme A Reductase, Reductase Kinase, and Reductase Kinase Kinase by Mevalonolactone," *Proceedings of the National Academy of Sciences of the United States of America* 81 (1984): 7293–7297.

Beg, Z.H., Stonik, J.A., and Brewer, H.B., Jr., "Human Hepatic 3-hydroxy-3-Methylglutaryl Coenzyme A Reductase: Evidence for the Regulation of Enzymic Activity by a Bicyclic Phosphorylation Cascade," *Biochemical and Biophysical Research Communications* 119 (1984): 488–498.

Chow, J.D., Higgins, M.J.P., and Rudney, H., "The Inhibitory Effect of ATP on HMG CoA Reductase," *Biochemical and Biophysical Research Communications* 63 (1975): 1077–1084.

Field, F.J., Henning, B., and Mathur, S.N., "In Vitro Regulation of 3-Hydroxy-3-Methylglutarylcoenzyme A Reductase and Acylcoenzyme A: Cholesterol Acyltransferase Activities by Phosphorylation-Dephosphorylation in Rabbit Intestine," *Biochimica et Biophysica Acta* 802 (1984): 9–16.

Gil, G., Calvet, V.E., Asins, G., et al., "Inactivation of Rat Liver HMG-CoA Reductase Phosphatases by Nucleotides," *Revista Espanola de Fisiologia* (Spanish) 39 (1983): 259–266.

Gil, G., Calvet, V.E., Ferrer, A., et al., "Inactivation and Reactivation of Rat Liver 3-Hydroxy-3-Methylglutaryl-CoA-Reductase Phosphatases: Effect of Phosphate, Pyrophosphate and Divalent Cations," *Hoppe-Seyler's Zeitschrift für Physiologische Chemie* 363 (1982): 1217–1224.

Harwood, H.J., Jr., Schneider, M., and Stacpoole, P.W., Regulation of Human Leukocyte Microsomal Hydroxymethylglutaryl-CoA Reductase Activity by a Phosphorylation and Dephosphorylation Mechanism," *Biochimica et Biophysica Acta* 805 (1984): 245–251.

Kumar, A.R., and Kurup, P.A., "Membrane Na+ K+ ATPase Inhibition Related Dyslipidemia and Insulin Resistance in Neuropsychiatric Disorders," *Indian Journal of Physiology and Pharmacology* 45 (2001): 296–304.

Rieder, vH., "[The effect of Magnesium on Serum Cholesterol Levels]," *Magnesium Bulletin* (German) 1 (1980): 56–60.

Schroepfer, G.J., Jr., Parish, E.J., Kandutsch, A.A., et al., "15 Beta-Methyl-5 Alpha,14 Beta-Cholest-7-ene-3 Beta,15 Alpha-Diol. Synthesis, Structure, and Inhibition of Sterol Synthesis in Animal Cells," *Biochemistry International* 15 (1987): 403–408.

Magnesium and HDL, LDL Cholesterol Levels

Davis, W.H., Leary, W.P., Reyes, A.J., et al., "Monotherapy with Magnesium Increases Abnormally Low High Density Lipoprotein Cholesterol: A Clinical Assay," *Current Therapeutic Research* 36 (1984): 341–344.

Djurhuus, M.S., Henriksen, J.E., Klitgaard, N.A., et al., "Effect of Moderate Improvement in Metabolic Control on Magnesium and Lipid Concentrations in Patients with Type 1 Diabetes," *Diabetes Care* 22 (1999): 546–554.

Djurhuus, M.S., Klitgaard, N.A., Pedersen, K.K., et al., "Magnesium Reduces Insulin-Stimulated Glucose Uptake and Serum Lipid Concentrations in type 1 Diabetes," *Metabolism* 50 (2001): 1409–1417.

Field, F.J., Henning, B., and Mathur, S.N., In Vitro Regulation of 3-Hydroxy-3-Methylglutarylcoenzyme A Reductase and Acylcoenzyme A: Cholesterol Acyltransferase Activities by Phosphorylation-Dephosphorylation in Rabbit Intestine," *Biochimica et Biophysica Acta* 802 (1984): 9–16.

Itoh, K., Kawasaka, T., and Nakamura, M., "The Effects of High Oral Magnesium Supplementation on Blood Pressure, Serum Lipids and Related Variables in Apparently Healthy Japanese Subjects," *The British Journal of Nutrition* 78 (1997): 737–750.

Rasmussen, H.S., Aurup, P., Goldstein, K., et al., "Influence of Magnesium Substitution Therapy on Blood Lipid Composition in Patients with Ischemic Heart Disease. A Double-Blind, Placebo Controlled Study," *Archives of Internal Medicine* 149 (1989): 1050–1053.

Singh, R.B., Rastogi, S.S., Sharma, V.K., et al., "Can Dietary Magnesium Modulate

Lipoprotein Metabolism?" *Magnesium and Trace Elements* 9 (1990): 255–264.

THE PLAQUE THEORY OF ARTERIOSCLEROSIS AND MAGNESIUM

Altura, B.M., and Altura, B.T., "Magnesium and Cardiovascular Biology: An Important Link between Cardiovascular Risk Factors and Atherogenesis," *Cellular and Molecular Biology Research* 41 (1995): 347–359.

Bloom, S., "Coronary Arterial Lesions in Mg-Deficient Hamsters," *Magnesium* 4 (1985): 82–95.

Enos, W.F., and Beyer, J.C., "Coronary Artery Disease in Younger Men," *Journal of the American Medical Association* 218 (1971): 1434.

Enos, W.F., Holmes, R.H., and Beyer, J., "Landmark Article, July 18, 1953: Coronary Disease among United States Soldiers Killed in Action in Korea. Preliminary Report. By William F. Enos, Robert H. Holmes and James Beyer," *Journal of the American Medical Association* 256 (1986): 2859–2862.

Gruberg, Edward P., and Raymond, Stephen A., *Beyond Cholesterol: Vitamin B_6, Arteriosclerosis, and Your Heart* (New York: St. Martin's Press, 1981).

Jellinek, H., and Takacs, E., "[Course of the Progression of Experimentally Induced Arteriosclerotic Vessel Wall Changes after Treatment with Magnesium Orotate]," *Arzneimittelforschung* 50 (2000): 1071–1077.

Orimo, H., and Ouchi, Y., "The Role of Calcium and Magnesium in the Development of Atherosclerosis. Experimental and Clinical Evidence," *Annals of the New York Academy of Sciences* 598 (1990): 444–457.

Rayssiguier, Y., "Role of Magnesium and Potassium in the Pathogenesis of Arteriosclerosis," *Magnesium* 3 (1984): 226–238.

Rigo, J., "The Relationship between Magnesium and the Vascular System," in *Proceedings of the First International Symposium on Magnesium (Vittel, France)*, ed. Jean Durlach, pp. 215–228.

Shechter, M., Bairey Merz, C.N., Paul-Labrador, M.J., et al., "Plasma Apolipoprotein B Levels Predict Platelet-Dependent Thrombosis in Patients with Coronary Artery Disease," *Cardiology* 92 (1999): 151–155.

Sherer, Y., Shoenfeld, Y., Shaish, A., et al., "Suppression of Atherogenesis in Female Low-Density Lipoprotein Receptor Knockout Mice Following Magnesium Fortification of Drinking Water: The Importance of Diet," *Pathobiology* 68 (2000): 93–98.

Stehbens, W.E., "Coronary Heart Disease, Hypercholesterolemia, and Atherosclerosis. II. Misrepresented Data," *Experimental and Molecular Pathology* 70 (2001): 120–139.

The Effect of Fat Intake on Magnesium Absorption

Connor, W.E., and Connor, S.L., "The Key Role of Nutritional Factors in the Prevention of Coronary Heart Disease," *Preventive Medicine* 1 (1972): 49–83.

Fourman, P., and Morgan, D.B., "Chronic Magnesium Deficiency," *The Proceedings of the Nutrition Society* 21 (1962): 34–41.

Hathaway, M.L., *Magnesium in Human Nutrition,* Home Economics Research Report No. 19 (Washington, D.C.: Agricultural Research Service, U.S. Department of Agriculture, 1962).

Irwin, M.I., and Wiese, H.F., "Variations in Linoleic Acid Content of Dietary Fat in Relation to Metabolism of Fat, Nitrogen and Minerals, and to Changes in Blood Lipids," *The Journal of Nutrition* 74 (1961): 217–225.

MacBeth, R.A.L., and Mabbott, J., "Magnesium Balance in the Postoperative Patient," *Surgery, Gynecology, and Obstetrics* 118 (1964): 748–760.

Ovesen, L., Chu, R., and Howard, L., "The Influence of Dietary Fat on Hejunostomy Output in Patients with Severe Short Bowel Syndrome," *American Journal of Clinical Nutrition* 38 (1983): 270–277.

Sawyer, M., Baumann, L., and Stevens, F., "Studies of Acid Production. II. The Mineral Loss during Acidosis," *The Journal of Biological Chemistry* 33 (1918): 103–109.

Seelig, M.S., "The Requirement of Magnesium by the Normal Adult," *American Journal of Clinical Nutrition* 14 (1964): 342–390.

How High Cholesterol Became the Enemy

Connor, W.E., Stone, D.B., and Hodges, R.E., "The Interrelated Effects of Dietary

Cholesterol and Fat upon Human Serum Lipid Levels," *Journal of Clinical Investigations* 43 (1964): 1691–1696.

Flynn, M.A., Nolph, G.B., Flynn, T.C., et al., "Effect of Dietary Egg on Human Serum Cholesterol and Triglycerides," *American Journal of Clinical Nutrition* 32 (1979): 1051–1057.

Frank, G.C., Berenson, G.S., and Webber, L.S., "Dietary Studies and the Relationship of Diet to Cardiovascular Disease Risk Factor Variables in 10-Year-Old Children—The Bogalusa Heart Study," *American Journal of Clinical Nutrition* 31 (1978): 328–340.

Gruberg, Edward P., and Raymond, Stephen A., *Beyond Cholesterol: Vitamin B_6, Arteriosclerosis, and Your Heart* (New York: St. Martin's Press, 1981).

Hooper, L., Summerbell, C.D., Higgins, J.P., et al., "Dietary Fat Intake and Prevention of Cardiovascular Disease: Systematic Review," *British Medical Journal* 322 (2001): 757–763.

Hulley, S.B., "A National Program for Lowering High Blood Cholesterol," *American Journal of Obstetrics and Gynecology* 158 (1988): 1561–1567.

Jellinek, H., and Takacs, E., "[Course of the Progression of Experimentally Induced Arteriosclerotic Vessel Wall Changes after Treatment with Magnesium Orotate]," *Arzneimittelforschung* (German) 50 (2000): 1071–1077.

Kahn, H.A., Medalie, J.H., Neufeld, H.N., et al., "Serum Cholesterol: Its Distribution and Association with Dietary and Other Variables in a Survey of 10,000 Men," *Israel Journal of Medical Sciences* 5 (1969): 1117–1127.

Kannel, W.B., McGee, D., and Gordon, T., "A General Cardiovascular Risk Profile: The Framingham Study, *The American Journal of Cardiology* 38 (1976): 46–51.

Katerndahl, D.A., and Lawler, W.R., "Variability in Meta-Analytic Results Concerning the Value of Cholesterol Reduction in Coronary Heart Disease: A Meta-Meta-Analysis," *American Journal of Epidemiology* 149 (1999): 429–441.

Kmietowicz, Z., "Cholesterol Screening Is Not Worth While," *British Medical Journal* 316 (1998): 725.

Kristenson, M., Zieden, B., Kucinskiene, Z., et al., "Antioxidant State and Mortality from Coronary Heart Disease in Lithuanian and Swedish Men: Concomitant Cross Sectional Study of Men Aged 50," *British Medical Journal* 314 (1997): 629–633.

Lamarche, B., Tchernof, A., Mauriege, P., et al., "Fasting Insulin and Apolipoprotein B Levels and Low-Density Lipoprotein Particle Size as Risk Factors for Ischemic Heart Disease," *Journal of the American Medical Association* 279 (1998): 1955–1961.

Mann, J.I., Appleby, P.N., Key, T.J., et al., "Dietary Determinants of Ischaemic Heart Disease in Health Conscious Individuals," *Heart* 78 (1997): 450–455.

Nichols, A.B., Ravenscroft, C., Lamphiear, D.E., et al., "Independence of Serum Lipid Levels and Dietary Habits. The Tecumseh Study," *Journal of the American Medical Association* 236 (1976): 1948–1953.

Parsons, R.S., "The Biochemical Changes Associated with Coronary Artery Disease Treated with Magnesium Sulphate," *Medical Journal of Australia* 1 (1958): 883–884.

Porter, M.W., Yamanaka, W., Carlson, S.D., et al., "Effect of Dietary Egg on Serum Cholesterol and Triglyceride of Human Males," *American Journal of Clinical Nutrition* 30 (1977): 490–495.

Smith, D., "Cardiovascular Disease: A Historic Perspective," *The Japanese Journal of Veterinary Research* 48 (2000): 147–166.

Stehbens, W.E., "Coronary Heart Disease, Hypercholesterolemia, and Atherosclerosis. I. False Premises," *Experimental and Molecular Pathology* 7- (2001): 103–119.

Stehbens, W.E., "Coronary Heart Disease, Hypercholesterolemia, and Atherosclerosis. II. Misrepresented Data," *Experimental and Molecular Pathology* 70 (2001): 120–139.

Steinberg, D., and Gotto, A.M., Jr., "Preventing Coronary Artery Disease by Lowering Cholesterol Levels: Fifty Years from Bench to Bedside," *Journal of the American Medical Association* 282 (1999): 2043–2050.

Stulb, S.C., McDonough, J.R., Greenberg, B.G., et al., "The Relationship of Nutrient Intake and Exercise to Serum Cholesterol Levels in White Males in Evans County, Georgia," *American Journal of Clinical Nutrition* 16 (1965): 328–242.

Szelenyi, I., "Physiological Interrelationship Between Magnesium and the Heart," in *Proceedings of the First International Symposium on Magnesium (Vittel, France),* ed. Jean Durlach, pp. 195–211.

Whyte, M., Nestel, P., and MacGregor, A., "Cholesterol Metabolism in Papua New Guineans," *European Journal of Clinical Investigation* 7 (1977): 53–60.

The True Benefit of a Low-Fat, Low-Cholesterol Diet

Atkins, Robert C, *Dr. Atkins' New Diet Revolution* (New York: Avon Books, 1992).

Bershon, I., and Oelofse, P., "Correlation of Serum-Magnesium and Serum-Cholesterol Levels in South Aftican Bantu and European Subjects," *Lancet* (1957): 1020–1021.

Booyens, J., de Waal, V.M., and Rademeyer, L.J., "The Effect of Dietary Maize Meal Supplementation on the Levels of Serum Cholesterol and Magnesium," *South African Medical Journal* 40 (1966): 237–239.

Dougherty, R.M., Fong, A.K., and Iacono, J.M., "Nutrient Content of the Diet When the Fat Is Reduced," *American Journal of Clinical Nutrition* 48 (1988): 970–979.

Elliot, B., Roeser, H.P., Warrell, A., et al., "Effect of a High Energy, Low Carbohydrate Diet on Serum Levels of Lipids and Lipoproteins," *Medical Journal of Australia* 1 (1981): 237–240.

Franklin, T.L., Kolasa, K.M., Griffin, K., et al., "Adherence to Very-Low-Fat Diet by a Group of Cardiac Rehabilitation Patients in the Rural Southeastern United States," *Archives of Family Medicine* 4 (1995): 551–554.

Hughes, K., "Diet and Coronary Heart Disease—A Review," *Annals of the Academy of Medicine, Singapore* 24 (1995): 224–229.

Kris-Etherton, P., Eissenstat, B., Jaax, S., et al., "Validation for MEDFICTS, a Dietary Assessment Instrument for Evaluating Adherence to Total and Saturated Fat Recommendations of the National Cholesterol Education Program Step 1 and Step 2 Diets," *Journal of the American Dietetic Association* 101 (2001): 81–86.

McCarron, D.A., Oparil, S., Chait, A., et al., "Nutritional Management of Cardiovascular Risk Factors. A Randomized Clinical Trial," *Archives of Internal Medicine* 157 (1997): 169–177.

Metz, J.A., Kris-Etherton, P.M., Morris, C.D., et al., "Dietary Compliance and Cardiovascular Risk Reduction with a Prepared Meal Plan Compared with a Self-Selected Diet," *American Journal of Clinical Nutrition* 66 (1997): 373–385.

Nieman, D.C., Underwood, B.C., Sherman, K.M., et al., "Dietary Status of Seventh-Day Adventist Vegetarian and Nonvegetarian Elderly Women," *Journal of the American Dietetic Association* 89 (1989): 1763–1769.

Ornish, Dean, *Dr. Dean Ornish's Program for Reversing Heart Disease,* reprint ed. (New York: Ivy Books, 1996).

Ornish, D., Scherwitz, L.W., Billings, J.H., et al., "Intensive Lifestyle Changes for Reversal of Coronary Heart Disease," *Journal of the American Medical Association* 280 (1998): 2001–2007.

"Ornish Lifestyle Modification Program Continues to Produce Impressive Outcomes for CHD," *Healthcare Demand and Disease Management* 3 (1997): 59–61.

Retzlaff, B.M., Dowdy, A.A., Walden, C.E., et al., "Changes in Vitamin and Mineral Intakes and Serum Concentrations among Free-Living men on Cholesterol-Lowering Diets: The Dietary Alternatives Study," *American Journal of Clinical Nutrition* 53 (1991): 890–898.

Retzlaff, B.M., Walden, C.E., McNeney, W.B., et al., "Nutritional Intake of Women and Men on the NCEP Step I and Step II Diets," *Journal of the American College of Nutrition* 16 (1997): 52–61.

Sacks, F.M., Ornish, D., Rosner, B., et al., "Plasma Lipoprotein Levels in Vegetarians. The Effect of Ingestion of Fats from Dairy Products," *Journal of the American Medical Association* 254 (1985): 1337–1341.

Schaefer, E.J., Lamon-Fava, S., Ausman, L.M., et al., "Individual Variability in Lipoprotein Cholesterol Response to National Cholesterol Education Program Step 2 Diets," *American Journal of Clinical Nutrition* 65 (1997): 823–830.

Walden, C.E., Retzlaff, B.M., Buck, B.L., et al., "Lipoprotein Lipid Response to the National Cholesterol Education Program step II Diet by Hypercholesterolemic and Combined Hyperlipidemic Women and Men," *Arteriosclerosis, Thrombosis, and Vascular Biology* 17 (1997): 375–382.

Willi, S.M., Oexmann, M.J., Wright, N.M., et al., "The Effects of a High-Protein, Low-Fat, Ketogenic Diet on Adolescents with Morbid Obesity: Body Composition, Blood Chemistries, and Sleep Abnormalities," *Pediatrics* 101 (1998): 61–77.

Problems with Low-Fat, Low-Cholesterol Diets

Knopp, R.H., Walden, C.E., Retzlaff, B.M., et al., "Long-Term Cholesterol-Lowering Effects of 4 Fat-Restricted Diets in Hypercholesterolemic and Combined Hyperlipidemic Men. The Dietary Alternatives Study," *Journal of the American Medical Association* 278 (1997): 1509–1515.

Knopp, R.H., Retzlaff, B., Walden, C., et al., "One-Year Effects of Increasingly Fat-Restricted, Carbohydrate-Enriched Diets on Lipoprotein Levels in Free-Living Subjects," *Proceedings of the Society for Experimental Biology and Medicine* 225 (2000): 191–199.

CHOLESTEROL-LOWERING DRUGS COMPARED WITH MAGNESIUM

The Effects of Statin Drugs

Aengevaeren, W.R., Uijen, G.J., Jukema, J.W., et al., "Functional Evaluation of Lipid-Lowering Therapy by Pravastatin in the Regression Growth Evaluation Statin Study (REGRESS)," *Circulation* 96 (1997): 429–435.

Aguilar-Salinas, C.A., Barrett, H., and Schonfeld, G., "Metabolic Modes of Action of the Statins in the Hyperlipoproteinemias," *Atherosclerosis* 141 (1998): 203–207.

Ballantyne, C.M., "Reducing Atherothrombotic Events in High-Risk Patients: Recent Data on Therapy with Statins and Fatty Acids," *Current Atherosclerosis Reports* 1 (1999): 6–8.

Blauw, G.J., Lagaay, A.M., Smelt, A.H., et al., "Stroke, Statins, and Cholesterol. A Meta-Analysis of Randomized, Placebo-Controlled, Double-Blind Trials with HMG-CoA Reductase Inhibitors," *Stroke* 28 (1997): 946–950.

Bucher, H.C., Griffith, L.E., and Guyatt, G.H., "Systematic Review on the Risk and Benefit of Different Cholesterol-Lowering Interventions," *Arteriosclerosis, Thrombosis, and Vascular Biology* 19 (1999): 187–195.

Chen, H., Ikeda, U., Shimpo, M., et al., "Direct Effects of Statins on Cells Primarily Involved in Atherosclerosis," *Hypertension Research* 23 (2000): 187–192.

Davignon, J., "Advances in Drug Treatment of Dyslipidemia: Focus on Atorvastatin," *Canadian Journal of Cardiology* 14 (1998) (Supplement B): 28B–38B.

de Groot, E., Jukema, J.W., van Boven, A.J., et al., "Effect of Pravastatin on Progression and Regression of Coronary Atherosclerosis and Vessel Wall Changes in Carotid and Femoral Arteries: A Report from the Regression Growth Evaluation Statin Study," *The American Journal of Cardiology* 76 (1995): 40C–46C.

Dotani, M.I., Elnicki, D.M., Jain, A.C., et al., "Effect of Preoperative Statin Therapy and Cardiac Outcomes after Coronary Artery Bypass Grafting," *The American Journal of Cardiology* 86 (2000): 1128–1130, A6.

Downs, J.R., Clearfield, M., Tyroler, H.A., et al., "Air Force/Texas Coronary Atherosclerosis Prevention Study (AFCAPS/TEXCAPS): Additional Perspectives on Tolerability of Long-Term Treatment with Lovastatin," *The American Journal of Cardiology* 87 (2001): 1074–1079.

Ellen, R.L., and McPherson, R., "Long-Term Efficacy and Safety of Fenofibrate and a Statin in the Treatment of Combined Hyperlipidemia," *The American Journal of Cardiology* 81 (1998): 60B–65B.

Faggiotto, A., and Paoletti, R., "Do Pleiotropic Effects of Statins Beyond Lipid Alterations Exist In Vivo? What Are They and How Do They Differ Between Statins?" *Current Atherosclerosis Reports* 2 (2000): 20–25.

Feher, M.D., Foxton, J., Banks, D., et al., "Long-Term Safety of Statin-Fibrate Combination Treatment in the Management of Hypercholesterolaemia in Patients with Coronary Artery Disease," *British Heart Journal* (1995): 74:14–7.

Finardi, G., Perani, G., Tramarin, R., et al., "[Effectiveness and Tolerability of Simvastatin in Subjects with Primary Hypercholesterolemia. Multicenter Study]," *La Clinica Terapeutica* (Italian) 142 (1993): 225–233.

Garnett, W.R., "A Review of Current Clinical Findings with Fluvastatin," *The American Journal of Cardiology* 78 (1996): 20–25.

GISSI (Gruppo Italiano per lo Studio della Sopravvivenza nell'Infarto Miocardico) Prevenzione Investigators, "Results of the Low-Dose (20 mg) Pravastatin GISSI Prevenzione Trial in 4271 Patients with Recent Myocardial Infarction: Do Stopped Trials Contribute to Overall Knowledge?," *Italian Heart Journal* 1 (2000): 810–820.

Hay, J.W., Yu, W.M., and Ashraf, T., "Pharmacoeconomics of Lipid-Lowering Agents for Primary and Secondary Prevention of Coronary Artery Disease," *Pharmacoeconomics* 15 (1999): 47–74.

Hebert, P.R., Gaziano, J.M., Chan, K.S., et al., "Cholesterol Lowering with Statin Drugs, Risk of Stroke, and Total Mortality. An Overview of Randomized Trials," *Journal of the American Medical Association* 278 (1997): 313–321.

Hunt, D., Young, P., Simes, J., et al., "Benefits of Pravastatin on Cardiovascular Events and Mortality in Older Patients with Coronary Heart Disease Are Equal to or Exceed Those Seen in Younger Patients: Results from the LIPID Trial," *Annals of Internal Medicine* 134 (2001): 931–940.

Jick, H., Zornberg, G.L., Jick, S.S., et al., "Statins and the Risk of Dementia," *Lancet* 356 (2000): 1627–1631.

Jukema, J.W., Bruschke, A.V., van Boven, A.J., et al., "Effects of Lipid Lowering by Pravastatin on Progression and Regression of Coronary Artery Disease in Symptomatic Men with Normal to Moderately Elevated Serum Cholesterol Levels. The Regression Growth Evaluation Statin Study (REGRESS)," *Circulation* 91 (1995): 2528–2540.

Koh, K.K., Son, J.W., Ahn, J.Y., et al., "Non-Lipid Effects of Statin on Hypercholesterolemic Patients Established to Have Coronary Artery Disease Who Remained Hypercholesterolemic while Eating a Step-II Diet," *Coronary Artery Disease* 12 (2001): 305–311.

LaRosa, J.C., He, J., and Vupputuri, S., "Effect of Statins on Risk of Coronary Disease: A Meta-Analysis of Randomized Controlled Trials," *Journal of the American Medical Association* 282 (1999): 2340–2346.

Magnani, G., Carinci, V., Magelli, C., et al., "Role of Statins in the Management of Dyslipidemia after Cardiac Transplant: Randomized Controlled Trial Comparing the Efficacy and the Safety of Atorvastatin with Pravastatin," *The Journal of Heart and Lung Transplantation* 19 (2000): 710–715.

McTaggart, F., Buckett, L., Davidson, R., et al., "Preclinical and Clinical Pharmacology of Rosuvastatin, a New 3-Hydroxy-3-Methylglutaryl Coenzyme A Reductase Inhibitor," *The American Journal of Cardiology* 87 (2001): 28B–32B.

Muck, W., "Clinical Pharmacokinetics of Cerivastatin," *Clinical Pharmacokinetics* 39 (2000): 99–116.

O'Neill, F.H., Patel, D.D., Knight, B.L., et al., "Determinants of Variable Response to Statin Treatment in Patients with Refractory Familial Hypercholesterolemia," *Arteriosclerosis, Thrombosis, and Vascular Biology* 21 (2001): 832–837.

Paulweber, B., "[Statins in Primary Prevention of Coronary Heart Disease]," *Wiener Medizinische Wochenschrift* 149 (1999): 129–138.

Pedersen, T., and Gaw, A., "Statins—Similarities and Differences," *American Journal of Managed Care* 7 (2001): S132–S137.

Peters, T.K., "Safety Profile of Fluvastatin," *British Journal of Clinical Practice* 77A (Supplement) (1996): 20–23.

Rauch, U., Osende, J.I., Chesebro, J.H., et al., "Statins and Cardiovascular Diseases: The Multiple Effects of Lipid-Lowering Therapy by Statins," *Atherosclerosis* 153 (2000): 181–189.

Rindone, J.P., "The Outcome of Very Low Dosages of Simvastatin in Patients with Hypercholesterolemia," *Pharmacotherapy* 19 (1999): 399–403.

Sanjad, S.A., al-Abbad, A., and al-Shorafa, S., "Management of Hyperlipidemia in Children with Refractory Nephrotic Syndrome: The Effect of Statin Therapy," *Journal of Pediatrics* 130 (1997): 470–474.

Schonfeld, G., Aguilar-Salina, C., and Elias, N., "Role of 3-Hydroxy-3-Methylglutaryl Aoenzyme A Reductase Inhibitors ('Statins') in Familial Combined Hyperlipidemia," *The American Journal of Cardiology* 81 (1998): 43B–46B.

Shviro, I., and Leitersdorf, E., "The Patient at Risk: Who Should We Be Treating?"

British Journal of Clinical Practice 77A (1996) (Supplement): 24–27.

Spieker, L.E., Noll, G., Hannak, M., et al., "Efficacy and Tolerability of Fluvastatin and Bezafibrate in Patients with Hyperlipidemia and Persistently High Triglyceride Levels," *The Journal of Cardiovascular Pharmacology* 35 (2000): 361–365.

Stein, E., "Cerivastatin in Primary Hyperlipidemia—A Multicenter Analysis of Efficacy and Safety," *Atherosclerosis* 139 (1998) (Supplement 1): S15–S22.

Stein, E.A., and Black, D.M., "Lipoprotein Changes with Statins," *Current Atherosclerosis Reports* 4 (2002): 14–18.

Stein, E.A., Illingworth, D.R., Kwiterovich, P.O., Jr., et al., "Efficacy and Safety of Lovastatin in Adolescent Males with Heterozygous Familial Hypercholesterolemia: A Randomized Controlled Trial," *Journal of the American Medical Association* 281 (1999): 137–144.

Stein, E.A., Lane, M., and Laskarzewski, P., "Comparison of Statins in Hypertriglyceridemia," *The American Journal of Cardiology* 81 (1998): 66B–69B.

Stein, E.A., "Extending Therapy Options in Treating Lipid Disorders: A Clinical Review of Cerivastatin, a Novel HMG–CoA Reductase Inhibitor," *Drugs* 56 (1998) (Supplement 1): 25–31; discussion, 33.

Stein, E.A., "New Statins and New Doses of Older Statins," *Current Atherosclerosis Reports* 3 (2001): 14–18.

Stenestrand, U., and Wallentin, L., "Early Statin Treatment Following Acute Myocardial Infarction and 1-Year Survival," *Journal of the American Medical Association* 285 (2001): 430–436.

Walter, D.H., Schachinger, V., Elsner, M., et al., "Effect of Statin Therapy on Restenosis after Coronary Stent Implantation," *The American Journal of Cardiology* 85 (2000): 962–968.

Williamson, D.R., and Pharand, C., "Statins in the Prevention of Coronary Heart Disease," *Pharmacotherapy* 18 (1998): 242–254.

The Effects of Magnesium Compared with Those of Statins

"Potassium, Magnesium, and Cardiovascular Morbidity. Proceedings of a Symposium. November 10, 1985, Washington, D.C.," *The American Journal of Medicine* 80 (1986): 1–36.

Agus, M.S., and Agus, Z.S., "Cardiovascular Actions of Magnesium," *Critical Care Clinics* 17 (2001): 175–186.

Bellosta, S., Ferri, N., Bernini, F., et al., "Non-Lipid-Related Effects of Statins. *Annals of Medicine* 32 (2000): 164–176.

Blumenthal, R.S., "Statins: Effective Antiatherosclerotic Therapy," *American Heart Journal* 139 (2000): 577–583.

Dawes, M., and Ritter, J.M., "Mg(2+) Induced Vasodilation in Human Forearm Vasculature is Inhibited by N(G)-Monomethyl-L-Arginine but Not by Indomethacin, *Journal of Vascular Research* 37 (2000): 276–281.

de Groot, E., Jukema, J.W., Montauban van Swijndregt, A.D., et al., "B-Mode Ultrasound Assessment of Pravastatin Treatment Effect on Carotid and Femoral Artery Walls and Its Correlations with Coronary Arteriographic Findings: A Report of the Regression Growth Evaluation Statin Study (REGRESS)," *Journal of the American College of Cardiology* 31 (1998): 1561–1567.

Dupuis, J., "Mechanisms of Acute Coronary Syndromes and the Potential Role of Statins," *Atherosclerosis* 2 (2001) (Supplement): 9–14.

Fonseca, F.A., Paiva, T.B., Silva, E.G., et al., "Dietary Magnesium Improves Endothelial Dependent Relaxation of Balloon Injured Arteries in Rats," *Atherosclerosis* 139 (1998): 237–242.

Fujita, T., Ito, Y., Ando, K., et al., "Attenuated Vasodilator Responses to Mg2+ in Young Patients with Borderline Hypertension," *Circulation* 82 (1990): 384–393.

Gyamlani, G., Parikh, C., and Kulkarni, A.G., "Benefits of Magnesium in Acute Myocardial Infarction: Timing Is Crucial," *American Heart Journal* 139 (2000): 703.

Horner, S.M., "Efficacy of Intravenous Magnesium in Acute Myocardial Infarction in Reducing Arrhythmias and Mortality. Meta-Analysis of Magnesium in Acute Myocardial Infarction," *Circulation* 86 (1992): 774–779.

Hughes, A.D., "The Role of Isoprenoids in Vascular Smooth Muscle: Potential Benefits of Statins Unrelated to Cholesterol Lowering," *Journal of Human Hypertension* 10 (1996): 387–390.

Istvan, E.S., and Deisenhofer, J., "Structural Mechanism for Statin Inhibition of HMG–CoA Reductase," *Science* 292 (2001): 1160–1164.

Jellinek, H., and Takacs, E., "[Course of the Progression of Experimentally Induced Arteriosclerotic Vessel Wall Changes after Treatment with Magnesium Orotate]," *Arzneimittelforschung* 50 (2000): 1071–1077.

Laurant, P., and Touyz, R.M., "Physiological and Pathophysiological Role of Magnesium in the Cardiovascular System: Implications in Hypertension," *Journal of Hypertension* 18 (2000): 1177–1191.

Liao, F., Folsom, A.R., and Brancati, F.L., "Is Low Magnesium Concentration a Risk Factor for Coronary Heart Disease? The Atherosclerosis Risk in Communities (ARIC) Study," *American Heart Journal* 136 (1998): 480–490.

Luoma, H., Jauhiainen, M., Alakuijala, P., et al., "Seven Weeks Feeding of Magnesium and Fluoride Modifies Plasma Lipids of Hypercholesterolaemic Rats in Late Growth Phase," *Magnesium Research* 11 (1998): 271–282.

Maheswaran, R., Morris, S., Falconer, S., et al., "Magnesium in Drinking Water Supplies and Mortality from Acute Myocardial Infarction in North West England," *Heart* 82 (1999): 455–460.

Marier, J.R., and Neri, L.C., "Quantifying the Role of Magnesium in the Interrelationship between Human Mortality/Morbidity and Water Hardness," *Magnesium* 4 (1985): 53–59.

Miyagawa, K., Dohi, Y., Kojima, M., et al., "Magnesium Removal Impairs the Regulatory Role of Rat Endothelium," *Hypertension Research* 23 (2000): 23:669–675.

Moghadasian, M.H., Mancini, G.B., and Frohlich, J.J., "Pharmacotherapy of Hypercholesterolaemia: Statins in Clinical Practice," *Expert Opinion on Pharmacotherapy* 1 (2000): 683–695.

Neutra, R.R., "Epidemiology vs. Physiology? Drinking Water Magnesium and Cardiac Mortality," *Epidemiology* 10 (1999): 4–6.

Piepho, R.W., "The Pharmacokinetics and Pharmacodynamics of Agents Proven to Raise High-Density Lipoprotein Cholesterol," *The American Journal of Cardiology* 86 (2000): 35L–40L.

Raiteri, M., Arnaboldi, L., Quarato, P., et al., "[The Pharmacology of the Statins: The Evidence of a Direct Antiatherosclerotic Action]," *Annali Italiani di Medicina Interna* 10 (1995) (Supplement): 35S–42S.

Rayssiguier, Y., "Magnesium and Lipid Interrelationships in the Pathogenesis of Vascular Diseases," *Magnesium Bulletin* 3 (1981): 165–177.

Rayssiguier, Y., "Magnesium, Lipids and Vascular Diseases. Experimental Evidence in Animal Models," *Magnesium* 5 (1986): 182–190.

Rayssiguier, Y., and Gueux, E., "Magnesium and Lipids in Cardiovascular Disease," *Journal of the American College of Nutrition* 5 (1986): 507–519.

Rayssiguier, Y., Noe, L., Etienne, J., et al., "Effect of Magnesium Deficiency on Post-Heparin Lipase Activity and Tissue Lipoprotein Lipase in the Rat," *Lipids* 26 (1991): 182–186.

Rosenson, R.S., and Tangney, C.C., "Antiatherothrombotic Properties of Statins: Implications for Cardiovascular Event Reduction," *Journal of the American Medical Association* 279 (1998): 1643–1650.

Rubenowitz, E., Molin, I., Axelsson, G., et al., "Magnesium in Drinking Water in Relation to Morbidity and Mortality from Acute Myocardial Infarction," *Epidemiology* 11 (2000): 416–421.

Schwartz, G.G., Olsson, A.G., Ezekowitz, M.D., et al., "Effects of Atorvastatin on Early Recurrent Ischemic Events in Acute Coronary Syndromes: The Miracle Study: A Randomized Controlled Trial," *Journal of the American Medical Association* 285 (2001): 1711–1718.

Seelig, M.S., "Interrelationship of Magnesium and Congestive Heart Failure," *Wiener Medizinische Wochenschrift* (German) 150 (2000): 335–341.

Sessa, W.C., "Can Modulation of Endothelial Nitric Oxide Synthase Explain the Vasculoprotective Actions Of Statins?" *Trends in Molecular Medicine* 7 (2001): 189–191.

Shechter, M., Sharir, M., Labrador, M.J.,

et al., "Oral Magnesium Therapy Improves Endothelial Function in Patients with Coronary Artery Disease," *Circulation* 102 (2000): 2353–2358.

Sherer, Y., Shaish, A., Levkovitz, H., et al., "Magnesium Fortification of Drinking Water Suppresses Atherogenesis in Male LDL-Receptor-Deficient Mice," *Pathobiology* 67 (1999): 207–213.

Szabo, C., Hardebo, J.E., and Salford, L.G., "Role of Endothelium in the Responses of Human Intracranial Arteries to a Slight Reduction of Extracellular Magnesium," *Experimental Physiology* 77 (1992): 209–211.

Teragawa, H., Kato, M., Yamagata, T., et al., "The Preventive Effect of Magnesium on Coronary Spasm in Patients with Vasospastic Angina," *Chest* 118 (2000): 1690–1695.

Teragawa, H., Kato, M., Yamagata, T., et al., "Magnesium Causes Nitric Oxide Independent Coronary Artery Vasodilation in Humans," *Heart* 86 (2001): 212–216.

Thomas, M., and Mann, J., "Increased Thrombotic Vascular Events after Change of Statin," *Lancet* 352 (1998): 1830–1831.

Yang, Z.W., Gebrewold, A., Nowakowski, M., et al., "Mg(2+)-Induced Endothelium-Dependent Relaxation of Blood Vessels and Blood Pressure Lowering: Role of NO," *The American Journal of Physiology Regulatory, Integrative, and Comparative Physiology* 278 (2000): R628–R639.

Zheng, D., Upton, R.N., Ludbrook, G.L., et al., "Acute Cardiovascular Effects of Magnesium and Their Relationship to Systemic and Myocardial Magnesium Concentrations after Short Infusion in Awake Sheep," *The Journal of Pharmacological and Experimental Therapeutics* 297 (2001): 1176–1183.

The Issue of Side Effects

Black, D.M., Bakker-Arkema, R.G., and Nawrocki, J.W., "An Overview of the Clinical Safety Profile of Atorvastatin (Lipitor), a New HMG–CoA Reductase Inhibitor," *Archives of Internal Medicine* 158 (1998): 577–584.

Buajordet, I., Madsen, S., and Olsen, H., "[Statins—The Pattern of Adverse Effects with Emphasis on Mental Reactions. Data from a National and an International Database]," *Tidsskrift for den Norske Laegeforening* (Norwegian) 117 (1997): 3210–3213.

Chojnowska-Jezierska, J., "[Undesirable Drug Interactions of Hypolipemic Drugs]," *Polski Merkuriusz Lekarski* (Polist) 9 (2000): 618–620.

Ellen, R.L., and McPherson, R., "Long-Term Efficacy and Safety of Fenofibrate and a Statin in the Treatment of Combined Hyperlipidemia," *The American Journal of Cardiology* 81 (1998): 60B–65B.

Feely, J., McGettigan, P., and Kelly, A., "Growth in Use of Statins after Trials Is Not Targeted to Most Appropriate Patients," *Clinical Pharmacology and Therapeutics* 67 (2000): 438–441.

Franc, S., Bruckert, E., Giral, P., et al., "[Rhabdomyolysis in Patients with Preexisting Myopathy, Treated with Antilipemic Agents]," *Presse Medicale* (French) 26 (1997): 1855–1858.

Heerey, A., Barry, M., Ryan, M., et al., "The Potential for Drug Interactions with Statin Therapy in Ireland," *Irish Journal of Med Science* 169 (2000): 176–179.

Heuer, T., Gerards, H., Pauw, M., et al., "[Toxic Liver Damage Caused by HMG-CoA Reductase Inhibitor]," *Medezinische Klinik* (German) 95 (2000): 642–644.

Horlitz, M., Sigwart, U., and Niebauer, J., "[Statins Do Not Prevent Restenosis after Coronary Angioplasty: Where to Go from Here?]," *Herz* 9 (German) 26 (2001): 119–128.

Jeppesen, U., Gaist, D., Smith, T., et al., "Statins and Peripheral Neuropathy," *European Journal of Clinical Pharmacology* 54 (1999): 835–838.

Liebhaber, M.I., Wright, R.S., Gelberg, H.J., et al., "Polymyalgia, Hypersensitivity Pneumonitis and Other Reactions in Patients Receiving HMG-CoA Reductase Inhibitors: A Report of Ten Cases," *Chest* 115 (1999): 886–889.

Lupattelli, G., Palumbo, B., and Sinzinger, H., "Statin Induced Myopathy Does Not Show Up in MIBI Scintigraphy," *Nuclear Medicine Communications* 22 (2001): 575–578.

Oldemeyer, J.B., Lund, R.J., Koch, M, et al., "Rhabdomyolysis and Acute Renal Failure after Changing Statin-Fibrate Combinations," *Cardiology* 94 (2000): 127–128.

Reijneveld, J.C., Koot, R.W., Bredman, J.J., et al., "Differential Effects of 3-Hydroxy-3-Methylglutaryl-Coenzyme A Reductase Inhibitors on the Development of Myopathy in Young Rats," *Pediatric Research* 39 (1996): 1028–1035.

Saito, N., and Ogawa, Y., "[Drug Interactions of Lipid-Lowering Drugs and Precaution of Clinical Use]," *Nippon Rinsho. Japanese Journal of Medicine* 59 (2001) (Supplement 3): 690–695.

Short, Patricia, "Take Two Aspirin . . . Bayer's Drug Recall Shows How Trying to Do the Right Thing Isn't Always Enough," *Chemical and Engineering News* Vol. 79 No. 47 (19 November 2001), p. 12.

Simons, L.A., Simons, J., McManus, P., et al., "Discontinuation Rates for Use of Statins Are High," *British Medical Journal* 321 (2000): 1084.

Sinzinger, H., Lupattelli, G., and Chehne, F., "Increased Lipid Peroxidation in a Patient with CK-Elevation and Muscle Pain during Statin Therapy," *Atherosclerosis* 153 (2000): 255–256.

Tikkanen, M.J., "Statins: within-Group Comparisons, Statin Escape and Combination Therapy," *Current Opinion in Lipidology* 7 (1996): 385–388.

Other Issues—Cost

Maclaine, G.D., and Patel, H., "A Cost-Effectiveness Model of Alternative Statins to Achieve Target LDL-Cholesterol Levels," *International Journal of Clinical Practice* 55 (2001): 243–249.

Mansur, A.P., Mattar, A.P., Tsubo, C.E., et al., "[Prescription and Adherence to Statins of Patients with Coronary Artery Disease and Hypercholesterolemia]," *Arquivos Brasileiros de Cardiologia* (Portuguese) 76 (2001): 111–118.

Pharoah, P.D., and Hollingworth, W., "Cost Effectiveness of Lowering Cholesterol Concentration with Statins in Patients with and without Pre-Existing Coronary Heart Disease: Life Table Method Applied to Health Authority Population," *British Medical Journal* 312 (1996): 1443–1448.

OMEGA-3 AND OMEGA-6 FATTY ACIDS AND MAGNESIUM

Alfin-Slater, R.B., and Aftergood, L., "Fats and Other Lipids," in *Modern Nutrition in Health and Disease,* ed. Maurice E. Shils, James A. Olson, Moshe Shike, and Catherine A Ross (Philadelphia: Lippincott Williams & Wilkins, 1999): pp. 117–141.

Ballantyne, C.M., "Reducing Atherothrombotic Events in High-Risk Patients: Recent Data on Therapy with Statins and Fatty Acids," *Current Atherosclerosis Reports* 1 (1999): 6–8.

D'Almeida, A., Carter, J.P., Anatol, A., et al., "Effects of a Combination of Evening Primrose Oil (Gamma Linolenic Acid) and Fish Oil (Eicosapentaenoic + Docosahexaenoic Acid) versus Magnesium, and versus Placebo in Preventing Pre-Eclampsia," *Women Health* 19 (1992): 117–131.

Erasmus, Udo, *Fats that Heal, Fats that Kill* (Burnaby, BC, Canada: Alive Books, 1993) pp. 277–278.

Galland, L., "Impaired Essential Fatty Acid Metabolism in Latent Tetany," *Magnesium* 4 (1985): 333–338.

Hu, F.B., Manson, J.E., and Willett, W.C., "Types of Dietary Fat and Risk of Coronary Heart Disease: A Critical Review," *Journal of the American College of Nutrition* 20 (2001): 5–19.

Mahfouz, M.M., and Kummerow, F.A., "Effect of Magnesium Deficiency on Delta 6 Desaturase Activity and Fatty Acid Composition of Rat Liver Microsomes," *Lipids* 24 (1989): 727–732.

Mahfouz, M.M., Smith, T.L., and Kummerow, F.A., "Changes of Linoleic Acid Metabolism and Cellular Phospholipid Fatty Acid Composition in LLC–PK Cells Cultured at Low Magnesium Concentration," *Biochimica et Biophysica Acta* 1006 (1989): 70–74.

IMPROVING YOUR MAGNESIUM STATUS TO REDUCE THE DANGERS OF FAT AND CHOLESTEROL

Fraser, G.E., "Nut Consumption, Lipids, and Risk of a Coronary Event," *Clinical Cardiology* 22 (1999): III11–III15.

Rudin, Donald, and Felix, Clara, *Omega 3 Oils: To Improve Mental Health, Fight Degenerative Diseases, and Extend Your Life* (New York: Avery/Penguin Putnam, 1996).

Sirtori, C.R., Pazzucconi, F., Colombo, L., et al., "Double-Blind Study of the Addition of High-Protein Soya Milk v. Cows' Milk to the Diet of Patients with Severe Hypercholesterolaemia and Resistance to or Intolerance of Statins," *The British Journal of Nutrition* 82 (1999): 91–96.

Chapter Six

MAGNESIUM, STRESS, AND THE TYPE A PERSONALITY

STRESS MAGNESIUM REQUIREMENTS AND ROLE OF MAGNESIUM IN STRESS REACTIONS

Al-Ghamdi, S.M., Cameron, E.C., and Sutton, R.A., "Magnesium Deficiency: Pathophysiologic and Clinical Overview," *American Journal of Kidney Diseases* 24 (1994): 737–752.

Brundig, P., Borner, R.H., Schulz, E., et al., "[Modification of the Risk of Urolithiasis by Changes in Magnesium and Calcium Concentrations in the Urine as Affected by Stress Conditions]," *Zeitschrift für Urologie und Nephrologie* 78 (1985): 245–251.

Cernak, I., Savic, V., Kotur, J., et al., "Alterations in Magnesium and Oxidative Status during Chronic Emotional Stress," *Magnesium Research* 13 (2000): 29–36.

Classen, H.G., "Stress and Magnesium," *Artery* 9 (1981): 182–189.

Classen, H.G., Marquardt, P., Spath, M., et al., "Hypermagnesemia Following Exposure to Acute Stress," *Pharmacology* 5 (1971): 287–294.

Galland, L., "Magnesium, Stress and Neuropsychiatric Disorders," *Magnesium and Trace Elements* 10 (1991): 287–301.

Golf, S.W., Happel, O., Graef, V., et al., "Plasma Aldosterone, Cortisol and Electrolyte Concentrations in Physical Exercise after Magnesium Supplementation," *Journal of Clinical Chemistry and Clinical Biochemistry* 22 (1984): 717–721.

Henrotte, J.G., Franck, G., Santarromana, M., et al., "Tissue and Blood Magnesium Levels in Spontaneously Hypertensive Rats, at Rest and in Stressful Conditions," *Magnesium Research* 4 (1991): 91–96.

Konig, D., Weinstock, C., Keul, J., et al., "Zinc, Iron, and Magnesium Status in Athletes—Influence on the Regulation of Exercise-Induced Stress and Immune Function," *Exercise Immunology Review* 4 (1998): 2–21.

Okur, H., Kucukaydin, M., and Ustdal, K.M., "The Endocrine and Metabolic Response to Surgical Stress in the Neonate," *Journal of Pediatric Surgery* 30 (1995): 625–626.

Porta, S., Epple, A., Leitner, G., et al., "Impact of Stress and Triiodothyronine on Plasma Magnesium Fractions," *Life Sciences* 55 (1994): PL327–PL332.

Raab, W., "Myocardial Electrolyte Derangement: Crucial Feature of Pluricausal, So-Called Coronary Disease," *Annals of the New York Academy of Sciences* 147 (1969): 627–686.

Ramakrishnan, M., Schonthal, A.H., and Lee, A.S., "Endoplasmic Reticulum Stress-Inducible Protein GRP94 Is Associated with an Mg2+-Dependent Serine Kinase Activity Modulated by Ca2+ and GRP78/BiP," *Journal of Cellular Physiology* 170 (1997): 115–129.

Ryzen, E., Servis, K.L., and Rude, R.K., "Effect of Intravenous Epinephrine on Serum Magnesium and Free Intracellular Red Blood Cell Magnesium Concentrations Measured by Nuclear Magnetic Resonance," *Journal of the American College of Nutrition* 9 (1990): 114–119.

Seelig, M.S., "Consequences of Magnesium Deficiency on the Enhancement of Stress Reactions; Preventive and Therapeutic Implications (a Review)," *Journal of the American College of Nutrition* 13 (1994): 429–446.

Selye, H., "The Evolution of the Stress Concept. Stress and Cardiovascular Disease," *American Journal of Cardiology* 26 (1970): 289–299.

Vasku, J., Urbanek, E., and Dolezel, S., "[On the Irregular Course of the Alarm Reaction in Lympho-Epithelial and Lympho-Reticular Tissues under the Effect of K-Mg-Aspartate]," *Arzneimittelforschung* 16 (1966): 559–565.

Vink, R., and Cernak, I., "Regulation of Intracellular Free Magnesium in Central Nervous System Injury," *Frontiers in Bioscience* 5 (2000): D656–D665.

THE EFFECTS OF LOW MAGNESIUM COMBINED WITH STRESS

Altura, B.M., and Altura, B.T., "Magnesium and Cardiovascular Biology: An Important Link Between Cardiovascular Risk Factors and Atherogenesis," *Cellular and Molecular Biology Research* 41 (1995): 347–359.

Altura, B.M., Altura, B.T., Gebrewold, A., et al., "Extraaural Effects of Chronic Noise Exposure on Blood Pressure, Microcirculation and Electrolytes in Rats: Modulation by Mg2+," *Schriftenreihe des Vereins für Wasser-, Boden- und Lufthygiene* 88 (1993): 65–90.

Caddell, J., Kupiecki, R., Proxmire, D.L., et al., "Plasma Catecholamines in Acute Magnesium Deficiency in Weanling Rats," *The Journal of Nutrition* 116 (1986): 1896–1901.

Classen, H.G., "Stress and Magnesium," *Artery* 9 (1981): 182–189.

Classen, H.G., "Systemic Stress, Magnesium Status and Cardiovascular Damage," *Magnesium* 5 (1986): 105–110.

Gunther, T., "Biochemistry and Pathobiochemistry of Magnesium," *Artery* 9 (1981): 167–181.

Gunther, T., Ising, H., and Merker, H.J., "Electrolyte and Collagen Content of Rat Heart in Chronic Mg-Deficiency and Stress," *Journal of Clinical Chemistry and Clinical Biochemistry* 16 (1978): 293–297.

Joborn, H., Hjemdahl, P., Larsson, P.T., et al., "Effects of Prolonged Adrenaline Infusion and of Mental Stress on Plasma Minerals and Parathyroid Hormone," *Clinical Physiology* 10 (1990): 37–53.

Kaemmerer, K., and Kietzmann, M., "[Studies on Magnesium. 3. Effect of Magnesium Aspartate Hydrochloride on Stress Reactions in Magnesium-Deficient Animals]," *Zentralblatt für Veterinarmedizin. Reihe A* (German) 31 (1984): 334–339.

Kaemmerer K., Kietzmann M., and Kreisner M. [Studies on magnesium. 2. Effect of magnesium chloride and magnesium aspartate hydrochloride on stress reactions]. *Zentralblatt für Veterinarmedizin. Reihe A* (German) 31 (1984): 321–333.

Rasmussen, H.S., "Justification for Intravenous Magnesium Therapy in Acute Myocardial Infarction," *Magnesium Research* 1 (1988): 59–73.

Tanabe, K., Noda, K., Ozasa, A., et al., "The Relation of Physical and Mental Stress to Magnesium Deficiency in Patients with Variant Angina" (article in Japanese), *Journal of Cardiology* 22 (1992): 349–355.

Whyte, K.F., Addis, G.J., Whitesmith, R., et al., "Adrenergic Control of Plasma Magnesium in Man," *Clinical Science* 72 (1987): 135–138.

Wu, F., Altura, B.T., Gao, J., et al., " "Ferrylmyoglobin Formation Induced by Acute Magnesium Deficiency in Perfused Rat Heart Causes Cardiac Failure," *Biochimica et Biophysica Acta* 1225 (1994): 158–164.

How Adrenaline Release and Magnesium Deficit Reinforce Each Other

Durlach, J., "Recommended Dietary Amounts of Magnesium: Mg RDA," *Magnesium Research* 2 (1989): 195–203.

Galland, L., "Magnesium, Stress and Neuropsychiatric Disorders, *Magnesium and Trace Elements* 10 (1991): 287–301.

Hansen, O., and Johansson, B.W., "S-Mg Does Not Change Inversely to S-FFA during Acute Stress Situations," *Angiology* 40 (1989): 1011–1019.

Joborn, H., Hjemdahl, P., Larsson, P.T., et al., "Effects of Prolonged Adrenaline Infusion and of Mental Stress on Plasma Minerals and Parathyroid Hormone," *Clinical Physiology* 10 (1990): 37–53.

Leary, W.P., and Reyes, A.J., "Magnesium and Sudden Death," *South African Medical Journal* 64 (1983): 697–698.

Ryzen, E., Servis, K.L., and Rude, R.K., "Effect of Intravenous Epinephrine on Serum Magnesium and Free Intracellular Red Blood Cell Magnesium Concentrations Measured by Nuclear Magnetic Resonance," *Journal of the American College of Nutrition* 9 (1990): 114–119.

Salerno, D.M., Katz, A., Dunbar, D.N., et al., "Serum Electrolytes and Catecholamines after Cardioversion from Ventricular Tachycardia and Atrial Fibrillation," *Pacing and*

Clinical Electrophysiology 16 (1993): 1862–1871.

Seelig, M.S., "Consequences of Magnesium Deficiency on the Enhancement of Stress Reactions; Preventive and Therapeutic Implications (a Review)," *Journal of the American College of Nutrition* 13 (1994): 429–446.

Whyte, K.F., Addis, G.J., Whitesmith, R., et al., "Adrenergic Control of Plasma Magnesium in Man," *Clinical Science* 72 (1987): 135–138.

Damage to Magnesium Deficient Cells Caused by Stress

Altura, B.M., Gebrewold, A., Zhang, A., et al., "Magnesium Deficiency Exacerbates Brain Injury and Stroke Mortality Induced by Alcohol: a 31P–NMR In Vivo Study," *Alcohol* 15 (1998): 181–183.

Li, W., Zheng, T., Altura, B.T., et al., "Antioxidants Prevent Elevation in [Ca(2+)](i) Induced by Low Extracellular Magnesium in Cultured Canine Cerebral Vascular Smooth Muscle Cells: Possible Relationship to Mg(2+) Deficiency-Induced Vasospasm and Stroke," *Brain Research Bulletin* 52 (2000): 151–154.

THE EFFECT OF MAGNESIUM SUPPLEMENTS IN STRESS CONDITIONS

Classen, H.G., "Systemic Stress, Magnesium Status and Cardiovascular Damage," *Magnesium* 5 (1986): 105–110.

Classen, H.G., Fischer, G., Marx, J., et al., "Prevention of Stress-Induced Damage in Experimental Animals and Livestock by Monomagnesium-L-Aspartate Hydrochloride," *Magnesium* 6 (1987): 34–39.

Durlach, J., "Recommended Dietary Amounts of Magnesium: Mg RDA," *Magnesium Research* 2 (1989): 195–203.

Gartner, R.J., Ryley, J.W., and Beattie, A.W., "The Influence of Degree of Excitation on Certain Blood Constituents in Beef Cattle," *Australian Journal of Experimental Biology and Medical Science* 43 (1965): 713–724.

Kietzmann, M., Influence of Magnesium Gluconate on Stress Reactions in Rats," *Deutsche Tierarztliche Wochenschrift* 96 (1989): 292–293.

Niemack, E.A., "[Magnesium. Mineral—Trace Element—Therapeutic Substance? A Review]," *Schweizer Archiv für Tierheilkunde* (German) 127 (1985): 597–604.

Sair, R.A., Lister, D., Moody, W.G., et al., "Action of Curare and Magnesium on Striated Muscle of Stress-Susceptible Pigs," *The American Journal of Physiology* 218 (1970): 108–114.

HOW STRESS DEPLETES MAGNESIUM IN EVERYDAY LIFE

Stress of Surgery and Hospital Procedures

Allen, R.W., James, M.F., and Uys, P.C., "Attenuation of the Pressor Response to Tracheal Intubation in Hypertensive Proteinuric Pregnant Patients by Lignocaine, Alfentanil and Magnesium Sulphate," *British Journal of Anaesthesia* 66 (1991): 216–223.

Annoni, F., Bruttini, I., Donati, L., et al., "[Plasma and Erythrocyte Magnesium Concentration in the Postoperative Period. Relations between Calcium and Magnesium]," *Minerva Chirurgica* (Italian) 32 (1977): 323–332.

Cordova, A., "Variations of Serum Magnesium and Zinc after Surgery, and Postoperative Fatigue," *Magnesium Research* 8 (1995): 367–372.

Dickerson, R.N., and Brown, R.O., "Hypomagnesemia in Hospitalized Patients Receiving Nutritional Support," *Heart and Lung* 14 (1985): 561–569.

Greig, J.E., Keast, D,, Garcia-Webb, P., et al., "Inter-Relationships between Glutamine and Other Biochemical and Immunological Changes after Major Vascular Surgery," *British Journal of Biomedical Science* 53 (1996): 116–121.

Handwerker, S.M., Altura, B.T., Jones, K.Y., et al., "Maternal-Fetal Transfer of Ionized Serum Magnesium during the Stress of Labor and Delivery: A Human Study," *Journal of the American College of Nutrition* 14 (1995): 376–381.

Nakamura, M., Abe, S., Goto, Y., et al., "Sudden Sound-Induced Death in Magnesium-Deficient Rats after Repetitive Episodes of Seizures Result From Brain Dysfunction," *Magnesium Research* 8 (1995): 47–53.

Okur, H., Kucukaydin, M., and Ustdal

K,M., "The Endocrine and Metabolic Response to Surgical Stress in the Neonate," *Journal of Pediatric Surgery* 30 (1995): 626–630.

Olerich, M.A., and Rude, R.K., "Should We Supplement Magnesium in Critically Ill Patients?" *New Horizons* 2 (1994): 186–192.

Weissberg, N., Schwartz, G., Shemesh, O., et al., "Serum and Intracellular Electrolytes in Patients with and without Pain," *Magnesium Research* 4 (1991): 49–52.

Wilson, R.F., and Sibbald, W.J., "Fluid and Electrolyte Problems in the Emergency Department," *Journal of the American College of Emergency Physicians (JACEP)* 5 (1976): 339–346.

Critical Illness and Injury

Bergstrom, J.P., Larsson, J., Nordstrom, H., et al., "Influence of Injury and Nutrition on Muscle Water and Electrolytes: Effect of Severe Injury, Burns and Sepsis," *Acta Chirurgica Scandinavica* 153 (1987): 261–266.

Cunningham, J.J., Anbar, R.D., and Crawford, J.D., "Hypomagnesemia: A Multifactorial Complication of Treatment of Patients with Severe Burn Trauma," *(Journal of Parenteral and Enteral Nutrition (JPEN)* 11 (1987): 364–367.

Frankel, H., Haskell, R., Lee, S.Y., et al., "Hypomagnesemia in Trauma Patients," *World Journal of Surgery* 23 (1999): 966–969.

Handwerker, S.M., Altura, B.T., Jones, K.Y., et al., "Maternal-Fetal Transfer of Ionized Serum Magnesium during the Stress of Labor and Delivery: A Human Study," *Journal of the American College of Nutrition* 14 (1995): 376–381.

Hebert, P., Mehta, N., Wang, J., et al., "Functional Magnesium Deficiency in Critically Ill Patients Identified Using a Magnesium-Loading Test," *Critical Care Medicine* 25 (1997): 749–755.

Klein, G.L., Nicolai, M., Langman, C.B., et al., "Dysregulation of Calcium Homeostasis after Severe Burn Injury in Children: Possible Role of Magnesium Depletion," *Journal of Pediatrics* 131 (1997): 246–251.

Nakamura, M., Abe, S., Goto, Y., et al., "Sudden Sound-Induced Death in Magnesium-Deficient Rats after Repetitive Episodes of Seizures Result from Brain Dysfunction," *Magnesium Research* 8 (1995): 47–53.

Okur, H., Kucukaydin, M., and Ustdal, K.M., "The Endocrine and Metabolic Response to Surgical Stress in the Neonate," *Journal of Pediatric Surgery* 30 (1995): 626–630.

Olerich, M.A., and Rude, R.K., "Should We Supplement Magnesium in Critically Ill Patients?" *New Horizons* 2 (1994): 186–192.

Reinhart, R.A., "Magnesium Deficiency: Recognition and Treatment in the Emergency Medicine Setting," *The American Journal of Emergency Medicine* 10 (1992): 78–83.

Rubeiz, G.J., Thill-Baharozian, M., Hardie, D., et al., "Association of Hypomagnesemia and Mortality in Acutely Ill Medical Patients," *Critical Care Medicine* 21 (1993): 203–209.

Ryzen, E., "Magnesium Homeostasis in Critically Ill Patients," *Magnesium* 6 (1987): 258–259.

Ryzen, E., Servis, K.L., Rude, R.K., "Effect of Intravenous Epinephrine on Serum Magnesium and Free Intracellular Red Blood Cell Magnesium Concentrations Measured by Nuclear Magnetic Resonance," *Journal of the American College of Nutrition* 9 (1990): 114–119.

Ryzen, E., Wagers, P.W., Singer, F.R., et al., "Magnesium Deficiency in a Medical ICU Population," *Critical Care Medicine* 13 (1985): 19–21.

Salem, M., Munoz, R., and Chernow, B., "Hypomagnesemia in Critical Illness. A Common and Clinically Important Problem," *Critical Care Clinics* 7 (1991): 225–252.

Storm, W., and Zimmerman, J.J., "Magnesium Deficiency and Cardiogenic Shock after Cardiopulmonary Bypass," *The Annals of Thoracic Surgery* 64 (1997): 572–577.

Toffaletti, J., "Physiology and Regulation. Ionized Calcium, Magnesium and Lactate Measurements in Critical Care Settings," *American Journal of Clinical Pathology* 104 (1995): S88–S94.

Vink, R., and Cernak, I., "Regulation of Intracellular Free Magnesium in Central Nervous System Injury," *Frontiers in Bioscience* 5 (2000): D656–D665.

Weisinger, J.R., and Bellorin-Font, E.,

"Magnesium and Phosphorus," *Lancet* 352 (1998): 391–396.

Weissberg, N., Schwartz, G., Shemesh, O., et al., "Serum and Intracellular Electrolytes in Patients with and without Pain," *Magnesium Research* 4 (1991): 49–52.

Brain Injury from Trauma or Interference with Blood Supply

Altura, B.M., and Altura B.T., "Association of Alcohol in Brain Injury, Headaches, and Stroke with Brain-Tissue and Serum Levels of Ionized Magnesium: A Review of Recent Findings and Mechanisms of Action," *Alcohol* 19 (1999): 119–130.

Altura, B.M., Zhang, A., Cheng, T.P., et al., "Extracellular Magnesium Regulates Nuclear and Perinuclear Free Ionized Calcium in Cerebral Vascular Smooth Muscle Cells: Possible Relation to Alcohol and Central Nervous System Injury," *Alcohol* 23 (2001): 83–90.

Altura, B.T., Memon, Z.I., Zhang, A., et al., "Low Levels of Serum Ionized Magnesium Are Found in Patients Early after Stroke Which Result in Rapid Elevation in Cytosolic Free Calcium and Spasm in Cerebral Vascular Muscle Cells," *Neuroscience Letters* 230 (1997): 37–40.

Auer, R.N., "Non-Pharmacologic (Physiologic) Neuroprotection in the Treatment of Brain Ischemia," *Annals of the New York Academy of Sciences* 939 (2001): 271–282.

Cernak, I., Savic, V.J., Kotur, J., et al., "Characterization of Plasma Magnesium Concentration and Oxidative Stress Following Graded Traumatic Brain Injury in Humans," *Journal of Neurotrauma* 17 (2000): 53–68.

Cernak, I., and Vink, R., *Magnesium as a Regulatory Cation in Direct and Indirect Traumatic Brain Injury* (Belgrade, Yugoslavia: Institute for Medical Research, Military Medical Academy, 1998), pp. 12–14.

Cernak, I., and Vink, R., "Magnesium as a Regulatory Cation in Direct and Indirect Traumatic Brain Injury," *Magnesium Research* 12 (1999): 223–224.

Golf, S.W., Happel, O., Graef, V., et al., "Plasma Aldosterone, Cortisol and Electrolyte Concentrations in Physical Exercise after Magnesium Supplementation," *Journal of Clinical Chemistry and Clinical Biochemistry* 22 (1984): 717–721.

Heath, D.L., and Vink, R., "Blood-Free Magnesium Concentration Declines Following Graded Experimental Traumatic Brain Injury," *Scandinavian Journal of Clinical and Laboratory Investigation* 58 (1998): 161–166.

Heath, D.L., and Vink, R., "Neuroprotective Effects of $MgSO_4$ and $MgCl_2$ in Closed Head Injury: A Comparative Phosphorus NMR Study," *Journal of Neurotrauma* 15 (1998): 183–189.

Heath, D.L., and Vink, R., "Magnesium Sulphate Improves Neurologic Outcome Following Severe Closed Head Injury in Rats," *Neuroscience Letters* 228 (1997): 175–178.

Heath, D.L., and Vink, R., "Improved Motor Outcome in Response to Magnesium Therapy Received Up to 24 Hours after Traumatic Diffuse Axonal Brain Injury in Rats," *Journal of Neurosurgery* 90 (1999): 504–509.

Helpern, J.A., Vande-Linde, A.M., Welch, K.M., et al., "Acute Elevation and Recovery of Intracellular [Mg2+] Following Human Focal Cerebral Ischemia," *Neurology* 43 (1993): 1577–1581.

Lampl, Y., Geva, D., Gilad, R., et al., "Cerebrospinal Fluid Magnesium Level as a Prognostic Factor in Ischaemic Stroke," *Journal of Neurology* 245 (1998): 584–588.

Muir, K.W., "New Experimental and Clinical Data on the Efficacy of Pharmacological Magnesium Infusions in Cerebral Infarcts," *Magnesium Research* 11 (1998): 43–56.

Muir, K.W., "Magnesium for Neuroprotection in Ischaemic Stroke: Rationale for Use and Evidence of Effectiveness," *CNS Drugs* 15 (2001): 921–930.

Muir, K.W., "Magnesium in Stroke Treatment," *Postgraduate Medical Journal* 78 (2002): 641–645.

Raab, W., "Myocardial Electrolyte Derangement: Crucial Feature of Pluricausal, So-Called Coronary, Heart Disease (Dysionic Cardiopathy)," *Annals of the New York Academy of Sciences* 147 (1969): 627–686.

Selye, H., "The Evolution of the Stress Concept. Stress and Cardiovascular Disease," *The American Journal of Cardiology* 26 (1970): 289–299.

Thel, M.C., Armstrong, A.L., McNulty, S.E., et al., "Randomised Trial of Magnesium in I-Hospital Cardiac Arrest. Duke Internal Medicine Housestaff," *Lancet* 350 (1997): 1272–1276.

Vink, R., and Cernak, I., "Regulation of Intracellular Free Magnesium in Central Nervous System Injury," *Frontiers in Bioscience* 5 (2000): D656–D665.

Vink, R., and McIntosh, T.K., "Pharmacological and Physiological Effects of Magnesium on Experimental Traumatic Brain Injury," *Magnesium Research* 3 (1990): 163–169.

Yang, C.Y., Chiu, H.F., Chiu, J.F., et al., "Magnesium and Calcium in Drinking Water and Cerebrovascular Mortality in Taiwan," *Magnesium Research* 10 (1997): 51–57.

Type A Behavior

Altura, B.T., "Type-A Behavior and Coronary Vasospasm: A Possible Role of Hypomagnesemia," *Medical Hypotheses* 6 (1980): 753–757.

Durlach, J., "Recommended Dietary Amounts of Magnesium: Mg RDA," *Magnesium Research* 2 (1989): 195–203.

Friedman, M., and Rosenman, R.H., "Association of Specific Overt Behaviour Patterns with Blood and Cardiovascular Findings," *Journal of the American Medical Association* 169 (1959): 1286–1296.

Friedman, M., Thoresen, C.E., Gill, J.J., et al., "Feasibility of Altering Type A Behavior Pattern after Myocardial Infarction. Recurrent Coronary Prevention Project Study: Methods, Baseline Results and Preliminary Findings," *Circulation* 66 (1982): 83–92.

Henrotte, J.G., and Levy-Leboyer, C., "Is Type A Behavior Modulated by Genetic Factors Regulating Magnesium and Zinc Metabolism? Working Hypotheses and Preliminary Results," *Magnesium* 4 (1985): 295–302.

Henrotte, J.G., Plouin, P.F., Levy-Leboyer, C., et al., "Blood and Urinary Magnesium, Zinc, Calcium, Free Fatty Acids, and Catecholamines in Type A and Type B Subjects," *Journal of the American College of Nutrition* 4 (1985): 165–172.

Henrotte, J.G., "Type A Behavior and Magnesium Metabolism," *Magnesium* 5 (1986): 201–210.

Chronic Stress

Kerner, Fred, *Stress and Your Heart* (Lincoln, NE: iUniverse.com, 2000).

Selye, Hans, *Stress without Distress*, reissue edition (Philadelphia: Lippincott Williams & Wilkins, 1991).

Noise

Altura, B.M., Altura, B.T., Gebrewold, A., et al., "Noise-Induced Hypertension and Magnesium in Rats: Relationship to Microcirculation and Calcium," *Journal of Applied Physiology* 72 (1992): 194–202.

Altura, B.M., Altura, B.T., Gebrewold, A., et al., "Extraaural Effects of Chronic Noise Exposure on Blood Pressure, Microcirculation and Electrolytes in Rats: Modulation by Mg2+," *Schriftenreihe des Vereins für Wasser-, Boden- und Lufthygiene* 88 (1993): 65–90.

Belojevic, G., Kocijancic, R., and Stankovic, T., "[The Effect of a Preventive Health Care Program in a Textile Plant]," *Arhiv za Higijenu Rada i Toksikologiju* (Serbo–Croatian [Roman]) 42 (1991): 27–36.

Caddell, J., Kupiecki, R., Proxmire, D.L., et al., "Plasma Catecholamines in Acute Magnesium Deficiency in Weanling Rats," *The Journal of Nutrition* 116 (1986): 1896–1901.

Curio, I., and Michalak, R., "Results of a Low-Altitude Flight Noise Study in Germany: Acute Extraaural Effects," *Schriftenreihe des Vereins für Wasser-, Boden- und Lufthygiene* 88 (1993): 307–321.

Galland, L., "Magnesium, Stress and Neuropsychiatric Disorders," *Magnesium and Trace Elements* 10 (1991): 287–301.

Goto, Y., Nakamura, M., Abe, S., et al., "Physiological Correlates of Abnormal Behaviors in Magnesium-Deficient Rats," *Epilepsy Research* 15 (1993): 81–89.

Gunther, T., Ising, H., and Merker, H.J., "Electrolyte and Collagen Content of Rat Heart in Chronic Mg-Deficiency and Stress," *Journal of Clinical Chemistry and Clinical Biochemistry* 16 (1978): 293–297.

Gunther, T., Ising, H., Mohr-Nawroth,

F., et al., "Embryotoxic Effects of Magnesium Deficiency and Stress on Rats and Mice," *Teratology* 24 (1981): 225–233.

Ising, H., "Interaction of Noise-Induced Stress and Mg Decrease," *Artery* 9 (1981): 205–211.

Ising, H., Gunther, T., Merker, H.J., et al., "[Increase of Connective Tissue in Rat Hearts under Exposure to Noise and with Magnesium Deficiency,]" *Zentralblatt für Bakteriologie* (German) 162 (1976): 550–557.

Ising, H., Handrock, M., Gunther, T., et al., "Increased Noise Trauma in Guinea Pigs through Magnesium Deficiency," *Archives of Oto-Rhino-Laryngology* 236 (1982): 139–146.

Langley, W.F., and Mann, D., "Central Nervous System Magnesium Deficiency," *Archives of Internal Medicine* 151 (1991): 593–596.

Mocci, F., Canalis, P., Tomasi, P.A., et al., "The Effect of Noise on Serum and Urinary Magnesium and Catecholamines in Humans," *Occupational Medicine (Oxford, England)* 51 (2001): 56–61.

Nakamura, M., Abe, S., Goto, Y., et al., "Sudden Sound-Induced Death in Magnesium-Deficient Rats after Repetitive Episodes of Seizures Result from Brain Dysfunction," *Magnesium Research* 8 (1995): 47–53.

Nakamura, M., Abe, S., Goto, Y., et al., "In Vivo Assessment of Prevention of White-Noise-Induced Seizure in Magnesium-Deficient Rats by N-Methyl-D-Aspartate Receptor Blockers," *Epilepsy Research* 17 (1994): 249–256.

Wutzen, J., "[Selected Organopathies Caused by Experimental Magnesium Deficiency,]" *Polski Tygodnik Lekarski* (Polish) 44 (1989): 243–246.

Zdrojewicz, Z., Koziol, J., Januszewski, A., et al., "Evaluation of Magnesium, Zinc, Copper and Calcium Levels in Workers Exposed to Organic Solvents, Hydrogen Cyanide and Harmful Physical Factors]," *Medycyna Pracy* (Polish) 47 (1996): 217–225.

Heat and Exercise

Beller, G.A., Maher, J.T., Hartley, L.H., et al., "Changes in Serum and Sweat Magnesium Levels during Work in the Heat," *Aviation, Space, and Environmental Medicine* 46 (1975): 709–712.

Cordova, A., "Changes on Plasmatic and Erythrocytic Magnesium Levels after High-Intensity Exercises in Men," *Physiology and Behavior* 52 (1992): 819–821.

Hale, H.B., and Mefferd, R.B., Jr., "Influence of Chronic Heat Exposure and Prolonged Food Deprivation on Excretion of Magnesium, Phosphorus, Calcium, H+, and Ketones," technical report of the USAF School of Aerospace Medicine, SAM-TR-67-20 (1966): 1–11.

Hale, H.B., and Mefferd, R.B., Jr., "Influence of Chronic Heat Exposure and Prolonged Food Deprivation on Excretion of Magnesium, Phosphorus, Calcium, Hydrogen Ion and Ketones," *Aerospace Medicine* 39 (1968): 919–926.

Iyer, E.M., Dikshit, M.B., Banerjee, P.K., et al., "100% Oxygen Breathing during Acute Heat Stress: Effect on Sweat Composition," *Aviation, Space, and Environmental Medicine* 54 (1983): 232–235.

Konig, D., Weinstock, C., Keul, J., et al., "Zinc, Iron, and Magnesium Status in Athletes—Influence on the Regulation of Exercise-Induced Stress and Immune Function," *Exercise Immunology Review* 4 (1998): 2–21.

Porta, S., Epple, A., Leitner, G., et al., "Impact of Stress and Triiodothyronine on Plasma Magnesium Fractions," *Life Sciences* 55 (1994): PL327–PL332.

Rayssiguier, Y., Guezennec, C.Y., and Durlach, J., "New Experimental and Clinical Data on the Relationship between Magnesium and Sport," *Magnesium Research* 3 (1990): 93–102.

Sawka, M.N., and Montain, S.J., "Fluid and Electrolyte Supplementation for Exercise Heat Stress," *American Journal of Clinical Nutrition* 72 (2000): 564S–572S.

Stendig-Lindberg, G., "Sudden Death of Athletes: Is It Due to Long-Term Changes in Serum Magnesium, Lipids and Blood Sugar?" *Journal of Basic and Clinical Physiology and Pharmacology* 3 (1992): 153–164.

Stendig-Lindberg, G., Moran, D., and Shapiro, Y., "How Significant is Magnesium in Thermoregulation?" *Journal of Basic and Clinical Physiology and Pharmacology* 9 (1998): 73–85.

Stendig-Lindberg, G., Shapiro, Y., Epstein, Y., et al., "Changes in Serum Magnesium Concentration after Strenuous Exercise," *Journal of the American College of Nutrition* 6 (1987): 35–40.

Stendig-Lindberg, G., Wacker, W.E., et al., "Long Term Effects of Peak Strenuous Effort on Serum Magnesium, Lipids, and Blood Sugar in Apparently Healthy Young Men," *Magnesium Research* 4 (E1991): 59–65.

Emotional and Psychological Stress

Cernak, I., Savic, V., Kotur, J., et al., "Alterations in Magnesium and Oxidative Status during Chronic Emotional Stress," *Magnesium Research* 13 (2000): 29–36.

Hale, H.B., and Mefferd, R.B., Jr., "Influence of Chronic Heat Exposure and Prolonged Food Deprivation on Excretion of Magnesium, Phosphorus, Calcium, H+, and Ketones," technical report of the USAF School of Aerospace Medicine, SAM-TR-67-20 (1966): 1–11.

Hale, H.B., and Mefferd, R.B., Jr., "Influence of Chronic Heat Exposure and Prolonged Food Deprivation on Excretion of Magnesium, Phosphorus, Calcium, Hydrogen Ion and Ketones," *Aerospace Medicine* 39 (1968): 919–926.

Joborn, H., Hjemdahl, P., Larsson, P.T., et al., "Effects of Prolonged Adrenaline Infusion and of Mental Stress on Plasma Minerals and Parathyroid Hormone," *Clinical Physiology* 10 (1990): 37–53.

Langley, W.F., and Mann, D., "Central Nervous System Magnesium Deficiency," *Archives of Internal Medicine* 151 (1991): 593–596.

Mackenbach, J.P., Cavelaars, A.E., Kunst, A.E., et al., "Socioeconomic Inequalities in Cardiovascular Disease Mortality; An International Study," *European Heart Journal* 21 (2000): 1141–1151.

Ruddel, H., Schmieder, R., Langewitz, W., et al., "Impact of Antihypertensive Therapy on Blood Pressure Reactivity during Mental Stress," *Journal of Human Hypertension* 1 (1988): 259–265.

Rulli, V., Menotti, A., and Signoretti, P., "[Rehabilitation in Cardiology Today. The Predictive Value of Different Occupational Activities in Primary and Secondary Prevention]," *Minerva Cardioangiologica* (Italian) 27 (1979): 271–273.

Shah, J.H., Motto, G.S., Kukreja, S.C., et al., "Stimulation of the Secretion of Parathyroid Hormone during Hypoglycemic Stress," *The Journal of Clinical Endocrinology and Metabolism* 41 (1975): 692–696.

Siltanen, P., Lauroma, M., Nirkko, O., et al., "Psychological Characteristics Related to Coronary Heart Disease," *Journal of Psychosomatic Research* 19 (1975): 183–195.

Tanabe, K., Noda, K., Ozasa, A., et al., "The Relation of Physical and Mental Stress to Magnesium Deficiency in Patients with Variant Angina," *Journal of Cardiology* (Japanese) 22 (1992): 349–355.

Wutzen, J., "[Selected Organopathies Caused by Experimental Magnesium Deficiency,]" *Polski Tygodnik Lekarski* (Polish) 44 (1989): 243–246.

Oxidative Stress

Cernak I, Savic V, Kotur J, et al., "Alterations in Magnesium and Oxidative Status during Chronic Emotional Stress," *Magnesium Research* 13 (2000): 29–36.

Cernak, I., Savic, V.J., Kotur, J., et al., "Characterization of Plasma Magnesium Concentration and Oxidative Stress Following Graded Traumatic Brain Injury in Humans," *Journal of Neurotrauma* 17 (2000): 53–68.

Chugh, S.N., Kolley, T., Kakkar, R., et al., "A Critical Evaluation of Anti-Peroxidant Effect of Intravenous Magnesium in Acute Aluminium Phosphide Poisoning," *Magnesium Research* 10 (1997): 225–230.

Liu, B., and Hannun, Y.A., "Inhibition of the Neutral Magnesium-Dependent Sphingomyelinase by Glutathione," *The Journal of Biological Chemistry* 272 (1997): 16281–16287.

Poeggeler, B., Reiter, R.J., Tan, D.X., et al., "Melatonin, Hydroxyl Radical–mediated Oxidative Damage, and Aging: A Hypothesis," *Journal of Pineal Research* 14 (1993): 151–168.

Rayssiguier, Y., Durlach, J., Gueux, E., et al., "Magnesium and Ageing. I. Experimental Data: Importance of Oxidative Damage," *Magnesium Research* 6 (1993): 369–378.

Wu, F., Altura, B.T., Gao, J., et al., "Ferrylmyoglobin Formation Induced by Acute Magnesium Deficiency in Perfused Rat

Heart Causes Cardiac Failure," *Biochimica et Biophysica Acta* 1225 (1994): 158–164.

Zhou, Q., Olinescu, R.M., and Kummerow, F.A., "Influence of Low Magnesium Concentrations in the Medium on the Antioxidant System in Cultured Human Arterial Endothelial Cells," *Magnesium Research* 12 (1999): 19–29.

Stress Ulcers

Classen, H.G., "[Effect of the Current Magnesium Status on the Development of Stress Ulcers and Myocardial Necroses]," *Fortschritte der Medizin* (German) 99 (1981): 1303–1306.

Classen, H.G., "Stress and Magnesium with Special Regard to the Gastrointestinal Tract," in *Proceedings of the Fifth International Magnesium Symposium (Kyoto, Japan)*, ed. Y. Itokawa and J. Durlach (London, England: John Libbey & Company: 1988), pp. 271–278.

Estruch, R., Pedrol, E., Castells, A., et al., "Prophylaxis of Gastrointestinal Tract Bleeding with Magaldrate in Patients Admitted to a General Hospital Ward," *Scandinavian Journal of Gastroenterology* 26 (1991): 819–826.

Henrotte, J.G., Aymard, N., and Allix, M., "Effect of Pyridoxine and Magnesium on Stress-Induced Gastric Ulcers in Mice Selected for Low or High Blood Magnesium Levels," *Annals of Nutrition and Metabolism* 39 (1995): 285–290.

Kentrup, H., Skopnik, H., Wolter, L., et al., "[Antacids for Postoperative Prevention of Stress Ulcer in Infants: A Dose Finding Study]," *Klinische Padiatrie* (German) 208 (1996): 14–16.

Mangler, B., Fischer, G., and Classen, H.G., "The Influence of Magnesium-Deficiency on the Development of Gastric Stress Ulcers in Rats," *Magnesium Bulletin* 4 (1982): 9–12.

Martin, L.F., "Stress Ulcers Are Common after Aortic Surgery. Endoscopic Evaluation of Prophylactic Therapy," *The American Surgeon* 60 (1994): 169–174.

Mesmer, M., Fischer, G., and Classen, H.G., "[Inhibition of Stress Reactions by Magnesium. Beneficial Effects of Parenteral Magnesium Therapy on the Development of Stress Ulcers in Rats]," *Arzneimittelforschung* (German) 31 (1981): 389–391.

Chapter Seven
Magnesium and Genetics: Family History and Sex Differences

Genetic Variability in Nutritional Needs

Carpenter, Kenneth J., *The History of Scurvy and Vitamin C* (Cambridge, England: Cambridge University Press, 1987), p. 288.

Williams, R.J., and Deason, G., "Individuality in Vitamin C Needs." *Proceedings of the National Academy of Sciences of the United States of America* 57 (1967): 1638–1641.

Williams, R.J., and Pelton, R.B., "Individuality in Nutrition: Effects of Vitamin A-Deficient and Other Deficient Diets on Experimental Animals," *Proceedings of the National Academy of Sciences of the United States of America* 55 (1966): 126–134.

Genetics and Cardiovascular Disease

Schuster, H., "Phenotyping and Genotyping Patients with Cardiovascular Risk Factors," *Diabetic Medicine* 14 (1997) (Supplement 3): S57–S59.

Schuster, H., Lamprecht, A., Junghans, C., et al., "Approaches to the Genetics of Cardiovascular Disease through Genetic Field Work," *Kidney International* 53 (1998): 1449–1454.

Familial Differences in Cardiovascular Disease and in Genetic Handling of Magnesium

Keating, M., Dunn, C., Atkinson, D., et al., "Consistent Linkage of the Long-QT Syndrome to the Harvey Ras-1 Locus on Chromosome 11," *American Journal of Human Genetics* 49 (1991): 1335–1339.

Moss, A.J., and Robinson, J., "Clinical Features of the Idiopathic Long QT Syndrome," *Circulation* 85 (1992): I140–I144.

Napolitano, C., Priori, S.G., and Schwartz, P.J., "Torsade de Pointes. Mechanisms and Management," *Drugs* 47 (1994): 51–65.

Papaceit, J., Moral, V., Recio, J., et al., "[Severe Heart Arrhythmia Secondary to Magnesium Depletion. Torsade de Pointes]," *Revista Espanola de Anestesiologia y Reanimacion* (Spanish) 37 (1990): 28–31.

Perticone, F., and Marsico, S.A., "Familial Case of Permanent Form of Junctional Reciprocating Tachycardia: Possible Role of the HLA System," *Clinical Cardiology* 11 (1988): 345–348.

Pesonen, E., Norio, R., and Sarna, S., "Thickenings in the Coronary Arteries in Infancy as an Indication of Genetic Factors in Coronary Heart Disease," *Circulation* 51 (1975): 218–225.

Po, S.S., Wang, D.W., Yang, I.C., et al., "Modulation of HERG Potassium Channels by Extracellular Magnesium and Quinidine," *The Journal of Cardiovascular Pharmacology* 33 (1999): 181–185.

Schuster, H., "DNA Diagnosis of Familial Hypercholesterolemia," *European Journal of Medical Research* 3 (1998): 42–44.

Schuster, H., "High Risk/High Priority: Familial Hypercholesterolemia—A Paradigm for Molecular Medicine," *Atherosclerosis* 2 (2002) (Supplement): 27–30; discussion 30–32.

Schwartz, P.J., Moss, A.J., Vincent, G.M., et al., "Diagnostic Criteria for the Long QT Syndrome. An Update," *Circulation* 88 (1993): 782–784.

Vergopoulos, A., Knoblauch, H., and Schuster, H., "DNA Testing for Familial Hypercholesterolemia: Improving Disease Recognition and Patient Care," *American Journal of Pharmacogenomics* 2 (2002): 253–262.

Type A Personality

Henrotte, J.G., and Levy-Leboyer, C., "[Is type A Behavior Modulated by Genetic Factors Regulating Magnesium and Zinc Metabolism? Working Hypotheses and Preliminary Results]," *Magnesium* 4 (1985): 295–302.

Diabetes

Acton, R.T., Roseman, J.M., Bell, D.S., et al., "Genes within the Major Histocompatibility Complex Predict NIDDM in African-American Women in Alabama," *Diabetes Care* 17 (1994): 1491–1494.

Aitman, T.J., and Todd, J.A., "Molecular Genetics of Diabetes Mellitus," *Baillieres Clinical Endocrinology and Metabolism* 9 (1995): 631–656.

Dittmer, I., Woodfield, G., and Simpson, I., "Non-Insulin-Dependent Diabetes Mellitus in New Zealand Maori: A Relationship with Class I but not Class II Histocompatibility Locus Antigens," *The New Zealand Medical Journal* 111 (1998): 294–296.

Ghabanbasani, M.Z., Spaepen, M., Buyse, I., et al., "Increased and Decreased Relative Risk for Non-Insulin-Dependent Diabetes Mellitus Conferred by HLA class II and by CD4 Alleles," *Clinical Genetics* 47 (1995): 225–230.

Lostroh, A.J., and Krahl, M.E., "Magnesium, a Second Messenger for Insulin: Ion Translocation Coupled to Transport Activity," *Advances in Enzyme Regulation* 12 (1974): 73–81.

Martin, H.E., Mehl, J., and Wertman, M., "Clinical Studies of Magnesium Metabolism," *The Medical Clinics of North America* 36 (1952): 1157–1171.

Martin, H.E., and Wertman, M., "Serum Potassium, Magnesium and Calcium Levels in Diabetic Acidosis," *The Journal of Clinical Investigations* 26 (1947): 217–228.

Pandey, J.P., Zamani, M., and Cassiman, J.J., "Epistatic Effects of Genes Encoding Tumor Necrosis Factor-Alpha, Immunoglobulin Allotypes, and HLA Antigens on Susceptibility to Non-Insulin-Dependent (Type 2) Diabetes Mellitus," *Immunogenetics* 49 (1999): 860–864.

Rich, S.S., French, L.R., Sprafka, J.M., et al., "HLA-Associated Susceptibility to Type 2 (Non-Insulin-Dependent) Diabetes Mellitus: The Wadena City Health Study," *Diabetologia* 36 (1993): 234–238.

Thorsby, P., Undlien, D.E., Berg, J.P., et al., "[Diabetes Mellitus—A Complex Interaction between Heredity and Environment]," *Tidsskrift for den Norske Laegeforening* (Norwegian) 118 (1998): 2519–2524.

Tuomi, T., Carlsson, A., Li, H., et al., "Clinical and Genetic Characteristics of Type 2 Diabetes with and without GAD Antibodies," *Diabetes* 48 (1999): 150–157.

Tuomilehto-Wolf, E., Tuomilehto, J., Hitman, G.A., et al., "Genetic Susceptibility to Non-Insulin-Dependent Diabetes Mellitus and Glucose Intolerance Are Located in

HLA Region," *British Medical Journal* 307 (1993): 155–159.

Mitral Valve Prolapse

Bobkowski, W., Siwinska, A., Zachwieja, J., et al., "[Electrolyte Abnormalities and Ventricular Arrhythmias in Children with Mitral Valve Prolapse]," *Polski Merkuriusz Lekarski* (Polish) 11 (2001): 125–128.

Braun, W.E., Ronan, J., Schacter, B., et al., "HLA Antigens in Mitral Valve Prolapse," *Transplantation Proceedings* 9 (1977): 1869–1871.

Devereux, R.B., Jones, E.C., Roman, M.J., et al., "Prevalence and Correlates of Mitral Valve Prolapse in a Population-Based Sample of American Indians: The Strong Heart Study," *The American Journal of Medicine* 111 (2001): 679–685.

Disse, S., Abergel, E., Berrebi, A., et al., "Mapping of a First Locus for Autosomal Dominant Myxomatous Mitral-Valve Prolapse to Chromosome 16p11.2-p12.1," *American Journal of Human Genetics* 65 (1999): 1242–1251.

Durlach, J., Bac, P., Durlach, V., et al., "Neurotic, Neuromuscular and Autonomic Nervous Form of Magnesium Imbalance," *Magnesium Research* 10 (1997): 169–195.

Durlach, J., and Durlach, V., "Idiopathic Mitral Valve Prolapse and Magnesium: State of the Art," *Magnesium Bulletin* 8 (1986): 156–169.

Durlach, J., Henrotte, J.G., Lepage, V., et al., "HLA-Bw35 Antigen, and Blood Magnesium Level," in *First European Congress on Magnesium (Lisbon)*, ed. M.J. Halpern and J. Durlach (Basel, Switzerland: S. Karger AG, 1985) pp. 95–101.

Fauchier, J.P., Babuty, D., Fauchier, L., et al., "[Mitral Valve Prolapse, Arrhythmias and Sudden Death]," *Archives des Maladies du Coeur et des Vaisseaux* 93 (2000): 1541–1547.

Galland, L.D., Baker, S.M., McLellan, R.K., "Magnesium Deficiency in the Pathogenesis of Mitral Valve Prolapse," *Magnesium* 5 (1986): 165–174.

Kachru, R.B., Telischi, M., Cruz, J.B., et al., "The HLA Antigens and ABO Blood Groups in an American Black Population with Mitral Valve Prolapse," *Tissue Antigens* 14 (1979): 256–260.

Reba, A., Lutfalla, G., and Pailleret, J.J., "Latent Tetany Due to Magnesium Deficit and Billowing or Prolapse of the Mitral Valve?" *Magnesium Bulletin* 8 (1986): 268.

Reba, A.N., "Magnesium and Barlow's Syndrome: New Data," *Magnesium Research* 1 (1988): 119.

Simoes Fernandes, J., Pereira, T., Carvalho, J., et al., "Therapeutic Effect of a Magnesium Salt in Patients Suffering from Mitral Valvular Prolapse and Latent Tetany," *Magnesium* 4 (1985): 283–290.

Zeana, C., Briciu, M., Florescu, A., et al., "Considerations on the Pathogenesis of Mitral Valve Prolapse," *Médecine Interne* 23 (1985): 165–170.

Zeana, C.D., "Recent Data on Mitral Valve Prolapse and Magnesium Deficit," *Magnesium Research* 1 (1988): 203–211.

GENETIC CONTROL OF THE MAGNESIUM REQUIREMENT FOR HEALTH

Darlu, P., Defrise-Gussenhoven, E., Michotte, Y., et al., "Possible Linkage Relationship Between Genetic Markers and Blood Magnesium and Zinc. A Twin Study," *Acta Geneticae Medicae et Gemellologiae* 34 (1985): 109–112.

Darlu, P., Michotte, Y., Defrise-Gussenhoven, E., et al., "The Inheritance of Plasma and Red Blood Cell Magnesium and Zinc Levels Studied from Twin and Family Data," *Acta Geneticae Medicae et Gemellologiae* 30 (1981): 67–75.

Gattegno, L., Henrotte, J.G., and Benbunan, M., "Content of Red Blood Cell Sialic Acid in BW 35 Blood Donors. Relation to Magnesium Concentration and Pyruvate Kinase Activity," *Carbohydrate Research* 142 (1985): 115–122.

Henrotte, J.G., "[Erythrocyte Magnesium and HLA Groups]," *Comptes Rendus des Seances de l'Academie des Sciences. Serie D, Sciences Naturelles* 289 (1979): 445–447.

Henrotte, J.G., "The Variability of Human Red Blood Cell Magnesium Level According to HLA Groups," *Tissue Antigens* 15 (1980): 419–430.

Henrotte, J.G., "[Genetic Factors of Magnesium Metabolism Regulation in Man]," *Magnesium Bulletin* 3 (1981): 237–248.

Henrotte, J.G., "Genetic Regulation of Red Blood Cell Magnesium Content and Major Histocompatibility Complex," *Magnesium* 1 (1982): 69–80.

Henrotte, J.G., "Recent Advances on Genetic Factors Regulating Blood and Tissue Magnesium Concentrations; Relationship with Stress and Immunity," in *Magnesium in Health and Disease,* ed. Y. Itokawa and J. Durlach (London, England: John Libbey & Company: 1989), pp. 285–289.

Henrotte, J.G., "Genetic Regulation of Cellular Magnesium Content," in *Magnesium and the Cell,* ed. N.J. Birch (London, England: Academic Press Ltd., 1993), pp. 177–195.

Henrotte, J.G., Pla, M., and Dausset, J., "HLA- and H-2-Associated Variations of Intra- and Extracellular Magnesium Content," *Proceedings of the National Academy of Sciences of the United States of America* 87 (1990): 1894–1898.

Lalouel, J.M., Darlu, P., Henrotte, J.G., et al., "Genetic Regulation of Plasma and Red Blood Cell Magnesium Concentration in Man. II. Segregation Analysis," *American Journal of Human Genetics* 35 (1983): 938–950.

Santarromana, M., Delepierre, M., Feray, J.C., et al., "Correlation Between Total and Free Magnesium Levels in Human Red Blood Cells. Influence of HLA Antigens," *Magnesium Research* 2 (1989): 281–283.

Seelig, M.S., Nutritional Status and Requirements of Magnesium, with Consideration of Individual Differences and Prevention of Cardiovascular Disease," *Magnesium Bulletin* 8 (1986): 170–185.

Genetic Intestinal Magnesium Malabsorption

Aries, P.M., Schubert, M., Muller-Wieland, D., et al., "[Subcutaneous Magnesium Pump in a Patient with Combined Magnesium Transport Defect]," *Deutsche Medizinische Wochenschrift* (German) 125 (2000): 970–972.

Cole, D.E., Kooh, S.W., and Vieth, R:, "Primary Infantile Hypomagnesaemia: Outcome after 21 Years and Treatment with Continuous Nocturnal Nasogastric Magnesium Infusion," *European Journal of Pediatrics* 159 (2000): 38–43.

Friedman, M., Hatcher, G., and Watson, L., "Primary Hypomagnesemia with Secondary Hypocalcemia in an Infant," *Lancet* 1 (1967): 703–705.

Geven, W.B., Monnens, L.A., and Willems, J.L., "Magnesium Metabolism in Childhood," *Mineral and Electrolyte Metabolism* 19 (1993): 308–313.

Mettey, R., Guillard, O., Merle, P., et al., "Severe Selective Magnesium Malabsorption: Tests of Tolerance of Oral Magnesium Supplements," *Magnesium Research* 3 (1990): 291–295.

Nordio, S., Donath, A., Macagno, F., et al., "Chronic Hypomagnesemia with Magnesium Dependent Hypocalcemia I. A New Syndrome with Intestinal Malabsorption. II. Magnesium, Calcium and Strontium," *Acta Paediatrica Scandinavica* 60 (1971): 441–448, 449–455.

Paunier, L., and Radde, I.C., "Normal and Abnormal Magnesium Metabolism," *Bulletin of the Hospital for Sick Children (Toronto)* 14 (1965): 16–23.

Seelig, M.S, "Prenatal and Genetic Magnesium Deficiency in Cardiomyopathy: Possible Vitamin and Trace Mineral Interactions," in *Childhood Nutrition,* ed. Fima Lifshitz (Boca Raton FL: CRC Press, 1995), pp. 197–224.

Skyberg, D., Stromme, J.H., Nesbakken, R., et al., "Neonatal Hypomagnesemia with a Selective Malabsorption of Magnesium—A Clinical Entity," *Scandinavian Journal of Clinical Investigations* 21 (1968): 355–363.

Renal Magnesium Wastage

Bartter, F.C., Pronove, P., Gill, J.R., et al., "Hyperplasia of the Juxtaglomerular Complex with Hyperaldosteronism and Hypokalemic Alkalosis. A New Syndrome," *The American Journal of Medicine* 33 (1962): 811–828.Blomstrom-Lundqvist, C., Caidahl, K., Olsson, S.B., et al., "Electrocardiographic Findings and Frequency of Arrhythmias in Bartter's Syndrome," *British Heart Journal* 61 (1989): 274–279.

Cole, D.E., and Quamme, G.A., "Inherited Disorders of renal magnesium handling," *Journal of the American Society of Nephrology* 11 (2000): 1937–1947.

Gitelman, H.J., Graham, J.B., and Welt,

L.G., "A New Familial Disorder Characterized by Hypokalemia and Hypomagnesemia," *Transactions of the Association of American Physicians* 79 (1966): 221–235.

Gullner, H.G., Gill, J.R., Jr., and Bartter, F.C., "Correction of Hypokalemia by Magnesium Repletion in Familial Hypokalemic Alkalosis with Tubulopathy," *The American Journal of Medicine* 71 (1981): 578–582.

Kamel, K.S., Harvey, E., Douek, K., et al., "Studies on the Pathogenesis of Hypokalemia in Gitelman's Syndrome: Role of Bicarbonaturia and Hypomagnesemia," *American Journal of Nephrology* 18 (1998): 42–49.

Kantorovich, V., Adams, J.S., Gaines, J.E., et al., "Genetic Heterogeneity in Familial Renal Magnesium Wasting," *The Journal of Clinical Endocrinology and Metabolism* 87 (2002): 612–617.

Nakai, Y., Kono, T., Yoshimi, T., et al., "[Case of Bartter's Syndrome and the Study of Its Etiology]," *Nippon Rinsho. Japanese Journal of Medicine* 29 (1971): 788–800.

DIFFERENT MAGNESIUM NEEDS IN HEALTHY PEOPLE

Hathaway, M.L., *Magnesium in Human Nutrition,* Home Economics Research Report No. 19 (Washington, D.C.: Agricultural Research Service, U.S. Department of Agriculture, 1962).

Magnesium Balance Studies of Women and Men

Seelig, M.S., "The Requirement of Magnesium by the Normal Adult," *American Journal of Clinical Nutrition* 14 (1964): 342–390.

Differences between the Sexes in Utilizing Magnesium

Canto, J.G., Allison, J.J., Kiefe, C.I., et al., "Relation of Race and Sex to the Use of Reperfusion Therapy in Medicare Beneficiaries with Acute Myocardial Infarction," *The New England Journal of Medicine* 342 (2000): 1094–1100.

Ema, M., Gebrewold, A., Altura, B.T., et al., "Magnesium Sulfate Prevents Alcohol-Induced Spasms of Cerebral Blood Vessels: An In Situ Study on the Brain Microcirculation from Male versus Female Rats," *Magnesium and Trace Elements* 10 (1991): 269–280.

Heyden, S., "[Sex Differences in Cardiovascular Mortality of Diabetics]," *Deutsche Medizinische Wochenschrift* (German) 101 (1976): 789–793.

Liao, F., Folsom, A.R., and Brancati, F.L., "Is Low Magnesium Concentration a Risk Factor for Coronary Heart Disease? The Atherosclerosis Risk in Communities (ARIC) Study," *American Heart Journal* 136 (1998): 480–490.

Muneyvirci-Delale, O., Nacharaju, V.L., Altura, B.M., et al., "Sex Steroid Hormones Modulate Serum Ionized Magnesium and Calcium Levels throughout the Menstrual Cycle in Women," *Fertility and Sterility* 69 (1998): 958–962.

Phillips, G.B., Jing, T.Y., Resnick, L.M., et al., "Sex Hormones and Hemostatic Risk Factors for Coronary Heart Disease in Men with Hypertension," *Journal of Hypertension* 11 (1993): 699–702.

Rubenowitz, E., Axelsson, G., and Rylander, R., "Magnesium in Drinking Water and Death from Acute Myocardial Infarction," *American Journal of Epidemiology* 143 (1996): 456–462.

Rubenowitz, E., Axelsson, G., and Rylander, R., "Magnesium and Calcium in Drinking Water and Death from Acute Myocardial Infarction in Women," *Epidemiology* 10 (1999): 31–36.

Rubenowitz, E., Landin, K., and Wilhelmsen, L., "Skeletal Muscle Magnesium and Potassium by Gender and Hypertensive Status," *Scandinavian Journal of Clinical and Laboratory Investigation* 58 (1998): 47–54.

Zhang, A., Altura, B.T., and Altura, B.M., "Sexual Dimorphism of Vascular Smooth Muscle Responsiveness Is Dependent on Anions and Estrogen," *Steroids* 56 (1991): 524–526.

Estrogen and Magnesium Retention

Seelig, M.S., "Increased Need for Magnesium with the Use of Combined Oestrogen and Calcium for Osteoporosis Treatment," *Magnesium Research* 3 (1990): 197–215.

Estrogen and Blood Clotting

Agardh, C.D., Rasmussen, F., Nilsson-Ehle, P., et al., "Influence of Treatment with Diethylstilbestrol for Carcinoma of Prostate on Platelet Aggregation and Plasma Lipoproteins, *Urology* 28 (1986): 469–471.

Blackard, C.E., Doe, R.P., Mellinger, G.T., et al., "Incidence of Cardiovascular Disease and Death in Patients Receiving Diethylstilbestrol for Carcinoma of the Prostate," *Cancer* 26 (1970): 249–256.

Bruckert, E., and Turpin, G., "Estrogens and Progestins in Postmenopausal Women: Influence on Lipid Parameters and Cardiovascular Risk," *Hormone Research* 43 (1995): 100–103.

Buller, J.C., Kritz-Silverstein, D., Barrett-Connor, E., et al., "Type A Behavior Pattern, Heart Disease Risk Factors, and Estrogen Replacement Therapy in Postmenopausal Women: The Rancho Bernardo Study," *Journal of Women's Health* 7 (1998): 49–56.

Byar, D.P., and Corle, D.K., "Hormone Therapy for Prostate Cancer: Results of the Veterans Administration Cooperative Urological Research Group Studies," National Cancer Institute Monograph 7 (1988), pp. 165–170.

Durlach, J., "[Pills and Thrombosis (Platelets, Estrogens and Magnesium)]," *La Revue Francaise d'Endocrinologie Clinique, Nutrition, et Metabolisme* (French) 54 (1970): 45–54.

Eisen, M., Napp, H.E., and Vock, R., "Inhibition of Platelet Aggregation Caused by Estrogen Treatment in Patients with Carcinoma of the Prostate," *The Journal of Urology* 114 (1975): 93–97.

Henriksson, P., "Estrogen in Patients with Prostatic Cancer. An Assessment of the Risks and Benefits," *Drug Safety* 6 (1991): 47–53.

Henriksson, P., Blomback, M., Bratt, G., et al., "Effects of Oestrogen Therapy and Orchidectomy on Coagulation and Prostanoid Synthesis in Patients with Prostatic Cancer," *Medical Oncology and Tumor Pharmacotherapy* 6 (1989): 219–225.

Peterson, L.R., "Estrogen Replacement Therapy and Coronary Artery Disease," *Current Opinion in Cardiology* 13 (1998): 223–231.

Pines, A., Bornstein, N.M., and Shapira, I., "Menopause and Ischaemic Stroke: Basic, Clinical and Epidemiological Considerations. The Role of Hormone Replacement," *Human Reproduction Update* 8 (2002): 161–168.

"Risks and Benefits of Estrogen Plus Progestin in Healthy Postmenopausal Women: Principal Results from the Women's Health Initiative Randomized Controlled Trial," *Journal of the American Medical Association* 288 (2002): 321–333.

Rossouw, L., Press conference announcing termination of the Women's Health Initiative Study, 9 July 2002.

The Women's Health Initiative Study Group, "Design of the Women's Health Initiative Clinical Trial and Observational Study," *Controlled Clinical Trials* 19 (1998): 61–109.

Individual Differences in Manifestations of Magnesium Deficiency

Rude, R.K., "Magnesium Deficiency: A Cause of Heterogeneous Disease in Humans," *Journal of Bone Minereral Research* 13 (1998): 749–758.

CHAPTER EIGHT

MAGNESIUM AND OTHER HEART DISEASE RISK FACTORS

ALCOHOL

Alcoholism and Cardiovascular Disease

Abbott, L., Nadler, J., and Rude, R.K., "Magnesium Deficiency in Alcoholism: Possible Contribution to Osteoporosis and Cardiovascular Disease in Alcoholics," *Alcoholism, Clinical and Experimental Research* 18 (1994): 1076–1082.

Ajani, U.A., Gaziano, J.M., Lotufo, P.A., et al., "Alcohol Consumption and Risk of Coronary Heart Disease by Diabetes Status," *Circulation* 102 (2000): 500–505.

Alexander, C.S., "The Concept of Alcoholic Cyocardiopathy," *The Medical Clinics of North America* 52 (1968): 1183–1191.

Brigden, W., "Alcoholic Heart Disease," *British Medical Journal* 2 (1964): 1283–1289.

Brigden, W., "Alcoholic Cardiomyopathy," *British Journal of Hospital Medicine* 18 (1977): 122–125.

Bulloch, R.T., Pearce, M.B., Murphy, M.L., et al., "Myocardial Lesions in Idiopathic and Alcoholic Cardiomyopathy. Study by Ventricular Septal Biopsy," *The*

American Journal of Cardiology 29 (1972): 15–25.

Burch, G.E., and DePasquale, N.P., "Alcoholic Cardiomyopathy," *The American Journal of Cardiology* 23 (1969): 723–731.

Finn, P.R., and Pihl, R.O., "Risk for Alcoholism: A Comparison between Two Different Groups of Sons of Alcoholics on Cardiovascular Reactivity and Sensitivity to Alcohol," *Alcoholism, Clinical and Experimental Research* 12 (1988): 742–747.

Lieber, C.S., "Hepatic and Other Medical Disorders of Alcoholism: from Pathogenesis to Treatment," *Journal of Studies on Alcohol* 59 (1998): 9–25.

Miwa, K., Igawa, A., Miyagi, Y., et al., "Importance of Magnesium Deficiency in Alcohol-Induced Variant Angina," *The American Journal of Cardiology* 73 (1994): 813–816.

Pintar, K., Wolansky, B.M., Gubbay, E.R., "Alcoholic Cardiomyopathy," *Canadian Medical Association Journal* 93 (1965): 103–107.

Preedy, V.R., Reilly, M.E., Patel, V.B., et al., "Protein Metabolism in Alcoholism: Effects on Specific Tissues and the Whole Body," *Nutrition* 15 (1999): 604–608.

Stewart, S.H., Finn, P.R., and Pihl, R.O., "The Effects of Alcohol on the Cardiovascular Stress Response in Men at High Risk for Alcoholism: A Dose Response Study," *Journal of Studies on Alcohol* 53 (1992): 499–506.

Wahl, D., Paille, F., Pirollet, P., et al., "[Lipids and Lipoproteins in Chronic Alcoholism. Outcome after Alcohol Withdrawal]," *La Revue de Medicine Interne* 13 (1992): 97–102.

Moderate Drinking and Cardiovascular Disease

Agarwal, D.P., and Srivastava, L.M., "Does Moderate Alcohol Intake Protect against Coronary Heart Disease?" *Indian Heart Journal* 53 (2001): 224–230.

Cooper, H.A., Exner, D.V., and Domanski, M.J., "Light-to-Moderate Alcohol Consumption and Prognosis in Patients with Left Ventricular Systolic Dysfunction," *Journal of the American College of Cardiology* 35 (2000): 1753–1759.

Denke, M.A., "Nutritional and Health Benefits of Beer," *The American Journal of Medical Science* 320 (2000): 320–326.

Foppa, M., Fuchs, F.D., and Duncan, B.B., "Alcohol and Atherosclerosis," *Arquivos Brasileiros de Cardiologia* 76 (2001): 165–176.

German, J.B., and Walzem, R.L., "The Health Benefits of Wine," *Annual Review of Nutrition* 20 (2000): 561–593.

Kwasniewska, M., Kostka, T., and Drygas, W., "[Red Wine in Medicine: Panacea, Fashion or . . . Risk Factor?]. *Przeglad Lekarski* 57 (2000): 300–304.

Mukamal, K.J., Maclure, M., Muller, J.E., et al., "Prior Alcohol Consumption and Mortality Following Acute Myocardial Infarction," *Journal of the American Medical Association (JAMA)* 285 (2001): 1965–1970.

Papadakis, J.A., Ganotakis, E.S., and Mikhailidis, D.P., "Beneficial Effect of Moderate Alcohol Consumption on Vascular Disease: Myth or Reality?" *Journal of the Royal Society of Health* 120 (2000): 11–15.

Peele, S., and Brodsky, A., "Exploring Psychological Benefits Associated with Moderate Alcohol Use: A Necessary Corrective to Assessments of Drinking Outcomes?" *Drug and Alcohol Dependence* 60 (2000): 221–247.

Rotondo, S., Di Castelnuovo, A., and de Gaetano, G., "The Relationship between Wine Consumption and Cardiovascular Risk: From Epidemiological Evidence to Biological Plausibility," *Italian Heart Journal* 2 (2001): 1–8.

Samanek, M., "[Does Moderate Alcohol Drinking Decrease the Incidence and Mortality Rate in Ischemic Heart Disease?]" *Casopusi Lekaru Ceskych* (Czech) 139 (2000): 747–752.

Scanlan, M.F., Roebuck, T., Little, P.J., et al., "Effect of Moderate Alcohol upon Obstructive Sleep Apnoea," *The European Respiratory Journal* 16 (2000): 909–913.

Simons, L.A., McCallum, J., Friedlander, Y., et al., "Moderate Alcohol Intake Is Associated with Survival in the Elderly: The Dubbo Study," *The Medical Journal of Australia* 173 (2000): 121–124.

Solomon, C.G., Hu, F.B., Stampfer, M.J., et al., "Moderate Alcohol Consumption and Risk of Coronary Heart Disease among

Women with Type 2 Diabetes Mellitus," *Circulation* 102 (2000): 494–499.

Theobald, H., Bygren, L.O., Carstensen, J., et al., "A moderate Intake of Wine Is Associated with Reduced Total Mortality and Reduced Mortality from Cardiovascular Disease," *Journal of Studies on Alcohol* 61 (2000): 652–656.

Trevisan, M., Schisterman, E., Mennotti, A., et al., "Drinking Pattern and Mortality: The Italian Risk Factor and Life Expectancy Pooling Project," *Annals of Epidemiology* 11 (2001): 312–319.

Wahl, D., Paille, F., Pirollet, P., et al., "[Lipids and Lipoproteins in Chronic Alcoholism. Outcome after Alcohol Withdrawal]," *La Revue de Medicine Interne* 13 (1992): 97–102.

Wollin, S.D., and Jones, P.J., "Alcohol, Red Wine and Cardiovascular Disease," *The Journal of Nutrition* 131 (2001): 1401–1404.

TOBACCO

The Thermogenic Effect of Smoking

Green, J.H., and Muers, M.F., Comparisons between Basal Metabolic Rate and Diet-Induced Thermogenesis in Different Types of Chronic Obstructive Pulmonary Disease," *Clinical Science (London, England)* 83 (1992): 109–116.

Hofstetter, A., Schutz, Y., Jequier, E., et al., "Increased 24-Hour Energy Expenditure in Cigarette Smokers," *The New England Journal of Medicine* 314 (1986): 79–82.

Marks, B.L., and Perkins, K.A.," The Effects of Nicotine on Metabolic Rate," *Sports Medicine* 10 (1990): 277–285.

Nystrom, E., Lapidus, L., Petersen, K., et al., "[Does Metabolic Rate Slow Down after Smoking Cessation?]" *Lakartidningen* (Swedish) 90 (1993): 4307.

Perkins, K.A., "Metabolic Effects of Cigarette Smoking," *Journal of Applied Physiology* 72 (1992): 401–409.

Perkins, K.A., Epstein, L.H., Marks, B.L., et al., "The Effect of Nicotine on Energy Expenditure during Light Physical Activity," *The New England Journal of Medicine* 320 (1989): 898–903.

Perkins, K.A., Epstein, L.H., and Pastor, S., "Changes In Energy Balance Following Smoking Cessation and Resumption of Smoking in Women," *Journal of Consulting and Clinical Psychology* 58 (1990): 121–125.

Perkins, K.A., Epstein, L.H., Stiller, R.L., et al., "Acute Effects of Nicotine on Resting Metabolic Rate in Cigarette Smokers," *American Journal of Clinical Nutrition* 50 (1989): 545–550.

Perkins, K.A., Epstein, L.H., Stiller, R.L., et al., "Metabolic Effects of Nicotine after Consumption of a Meal in Smokers and Nonsmokers," *American Journal of Clinical Nutrition* 52 (1990): 228–233.

Robinson, S., and York, D.A., "The Effect of Cigarette Smoking on the Thermic Response to Feeding," *International Journal of Obesity* 10 (1986): 407–417.

Walker, J., Collins, L.C., Nannini, L., et al., "Potentiating Effects of Cigarette Smoking and Moderate Exercise on the Thermic Effect of a Meal," *International Journal of Obesity and Related Metabolic Disorders* 16 (1992): 341–347.

Warwick, P.M., and Baines, J., "Energy Expenditure in Free-Living Smokers and Nonsmokers: Comparison between Factorial, Intake-Balance, and Doubly Labeled Water Measures," *American Journal of Clinical Nutrition* 63 (1996): 15–21.

Warwick, P.M., and Busby, R., "Prediction of Twenty-Four-Hour Energy Expenditure in a Respiration Chamber in Smokers and Non-Smokers," *European Journal of Clinical Nutrition* 47 (1993): 600–603.

Warwick, P.M., Chapple, R.S., and Thomson, E.S., "The Effect of Smoking Two Cigarettes on Resting Metabolic Rate with and without Food," *International Journal of Obesity* 11 (1987): 229–237.

Warwick, P.M., Edmundson, H.M., and Thomson, E.S., "No Evidence for a Chronic Effect of Smoking on Energy Expenditure," *International Journal of Obesity and Related Metabolic Disorders* 19 (1995): 198–201.

Smoking and Magnesium

Attvall, S., Fowelin, J., Lager, I., et al., "Smoking Induces Insulin Resistance—a Potential Link with the Insulin Resistance Syndrome," *Journal of Internal Medicine* 233 (1993): 327–332.

Christiansen, E., and Madsbad, S., "[Smoking and Diabetes Mellitus]," *Ugeskrift for Laeger* (Danish) 151 (1989): 3050–3053.

Eliasson, B., Hjalmarson, A., Kruse, E., et al., "Effect of Smoking Reduction and Cessation on Cardiovascular Risk Factors," *Nicotine and Tobacco Research* 3 (2001): 249–255.

Facchini, F.S., Hollenbeck, C.B., Jeppesen, J., et al., "Insulin Resistance and Cigarette Smoking," *Lancet* 339 (1992): 1128–1130.

Li, W., Zheng, T., Altura, B.T., et al., "Magnesium Modulates Contractile Responses of Rat Aorta to Thiocyanate: A possible Relationship to Smoking-Induced Atherosclerosis," *Toxicology and Applied Pharmacology* 157 (1999): 77–84.

Loft, S., Astrup, A., Buemann, B., et al., "Oxidative DNA Damage Correlates with Oxygen Consumption in Humans," *The FASEB Journal* 8 (1994): 534–537.

Menditto, A., Morisi, G., Alimonti, A., et al., "Association of Serum Copper and Zinc with Serum Electrolytes and with Selected Risk Factors for Cardiovascular Disease in Men Aged 55–75 years. NFR Study Group," *Journal of Trace Elements and Electrolytes in Health and Disease* 7 (1993): 251–253.

Rajala, U., Laakso, M., Paivansalo, M., et al., "Low Insulin Sensitivity Measured by Both Quantitative Insulin Sensitivity Check Index and Homeostasis Model Assessment Method as a Risk Factor of Increased Intima-Media Thickness of the Carotid Artery," *Journal of Clinical Endocrinology and Metabolism* 87 (2002): 5092–5097.

Reaven, Gerald, Strom, Terry Kristen, and Fox, Barry, *Syndrome X: The Silent Killer* (New York: Simon & Schuster, 2000).

Srikumar, T.S., Kallgard, A., Lindeberg, S., et al., "Trace Element Concentrations in Hair of Subjects from Two South Pacific Islands, Atafu (Tokelau) and Kitava (Papua New Guinea)," *Journal of Trace Elements and Electrolytes in Health and Disease* 8 (1994): 21–26.

Touitou, Y., Godard, J.P., Ferment, O., et al., "Prevalence of Magnesium and Potassium Deficiencies in the Elderly," *Clinical Chemistry* 33 (1987): 518–523.

Touitou, Y., Touitou, C., Bogdan, A., et al., "Physiopathological Changes of Magnesium Metabolism with Aging," in *Magnesium in Health and Disease,* ed. Y. Itokawa and J. Durlach (London, England: John Libbey & Company, 1989) pp. 103–110.

Smoking and Weight

Chyou, P.H., Burchfiel, C.M., Yano, K., et al., "Obesity, Alcohol Consumption, Smoking, and Mortality," *Annals of Epidemiology* 7 (1997): 311–317.

Dallosso, H.M., and James, W.P., "The Role of Smoking in the Regulation of Energy Balance," *International Journal of Obesity* 8 (1984): 365–375.

Hatsukami, D., Hughes, J.R., and Pickens, R., "Characterization of Tobacco Withdrawal: Physiological and Subjective Effects," National Institute on Drug Abuse (NIDA) Research Monograph 53 (1985): 56–67.

Jarry, J.L., Coambs, R.B., Polivy, J., et al., "Weight Gain after Smoking Cessation in Women: The Impact of Dieting Status," *Internatoinal Journal of Eating Disorders* 24 (1998): 53–64.

Kawachi, I., Troisi, R.J., Rotnitzky, A.G., et al., "Can Physical Activity Minimize Weight Gain in Women after Smoking Cessation?" *American Journal of Public Health* 86 (1996): 999–1004.

Moffatt, R.J., and Owens, S.G., "Cessation from Cigarette Smoking: Changes in Body Weight, Body Composition, Resting Metabolism, and Energy Consumption," *Metabolism* 40 (1991): 465–470.

Stamford, B.A., Matter, S., Fell, R.D., et al., "Effects of Smoking Cessation on Weight Gain, Metabolic Rate, Caloric Consumption, and Blood Lipids," *American Journal of Clinical Nutrition* 43 (1986): 486–494.

Tonstad, S., Gorbitz, C., Sivertsen, M., et al., "Under-Reporting of Dietary Intake by Smoking and Non-Smoking Subjects Counselled for Hypercholesterolaemia," *Journal of Internal Medicine* 245 (1999): 337–344.

COCAINE

Altura, B.M., Gebrewold, A., Altura, B.T., et al., "Magnesium Protects against Cocaine-Induced Hemorrhagic Stroke in a

Rat Model: A 31P-NMR In-Vivo Study," *Frontiers in Bioscience* 2 (1997): a9–a12.

Altura, B.M., and Gupta, R.K., "Cocaine Induces Intracellular Free Mg Deficits, Ischemia and Stroke as Observed by In-Vivo 31P–NMR of the Brain," *Biochimica et Biophysica Acta* 1111 (1992): 271–274.

Altura, B.M., Zhang, A., Cheng, T.P., et al., "Cocaine Induces Rapid Loss of Intracellular Free Mg2+ in Cerebral Vascular Smooth Muscle Cells," *European Journal of Pharmacology* 246 (1993): 299–301.

Bauman, J.L., and DiDomenico, R.J., "Cocaine-Induced Channelopathies: Emerging Evidence on the Multiple Mechanisms of Sudden Death," *Journal of Cardiovascular Pharmacology and Therapeutics* 7 (2002): 195–202.

Billman, G.E., "Effect of Calcium Channel Antagonists on Cocaine-Induced Malignant Arrhythmias: Protection against Ventricular Fibrillation," *The Journal of Pharmacological and Experimental Therapeutics* 266 (1993): 407–416.

Brecklin, C.S., and Bauman, J.L., "Cardiovascular Effects of Cocaine: Focus on Hypertension," *Journal of Clinical Hypertension (Greenwich)* 1 (1999): 212–217.

Ferdinand, K.C., "Substance Abuse and Hypertension," *Journal of Clinical Hypertension (Greenwich)* 2 (2000): 37–40.

Galasko, G.I., "Cocaine, a Risk Factor for Myocardial Infarction," *Journal of Cardiovascular Risk* 4 (1997): 185–190.

Gamouras, G.A., Monir, G., Plunkitt, K., et al., "Cocaine Abuse: Repolarization Abnormalities and Ventricular Arrhythmias," *The American Journal of Medical Science* 320 (2000): 9–12.

Golbe, L.I., and Merkin, M.D., "Cerebral Infarction in a User of Free-Base Cocaine ('Crack')," *Neurology* 36 (1986): 1602–1604.

Huang, Q.F., Gebrewold, A., Altura, B.T., et al., "Cocaine-Induced Cerebral Vascular Damage Can Be Ameliorated by Mg2+ in Rat Brain," *Neuroscience Letters* 109 (1990): 113–116.

Jacobsen, T.N., Grayburn, P.A., Snyder, R.W., et al., "Effects of Intranasal Cocaine on Sympathetic Nerve Discharge in Humans," *Journal of Clinical Investigations* 99 (1997): 628–634.

Mittleman, M.A., Mintzer, D., Maclure, M., et al., "Triggering of Myocardial Infarction by Cocaine," *Circulation* 99 (1999): 2737–2741.

Qureshi, A.I., Suri, M.F., Guterman, L.R., et al., "Cocaine Use and the Likelihood of Nonfatal Myocardial Infarction and Stroke: Data from the Third National Health and Nutrition Examination Survey," *Circulation* 103 (2001): 502–506.

Singh, N., Singh, H.K., Singh, P.P., et al., "Cocaine-Induced Torsades de Pointes in Idiopathic Long Q-T Syndrome," *American Journal of Therapeutics* 8 (2001): 299–302.

Steinhauer, J.R., and Caulfield, J.B., "Spontaneous Coronary Artery Dissection Associated with Cocaine Use: A Case Report and Brief Review," *Cardiovascular Pathology* 10 (2001): 141–145.

Vasica, G., and Tennant, C.C., "Cocaine Use and Cardiovascular Complications," *The Medical Journal of Australia* 177 (2002): 260–262.

Vongpatanasin, W., Mansour, Y., Chavoshan, B., et al., "Cocaine Stimulates the Human Cardiovascular System Via a Central Mechanism of Action," *Circulation* 100 (1999): 497–502.

Weaver, K., Merrell, C.L., and Griffin, G., "Effect of Magnesium on Cocaine-Induced, Catecholamine-Mediated Platelet and Vascular Response in Term Pregnant Ewes," *American Journal of Obstetrics and Gynecology* 161 (1989): 1331–1337.

HOMOCYSTEINE

Donner, M.G., Schwandt, P., and Richter, W.O., "[Homocysteine and Coronary Heart Disease. Is Slight or Moderate Homocysteinemia Related to Increased Risk of Coronary Heart Disease?]" *Fortschritte der Medizin* (German) 115 (1997): 24–30.

Engman, M., "Homocysteinemia: New Information About an Old Risk Factor for Vascular Disease," *Journal of Insurance Medicine* 30 (1998): 231–236.

Glueck, C.J., Shaw, P., Lang, J.E., et al., "Evidence That Homocysteine Is an Independent Risk Factor for Atherosclerosis in Hyperlipidemic Patients," *The American Journal of Cardiology* 75 (1995): 132–136.

Guba, S.C., Fonseca, V., and Fink, L.M.,

"Hyperhomocysteinemia and Thrombosis," *Seminars in Thrombosis and Hemostasis* 25 (1999): 291–309.

Li, W., Zheng, T., Wang, J., et al., "Extracellular Magnesium Regulates Effects of Vitamin B_6, B_{12} and Folate on Homocysteinemia-Induced Depletion of Intracellular Free Magnesium Ions in Canine Cerebral Vascular Smooth Muscle Cells: Possible Relationship to [Ca2+]i, Atherogenesis and Stroke," *Neuroscience Letters* 274 (1999): 83–86.

Marci, M., Raffa, S., Lozzi, A., et al., "Relationships Between Serum Hyperhomocysteinemia and Carotid Atherosclerosis in Geriatric Patients," *Minerva Cardioangiologica* (Italian) 47 (1999): 339–345.

Nehler, M.R., Taylor, L.M., Jr., and Porter, J.M., "Homocysteinemia as a Risk Factor for Atherosclerosis: A Review," *Cardiovascular Surgery* 5 (1997): 559–567.

O.K., Lynn, E.G., Chung, Y.H., et al., "Homocysteine Stimulates the Production and Secretion of Cholesterol in Hepatic Cells," *Biochimica et Biophysica Acta* 1393 (1998): 317–324.

Potena, L., Grigioni, F., Magnani, G., et al., "Increasing Plasma Homocysteine during Follow-Up in Heart Transplant Recipients: Effects of Folate and Renal Function," *Italian Heart Journal* 1 (2000): 344–348.

Prasad, K., "Homocysteine, a Risk Factor for Cardiovascular Disease," *International Journal of Angiology* 8 (1999): 76–86.

Reis, R.P., Azinheira, J., Reis, H.P., et al., "[Prognosis Significance of Blood Homocysteine after Myocardial Infarction]," *Revista Portuguesa de Cardiologia* (Portuguese) 19 (2000): 581–585.

Reis, R.P., Azinheira, J., Reis, H.P., et al., "[Homocysteinemia as a Risk Factor for Cerebrovascular Disorders. The Role of Age and Homocysteine Levels]," *Acta Medica Portuguesa* 9 (1996): 15–20.

Reis, R.P., Azinheira, J., Reis, H.P., et al., "[The effect of sex and menopause on basal blood levels of homocysteine and after methionine loading]. *Revista Portuguesa de Cardiologia* 18 (1999): 155–159.

Robinson, K., Mayer, E., Jacobsen, D.W., "Homocysteine and Coronary Artery Disease," *Cleveland Clinical Journal of Medicine* 61 (1994): 438–450.

Robinson, K., Mayer, E.L., Miller, D.P., et al., "Hyperhomocysteinemia and Low Pyridoxal Phosphate. Common and Independent Reversible Risk Factors for Coronary Artery Disease," *Circulation* 92 (1995): 2825–2830.

Salardi, S., Cacciari, E., Sassi, S., et al., "Homocysteinemia, Serum Folate and Vitamin B_{12} in Very Young Patients with Diabetes Mellitus Type 1," *Journal of Pediatric Endocrinology and Metabolism* 13 (2000): 1621–1627.

Selhub, J., Jacques, P.F., Wilson, P.W., et al., "Vitamin Status and Intake as Primary Determinants of Homocysteinemia in an Elderly Population," *Journal of the American Medical Association (JAMA)* 270 (1993): 2693–2698.

Stampfer, M.J., and Malinow, M.R., "Can Lowering Homocysteine Levels Reduce Cardiovascular Risk?" *The New England Journal of Medicine* 332 (1995): 328–329.

Ubbink, J.B., Vermaak, W.J., Bennett, J.M., et al., "The Prevalence of Homocysteinemia and Hypercholesterolemia in Angiographically Defined Coronary Heart Disease," *Klinische Wochenschrift* 69 (1991): 527–534.

Chapter Nine

ARE WE REALLY LOW IN MAGNESIUM?

THE MODERN DIET: LOW IN MAGNESIUM

See also Chapter 5 References for the effect of dietary saturated fat on magnesium absorption.

Ericsson, Y., Angmar-Mansson, B., and Flores, M., "Urinary Mineral Ion Loss After Sugar Ingestion," *Bone and Mineral* 9 (1990): 233–237.

Karppanen, H., "Ischaemic Heart Disease. An Epidemiological Perspective with Special Reference to Electrolytes," *Drugs* 28 (1984) (Supplement 1): 17–27.

Li, M.K., Kavanagh, J.P., Prendiville, V., et al., "Does Sucrose Damage Kidneys?" *British Journal of Urology* 58 (1986): 353–357.

Lindeman, R.D., Adler, S., Yiengst, M.J., et al., "Influence of Various Nutrients on

Urinary Divalent Cation Excretion," *The Journal of Laboratory and Clinical Medicine* 70 (1967): 236–245.

Lindeman, R.D., "Influence of Various Nutrients and Hormones on Urinary Divalent Cation Excretion," *Annals of the New York Academy of Sciences* 162 (1969): 802–809.

Marier, J.R., "Magnesium Content of the Food Supply in the Modern-Day World," *Magnesium* 5 (1986): 1–8.

Marier, J.R., "Quantitative Factors Regarding Magnesium Status in the Modern-Day World," *Magnesium* 1 (1982): 3–15.

Marier, J.R., "Role of Environmental Magnesium in Cardiovascular Diseases," *Magnesium* 1 (1982): 266–276.

Meyer, F.L., Cooper, K., and Bolick, M., "Nitrogen and Mineral Excretion after Carbohydrate Test Meals," *American Journal of Clinical Nutrition* 25 (1972): 677–683.

Oberleas, D., "A New Perspective of Trace Element Deficiencies," *Trace Elements in Medicine* 12 (2002): 3.

Pennington, J.A.T., Young, B.E., and Wilson, D.B., "Nutritional Elements in U.S. Diets: Results from the Total Diet Study, 1982–1986," *Journal of the American Dietetic Association* 89 (1989): 659–664.

Preuss, H.G., Memon, S., Dadgar, A., et al., "Effects of High Sugar Diets on Renal Fluid, Electrolyte and Mineral Handling in Rats: Relationship to Blood Pressure," *Journal of the American College of Nutrition* 13 (1994): 73–82.

Scholz, R.W., and Featherston, W.R., "Influence of Dietary Carbohydrates on Magnesium Utilization in the Chick," *The Journal of Nutrition* 91 (1967): 223–230.

Schroeder, H.A., "Losses of Vitamins and Trace Minerals Resulting from Processing and Preservation of Foods," *American Journal of Clinical Nutrition* 24 (1971): 562–573.

Seelig, M.S., "The Requirement of Magnesium by the Normal Adult," *American Journal of Clinical Nutrition* 14 (1964): 342–390.

Sharief, N., and Macdonald, I., "Differences in the Metabolic Rate Following Ingestion of Sucrose and Glucose in Man," *The Proceedings of the Nutrition Society* 39 (1980): 42A.

BUT I TAKE A MULTIVITAMIN SUPPLEMENT EVERY DAY!

Rosanoff, A., "Magnesium is Below RDA Levels in Common Multivitamin/Mineral Supplements: A Survey," unpublished survey (2002).

WATER SUPPLIES: LOW IN MAGNESIUM

Azoulay, A., Garzon, P., and Eisenberg, M.J., "Comparison of the Mineral Content of Tap Water and Bottled Waters," *Journal of General Internal Medicine* 16 (2001): 168–175.

Bloom, S., and Peric-Golia, L., "Geographic Variation in the Incidence of Myocardial Calcification Associated with Acute Myocardial Infarction, *Human Pathology* 20 (1989): 726–731.

Feder, G.L., and Hopps, H.C., "Variations in Drinking Water Quality and the Possible Effects on Human Health," *Trace Substances and Environmental Health* 15 (1981): 96–103.

Hankin, J.H., Margen, S., and Goldsmith, N.F., "Contribution of Hard Water to Calcium and Magnesium Intakes of Adults," *Journal of the American Dietetic Association* 56 (1970): 212–224.

Hopps, H.C., and Feder, G.L., "Chemical Qualities of Water That Contribute to Human Health in a Positive Way," *The Science of the Total Environment* 54 (1986): 207–216.

Marx, A., and Neutra, R.R., "Magnesium in Drinking Water and Ischemic Heart Disease," *Epidemiologic Reviews* 19 (1997): 258–272.

Masironi, R., "Cardiovascular Mortality in Relation to Radioactivity and Hardness of Local Water Supplies in the USA," *Bulletin of the World Health Organization* 43 (1970): 687–697.

Neutra, RR., "Epidemiology vs. Physiology? Drinking Water Magnesium and Cardiac Mortality," *Epidemiology* 10 (1999): 4–6.

Robinson, J., "Industrial Water Treatment," in *Kirk-Othmer Encyclopedia of Chemical Technology,* 4th ed. Vol. 25 (New York: John Wiley & Sons, 1998) pp. 487–526.

Rubenowitz, E., Axelsson, G., Rylander, R., "Magnesium in Drinking Water and

Body Magnesium Status Measured Using an Oral Loading Test," *Scandinavian Journal of Clinical and Laboratory Investigation* 58 (1998): 423–428.

Schroeder, H.A., "Municipal Drinking Water and Cardiovascular Death Rates," *Journal of the American Medical Association (JAMA)* 195 (1966): 81–85.

Seelig, M.S, "Epidemiology of Water Magnesium; Evidence of Contributions to Health," in *Advances in Magnesium Research: Nutrition and Health: Proceedings of the Ninth International Symposium on Magnesium (Vichy, France)*, ed. Yves Rayssiguier, André Mazur, and Jean Durlach, (London, England: John Libbey & Company, 2001), pp. 211–218.

Sharrett, A.R., "The Role of Chemical Constituents of Drinking Water in Cardiovascular Diseases," *American Journal of Epidemiology* 110 (1979): 401–419.

MEDICATIONS

Seelig M.S., and Altura, B.M., "How Best to Determine Magnesium Requirement: Need to Consider Cardiotherapeutic Drugs That Affect Its Retention," *Journal of the American College of Nutrition* 16 (1997): 4–6.

CALCIUM SUPPLEMENTS

Bendich, A., Leader, S., and Muhuri, P., "Supplemental Calcium for the Prevention of Hip Fracture: Potential Health-Economic Benefits," *Clinical Therapeutics* 21 (6) (June 1999):1058–1072.

Dawson-Hughes, B., Harris, S.S., Dallal, G.E., et al., "Calcium Supplement and Bone Medication Use in a U.S. Medicare Health Maintenance Organization," *Osteoporosis International* 13 (8) (August 2002): 657–662.

Devine, A., Dick, I.M., Heal, S.J., et al., "A 4-Year Follow-Up Study of the Effects of Calcium Supplementation on Bone Density in Elderly Postmenopausal Women," *Osteoporosis International* 7 (1) (1997): 23–28.

Shils, Maurice E., "Magnesium," in *Modern Nutrition in Health and Disease*, ed. Maurice E. Shils, James A. Olson, Moshe Shike, and Catherine A. Ross (Philadelphia: Lippincott Williams & Wilkins, 1999), pp. 173–175.

Karppanen, H., Pennanen, R., and Passinen, L., "Minerals, Coronary Heart Disease and Sudden Coronary Death," *Advances in Cardiology* 25 (1978): 9–24.

Tranquilli, A.L., Lucino, E., Garzetti, G.G., et al., "Calcium, Phosphorus and Magnesium Intakes Correlate with Bone and Mineral Content in Postmenopausal Women," *Gynecological Endocrinology* 8 (1994): 55–58.

Zhang, A., Cheng, T.P., and Altura, B.M., "Magnesium Regulates Intracellular Free Ionized Calcium Concentration and Cell Geometry in Vascular Smooth Muscle Cells," *Biochimica et Biophysica Acta* 1134 (1992): 25–29.

STUDY RESULTS

Altura, B.M., and Altura B.T., "Cardiovascular Risk Factors and Magnesium: Relationships to Atherosclerosis, Ischemic Heart Disease and Hypertension," *Magnesium and Trace Elements* 10 (1991): 182–192.

Nadler, J.L., and Rude, R.K., "Disorders of Magnesium Metabolism," *Endocrinology and Metabolism Clinics of North America* 24 (1995): 623–641.

Pennington, J.A., and Schoen, S.A., "Total Diet Study: Estimated Dietary Intakes of Nutritional Elements, 1982–1991," *International Journal for Vitamin and Nutrition Research* 66 (1996): 350–362.

Pennington, J.A., Young, B.E., Wilson, D.B., et al., "Mineral Content of Foods and Total Diets: The Selected Minerals in Foods Survey, 1982 to 1984," *Journal of the American Dietetic Association* 86 (1986): 876–891.

Vir, S.C., and Love, A.H., "Nutritional Status of Institutionalized and Noninstitutionalized Aged in Belfast, Northern Ireland," *American Journal of Clinical Nutrition* 32 (1979): 1934–1947.

Chapter Ten

Do You Need More Magnesium?

Why Can't I Just Get a Blood Test for Magnesium?

Altura, B.M., "Basic Biochemistry and Physiology of Magnesium: A Brief Review," *Magnesium and Trace Elements* 10 (1991): 167–171.

Altura, B.T., and Altura, B.M., "A Method for Distinguishing Ionized, Complexed and Protein-Bound Mg in Normal and Diseased Subjects," *Scandinavian Journal of Clinical and Laboratory Investigation* 217 (1994) (Supplement): 83–87.

Altura, B.T., Wilimzig, C., Trnovec, T., et al., "Comparative Effects of a Mg-Enriched Diet and Different Orally Administered Magnesium Oxide Preparations on Ionized Mg, Mg Metabolism and Electrolytes in Serum of Human Volunteers," *Journal of the American College of Nutrition* 13 (1994): 447–454.

Elin, R.J., "Assessment of Magnesium Status," in *Magnesium in Health and Disease,* ed. Y. Itokawa and J. Durlach (London, England: John Libbey & Company, 1989), pp. 137–146.

Elin, R.J., "Laboratory Tests for the Assessment of Magnesium Status in Humans," *Magnesium and Trace Elements* 10 (1991): 172–181.

Handwerker, S.M., Altura, B.T., Chi, D.S., et al., "Serum Ionized Magnesium Levels During Intravenous $MgSO_4$ therapy of Preeclamptic Women," *Acta Obstetricia et Gynecolica Scandinavica* 74 (1995): 517–519.

Handwerker, S.M., Altura, B.T., Royo, B., et al., "Ionized Magnesium and Calcium Levels in Umbilical Cord Serum of Pregnant Women with Transient Hypertension during Labor," *American Journal of Hypertension* 6 (1993): 542–545.

Mauskop, A., Altura, B.T., Cracco, R.Q., et al., "Deficiency in Serum Ionized Magnesium but Not Total Magnesium in Patients with Migraines. Possible Role of ICa2+/IMg2+ Ratio," *Headache* 33 (1993): 135–138.

Memon, Z.I., Altura, B.T., Benjamin, J.L., et al., "Predictive Value of Serum Ionized but Not Total Magnesium Levels in Head Injuries," *Scandinavian Journal of Clinical and Laboratory Investigation* 55 (1995): 671–677.

Resnick, L.M., Altura, B.T., Gupta, R.K., et al., "Intracellular and Extracellular Magnesium Depletion in Type 2 (Non-Insulin-Dependent) Diabetes Mellitus," *Diabetologia* 36 (1993): 767–770.

Ryzen, E., Nelson, T.A., and Rude, R.K., Low Blood Mononuclear Cell Magnesium Content and Hypocalcemia in Normomagnesemic Patients," *The Western Journal of Medicine* 147 (1987): 549–553.

Seelig, M.S., and Altura, B.M., "How Best to Determine Magnesium Status: A New Laboratory Test Worth Trying," *Nutrition* 13 (1997): 376–377.

Standing Committee on the Scientific Evaluation of Dietary Reference Intakes, Food and Nutrition Board, Institute of Medicine, "Dietary Reference Intakes for Calcium, Phosphorus, Magnesium, Vitamin D, and Fluoride (Washington, D.C.: National Academy of Sciences, 1997).

How Magnesium Researchers Assess Magnesium Status

Resnick, L.M., personal communication, 2002.

Cellular Free Magnesium via NMR

Rude, R.K., Stephen A, and Nadler J., "Determination of Red Blood Cell Intracellular Free Magnesium by Nuclear Magnetic Resonance as an Assessment of Magnesium Depletion," *Magnesium and Trace Elements* 10 (1991): 117–121.

Ryzen, E., Servis, K.L., DeRusso, P., et al., "Determination of Intracellular Free Magnesium by Nuclear Magnetic Resonance in Human Magnesium Deficiency," *Journal of the American College of Nutrition* 8 (1989): 580–587.

Magnesium Load Testing

Caddell, J.L., "The Magnesium Load Test: I. A Design for Infants," *Clinical Pediatrics* 14 (1975): 449–451, 457–459, 518–519.

Caddell, J.L., and Reed, G.F., "Validity of

the Parenteral Magnesium Load Test for Mature Mammals," *Magnesium* 8 (1989): 65–70.

Cohen, L., and Laor, A., "Correlation Between Bone Magnesium Concentration and Magnesium Retention in the Intravenous Magnesium Load Test," *Magnesium Research* 3 (1990): 271–274.

Holm, C.N., Jepsen, J.M., Sjogaard, G., et al., "A Magnesium Load Test in the Diagnosis of Magnesium Deficiency," *Human Nutrition. Clinical Nutrition* 41 (1987): 301–306.

Martin, B.J., "The Magnesium Load Test: Experience in Elderly Subjects," *Aging (Milano)* 2 (1990): 291–296.

Nicar, M.J., and Pak, C.Y., "Oral Magnesium Load Test for the Assessment of Intestinal Magnesium Absorption. Application in Control Subjects, Absorptive Hypercalciuria, Primary Hyperparathyroidism, and Hypoparathyroidism," *Mineral and Electrolyte Metabolism* 8 (1982): 44–51.

Rubenowitz, E., Axelsson, G., and Rylander, R., "Magnesium in Drinking Water and Body Magnesium Status Measured Using an Oral Loading Test," *Scandinavian Journal of Clinical and Laboratory Investigation* 58 (1998): 423–428.

Ryzen, E., Elbaum, N., Singer, F.R., et al., "Parenteral Magnesium Tolerance Testing in the Evaluation of Magnesium Deficiency," *Magnesium* 4 (1985): 137–147.

Trauninger, A., Pfund, Z., Koszegi, T., et al., "Oral Magnesium Load Test in Patients with Migraine," *Headache* 42 (2002): 114–119.

Ionized Magnesium

Altura, B.T., and Altura, B.M., "Measurement of Ionized Magnesium in Whole Blood, Plasma and Serum with a New Ion-Selective Electrode in Healthy and Diseased Human Subjects," *Magnesium and Trace Elements* 10 (1991): 90–98.

Altura, B.T., Bertschat, F., Jeremias, A., et al., "Comparative Findings on Serum IMg2+ of Normal and Diseased Human Subjects with the NOVA and KONE ISE's for Mg2+," *Scandinavian Journal of Clinical and Laboratory Investigation* 217 (1994) (Supplement): 77–81.

Altura, B.T., Burack, J.L., Cracco, R.Q., et al., "Clinical Studies with the NOVA ISE for IMg2+," *Scandinavian Journal of Clinical and Laboratory Investigation* 217 (1994) (Supplement): 53–67.

Altura, B.T., Shirey, T.L., Young, C.C., et al., "Characterization of a New Ion Selective Electrode for Ionized Magnesium in Whole Blood, Plasma, Serum, and Aqueous Samples," *Scandinavian Journal of Clinical and Laboratory Investigation* 217 (1994) (Supplement): 21–36.

Altura, B.T., Shirey, T.L., Young, C.C., et al., "A New Method for the Rapid Determination of Ionized Mg2+ in Whole Blood, Serum and Plasma," *Methods and Findings in Experimental and Clinical Pharmacology* 14 (1992): 297–304.

Altura, B.T., Wilimzig, C., Trnovec, T., et al., "Comparative Effects of a Mg-Enriched Diet and Different Orally Administered Magnesium Oxide Preparations on Ionized Mg, Mg Metabolism and Electrolytes in Serum of Human Volunteers," *Journal of the American College of Nutrition* 13 (1994): 447–454.

Exatest

Intracellular Diagnostics, Inc., published research and references, 2003.

Silver, B.B., Haigney, M.C.P., Schulman, S.P., et al., "A Unique Non-Invasive Intracellular Magnesium Assay Correlating with Cardiac Tissues, Arrhythmias, and Therapeutic Intervention," Presentation to the Seventh International Symposium on Magnesium, Athens, Greece, 1997.

Silver, B.B., www.exatest.com/Research.htm.

Chapter Eleven

Making Sure You Have Enough Magnesium

Donangelo, C.M., Woodhouse, L.R., King, S.M., et al., "Supplemental Zinc Lowers Measures of Iron Status in Young Women with Low Iron Reserves," *The Journal of Nutrition* 132 (2002): 1860–1864.

Durlach, J., "Recommended Dietary Amounts of Magnesium: Mg RDA," *Magnesium Research* 2 (1989): 195–203.

Haynes, R.B., Kris-Etherton, P., McCarron, D.A., et al., "Nutritionally Complete

Prepared Meal Plan to Reduce Cardiovascular Risk Factors: A Randomized Clinical Trial," *Journal of the American Dietetic Association* 99 (1999): 1077–1083.

Hu, F.B., Rimm, E.B., Stampfer, M.J., et al., "Prospective Study of Major Dietary Patterns and Risk of Coronary Heart Disease in Men," *American Journal of Clinical Nutrition* 72 (2000): 912–921.

Kaski, J.C., and Smith, D.A., "The Management of Chronic Ischemic Heart Disease in the Elderly," *The American Journal of Geriatric Cardiology* 9 (2000): 145–150.

Liu, S., Manson, J.E., Lee, I.M., et al., "Fruit and Vegetable Intake and Risk of Cardiovascular Disease: The Women's Health Study," *American Journal of Clinical Nutrition* 72 (2000): 922–928.

Sanjuliani, A.F., de Abreu Fagundes, V.G., and Francischetti, E.A., "Effects of Magnesium on Blood Pressure and Intracellular Ion Levels of Brazilian Hypertensive Patients," *International Journal of Cardiology* 56 (1996): 177–183.

Shimokata, H., and Kuzuya, F., "[Aging, Basal Metabolic Rate, and Nutrition]," *Nippon Ronen Igakkai Zasshi* (Japanese) 30 (1993): 572–576.

Daubresse, J.C., "[Atherosclerosis and Nutrition]," *Revue Medicale de Bruxelles* (French) 21 (2000): A359–A362.

Sinatra, S.T., and DeMarco, J., Free Radicals, Oxidative Stress, Oxidized Low Density Lipoprotein (LDL), and the Heart: Antioxidants and Other Strategies to Limit Cardiovascular Damage," *Connecticut Medicine* 59 (1995): 579–588.

Singh, R.B., Niaz, M.A., Ghosh, S., et al., "Effect on Mortality and Reinfarction of Adding Fruits and Vegetables to a Prudent Diet in the Indian Experiment of Infarct Survival (IEIS)," *Journal of the American College of Nutrition* 12 (1993): 255–261.

Touitou, Y., Godard, J.P., Ferment, O., et al., "Prevalence of Magnesium and Potassium Deficiencies in the Elderly," *Clinical Chemistry* 33 (1987): 518–523.

Wutzen, J., "Selected Organopathies Caused by Experimental Magnesium Deficiency," *Polski Tygodnik Lekarski* 44 (1989): 243–246.

Chapter Twelve

Conclusion: Magnesium—Silent Guardian of Our Hearts and Arteries

Early Studies of Cardiovascular Damage Due to Magnesium Deficiency and of the Curative Effects of Magnesium

Berliner, K., "The Effect of Calcium Injections on the Human Heart," *The American Journal of the Medical Sciences* 191 (1963): 117–121.

Bernstein, M., and Simkins, S., "The Use of Magnesium Sulfate in the Measurement of Circulation Time," *American Heart Journal* 17 (1939): 218–237.

Bower, J.O., and Mengle, H.A.K., "Additive Effects of Calcium and Digitalis; Warning with Report of 2 Cases," *Journal of the American Medical Association* 106 (1936): 1151–1153.

Boyd, L.J., and Scherf, D., "Magnesium Sulfate in Paroxysmal Tachycardia," *The American Journal of the Medical Sciences* 206 (1943): 43–48.

Duncan, C.W., Huffman, C.F., and Robinson, C.W., "Magnesium Studies in Calves. I. Tetany Produced by a Ration of Milk or Milk with Various Supplements," *The Journal of Biological Chemistry* 108 (1935): 35–44.

Golden, J.S., and Brams, W.A., "Mechanism of Toxic Effects from Combined Use of Calcium and Digitalis," *Annals of Internal Medicine* 11 (1938): 1084–1088.

Huffman, C.F., Robinson, C.S., Winter, O.B., et al., "The Effect of Low Calcium, High Magnesium Diets on Growth and Metabolism of Calves," *The Journal of Nutrition* 2 (1930): 471–483.

Kruse, H.D., Orent, E.R., and McCollum, E.V., "Studies on Magnesium Deficiency in Animals," *The Journal of Biological Chemistry* 96 (1932): 519–539.

Lazard, E.M., "An Analysis of 575 Cases of Eclamptic and Pre-Eclamptic Toxemias Treated by Intravenous Injections of Magnesium Sulphate," *American Journal of Obstetrics and Gynecology* 26 (1933): 647–656.

Lehr, D., "Experimental Cardiovascular

Necrosis: Mechanisms of Production and Prevention," *Proceedings of the Rudolf Virchow Medical Society in the City of New York 1962* 21 (1963): 157–166.

Lloyd, W.D.M., "Danger of Intravenous Calcium Therapy," *British Medical Journal* 1 (1928): 662–669.

Miller, J.R., and Van Dellen, T.R., "Electrocardiographic Changes Following the Intravenous Administration of Magnesium Sulfate: An Experimental Study in Dogs," *The Journal of Laboratory and Clinical Medicine* 23 (1938): 914–918.

Moore, L.B., Hallman, E.T., and Sholl, L.B., "Cardiovascular and Other Lesions in Calves Fed Diets Low in Magnesium," *Archives of Pathology* 26 (1938): 820–838.

Schmidt, C.L.A., and Greenberg, D.M., "Occurrence, Transport, and Regulation of Calcium, Magnesium, and Phosphorus in the Animal Organism," *Physiological Reviews* 15 (1935): 297–434.

Seekles, L., Sjollema, B., and Vanderkay, J.C., *Tijdschrift voor Diergeneeskunde* (Dutch) 57 (1930): 1229.

Sjollema, B., "Nutritional and Metabolic Disorders in Cattle," *Nutrition Abstracts and Reviews* 1 (1932): 621–632.

Sjollema, B., and Seekles, L., "[Low Blood Magnesium in Tetany]," *Klinische Wochenschrift* (German) 11 (1932): 989.

Szekely, P., "The Action of Magnesium on the Heart," *British Heart Journal* 8 (1946): 115–124.

Wilkins, W.E., and Cullen, G.E., "Electrolytes in Human Tissue. III. A Comparison of Normal Hearts with Hearts Showing Congestive Heart Failure," *The Journal of Clinical Investigation* 12 (1933): 1063–1074.

Zwillinger, L., "[Effect of Magnesium on the Heart]," *Klinische Wochenschrift* (German) 14 (1935): 1429–1433.

MITRAL VALVE PROLAPSE AND MAGNESIUM

Bobkowski, W., Siwinska, A., Zachwieja, J., et al., "[Electrolyte Abnormalities and Ventricular Arrhythmias in Children with Mitral Valve Prolapse]," *Polski Merkuriusz Lek* (Polish)11 (2001): 125–128.

Coghlan, H.C., and Natello, G., "Erythrocyte Magnesium in Symptomatic Patients with Primary Mitral Valve Prolapse: Relationship to Symptoms, Mitral Leaflet Thickness, Joint Hypermobility and Autonomic Regulation," *Magnesium and Trace Elements* 10 (1991): 205–214.

Cohen, L., Bitterman, H., Grenadier, E., et al., "Idiopathic Magnesium Deficiency in Mitral Valve Prolapse," *The American Journal of Cardiology* 57 (1986): 486–487.

Durlach, J., and Durlach, V., "Idiopathic Mitral Valve Prolapse and Magnesium: State of the Art," *Magnesium Bulletin* 8 (1986): 156–169.

Durlach, J., Lutfalla, G., Poenaru, S., et al., "Latent Tetany and Mitral Valve Prolapse Due to Chronic Primary Magnesium Deficit," *Magnesium Deficiency Physiopathology and Treatment Implications,* ed. M.J. Halpern and J. Durlach (Basel, Switzerland: S. Karger AG, 1985), 102–112.

Frances, Y., Collet, F., and Luccioni, R., "Long-Term Follow-Up of Mitral Valve Prolapse and Latent Tetany. Preliminary Data," *Magnesium* 5 (1986): 175–181.

Galland, L., "Latent Tetany—A Cross-Cultural Confirmation," *Magnesium* 4 (1985): 204.

Galland, L.D., Baker, S.M., and McLellan, R.K., "Magnesium Deficiency in the Pathogenesis of Mitral Valve Prolapse," *Magnesium* 5 (1986): 165–174.

Gerard, R., Luccioni, R., Gatau-Pelanchon, J., et al., "[Mitral Valve Prolapse and Spasmophilia in the Adult]," *Archives des Maladies du Coeur et des Vaisseaux* (French) 72 (1979): 715–720.

Lichodziejewska, B., Klos, J., Rezler, J., et al., "Clinical Symptoms of Mitral Valve Prolapse Are Related to Hypomagnesemia and Attenuated by Magnesium Supplementation," *The American Journal of Cardiology* 79 (1997): 768–772.

Martynov, A.I., Stepura, O.B., Shekhter, A.B., et al., "[New Approaches to the Treatment of Patients with Idiopathic Mitral Valve Prolapse]," *Terapevticheskii arkhiv* (Russian) 72 (2000): 67–70.

Simoes Fernandes, J., Pereira, T., Carvalho, J., et al., "Therapeutic Effect of a Magnesium Salt in Patients Suffering from Mitral Valvular Prolapse and Latent Tetany," *Magnesium* 4 (1985): 283–290.

Zeana, C.D., "Recent Data on Mitral

Valve Prolapse and Magnesium Deficit," *Magnes Research* 1 (1988): 203–211.

MAGNESIUM, COLLAGEN, AND ELASTIN

Arnold, R.M., and Fincham, H., "Cardiovascular and Pulmonary Calcification Apparently Associated with Dietary Imbalance in Jamaica," *Journal of Comparative Pathology* 60 (1950): 51–66.

Durlach, J., and Durlach, V., "Idiopathic Mitral Valve Prolapse and Magnesium: State of the Art," *Magnesium Bulletin* 8 (1986): 156–169.

Galland, L., "Magnesium Deficiency in Mitral Valve Prolapse," in *Magnesium Deficiency Physiopathology and Treatment Implications,* ed. M.J. Halpern and J. Durlach (Basel, Switzerland: S. Karger AG, 1985), 117–119.

Galland, L.D., Baker, S.M., and McLellan, R.K., "Magnesium Deficiency in the Pathogenesis of Mitral Valve Prolapse," *Magnesium* 5 (1986): 165–174.

Moore, L.B., Hallman, E.T., and Sholl, L.B., "Cardiovascular and Other Lesions in Calves Fed Diets Low in Magnesium," *Archives of Pathology* 26 (1938): 820–838.

Muller, W., Iffland, R., and Firsching, R., "Relationship between Magnesium and Elastic Fibres," *Magnesium Research* 6 (1993): 215–222.

Rayssiguier, Y., "Magnesium and Lipid Interrelationships in the Pathogenesis of Vascular Diseases," *Magnesium Bulletin* 3 (1981): 165–177.

Rayssiguier, Y., "Role of Magnesium and Potassium in the Pathogenesis of Arteriosclerosis," *Magnesium* 3 (1984): 226–238.

Rayssiguier, Y., Chevalier, F., Bonnet, M., et al., "Influence of Magnesium Deficiency on Liver Collagen after Carbon Tetrachloride or Ethanol Administration to Rats," *The Journal of Nutrition* 115 (1985): 1656–1662.

Shivakumar, K., and Kumar, B.P., "Magnesium Deficiency Enhances Oxidative Stress and Collagen Synthesis in Vivo in the Aorta of Rats," *The International Journal of Biochemistry and Cell Biology* 29 (1997): 1273–1278.

Vitale, J.J., Hellerstein, E.E., Nakamura, M., et al., "Effects of Magnesium-Deficient Diet upon Puppies," *Circulation Research* 9 (1961): 387–394.

Vitale, J.J., Velez, H., Guzman, C., et al., "Magnesium Deficiency in the Cebus Monkey," *Circulation Research* 12 (1963): 642–650.

MAGNESIUM STUDIES AND DIET: PROPHYLACTIC STUDIES IN FINLAND

Isomaa, B., Almgren, P., Tuomi, T., et al., "Cardiovascular Morbidity and Mortality Associated with the Metabolic Syndrome," *Diabetes Care* 24 (2001): 683–689.

Karppanen, H., Pennanen, R., and Passinen, L., "Minerals, Coronary Heart Disease and Sudden Coronary Death," *Advances in Cardiology* 25 (1978): 9–24.

Karppannen, H., Mervaala, E., and Pihkala, E., "Regulations and Health Policies in Finland," presentation on invitation of the French Ministry of Health, January 2002.

Lehto, S., Ronnemaa, T., Pyorala, K., et al., "Cardiovascular Risk Factors Clustering with Endogenous Hyperinsulinaemia Predict Death from Coronary Heart Disease in Patients with Type II Diabetes," *Diabetologia* 43 (2000): 148–155.

Lempiainen, P., Mykkanen, L., Pyorala, K., et al., "Insulin Resistance Syndrome Predicts Coronary Heart Disease Events in Elderly Nondiabetic Men," *Circulation* 100 (1999): 123–128.

Pekka, P., Pirjo, P., and Ulla, U., "Influencing Public Nutrition for Noncommunicable Disease Prevention: From Community Intervention to National Programme—Experiences from Finland," *Public Health Nutrition* 5 (2002): 245–251.

Pietinen, P., Lahti-Koski, M., Vartiainen, E., et al., "Nutrition and Cardiovascular Disease in Finland since the Early 1970s: A Success Story," *The Journal of Nutrition, Health and Aging* 5 (2001): 150–154.

Pietinen, P., Vartiainen, E., Seppanen, R., et al., "Changes in Diet in Finland from 1972 to 1992: Impact on Coronary Heart Disease Risk," *Preventive Medicine* 25 (1996): 243–250.

Appendix A
Magnesium Questionnaire

FRUITS AND VEGETABLES

Hu, F.B., Rimm, E.B., Stampfer, M.J., et al., "Prospective Study of Major Dietary Patterns and Risk of Coronary Heart Disease in Men," *The American Journal of Clinical Nutrition* 72 (2000): 912–921.

Liu, S., Manson, J.E., Lee, I.M., et al., "Fruit and Vegetable Intake and Risk of Cardiovascular Disease: The Women's Health Study," *The American Journal of Clinical Nutrition* 72 (2000): 922–928.

CALCIUM

Heath, H., III, and Callaway, C.W., "Calcium Tablets for Hypertension?" *Annals of Internal Medicine* 103 (1985): 946–947.

Heggtveit, H.A., "Myopathy in Experimental Magnesium Deficiency," *Annals of the New York Academy of Sciences* 162 (1969): 758–765.

Orwoll, E.S., "The Milk-Alkali Syndrome: Current Concepts," *Annals of Internal Medicine* 97 (1982): 242–248.

Roe, D.A., "Diet, Nutrition, and Drug Reactions," in *Modern Nutrition in Health and Disease,* ed. Maurice E. Shils, James A. Olson, and Moshe Shike (Philadelphia: Lippincott Williams & Wilkins, 1994), 1411–1412.

Seelig, M.S., "Epidemiologic Data on Magnesium Deficiency-Associated Cardiovascular Disease and Osteoporosis: Consideration of Risks of Current Recommendations for High Calcium Intake," in *Advances in Magnesium Research: Nutrition and Health: Proceedings of the Ninth International Symposium on Magnesium (Vichy, France),* ed. Yves Rayssiguier, André Mazur, and Jean Durlach (London, England: John Libbey & Company, 2001), 177–190.

Shils, Maurice E., "Magnesium," in *Modern Nutrition in Health and Disease,* ed. Maurice E. Shils, James A. Olson, and Moshe Shike (Philadelphia: Lippincott Williams & Wilkins, 1994), 173–175.

Standing Committee on the Scientific Evaluation of Dietary Reference Intakes, Food, and Nutrition Board, Institute of Medicine, "Dietary Reference Intakes for Calcium, Phosphorus, Magnesium, Vitamin D, and Fluoride" (Washington, D.C.: National Academy of Sciences, 1997).

Wacker, W.E., and Williams, R.J., "Magnesium-Calcium Balances and Steady States of Biological Systems," *Journal of Theoretical Biology* 20 (1968): 65–78.

Watson, R.C., Grossman, H., and Meyers, M.A., "Radiologic Findings in Nutritional Disturbances," *Modern Nutrition in Health and Disease,* ed. Maurice E. Shils, James A. Olson, and Moshe Shike (Philadelphia: Lippincott Williams & Wilkins, 1994), 869, 871.

Whang, R., Oliver, J., Welt, L.G., et al., "Renal Lesions and Disturbance of Renal Function in Rats with Magnesium Deficiency," *Annals of the New York Academy of Sciences* 162 (1969): 766–774.

Whang, R., and Whang, D.D., "Update: Mechanisms by which Magnesium Modulates Intracellular Potassium," *Journal of the American College of Nutrition* 9 (1990): 84–85.

PHOSPHORUS

Andress, D.L., Vannatta, J.B., and Whang, R., "Treatment of Refractory Hypophosphatemia," *Southern Medical Journal* 75 (1982): 766–767.

Bell, R.R., Draper, H.H., Tzeng, D.Y., et al., "Physiological Responses of Human Adults to Foods Containing Phosphate Additives," *The Journal of Nutrition* 107 (1977): 42–50.

Calvo, M.S., "Dietary Phosphorus, Calcium Metabolism, and Bone," *The Journal of Nutrition* 123 (1993): 1627–1633.

Calvo, M.S., "The Effects of High Phosphorus Intake on Calcium Homeostasism," *Advances in Nutritional Research* 9 (1994): 183–207.

Calvo, M.S., and Park, Y.K., "Changing Phosphorus Content of the U.S. Diet: Potential for Adverse Effects on Bone," *The Journal of Nutrition* 126 (1996): 1168S–1180S.

Chonan, O., Takahashi, R., Kado, S., et al., "Effects of Calcium Gluconate on the Utilization of Magnesium and the Nephrocalcinosis in Rats Fed Excess Dietary Phosphorus and Calcium," *Journal of Nutritional*

Science and Vitaminology 42 (1996): 313–323.

El-Shaarawy, M.I., and Reith, J.F., "On the Phosphate Problem," *Pahlavi Medical Journal* 7 (1976): 195–213.

Franz, K.B., "Influence of Phosphorus on Intestinal Absorption of Calcium and Magnesium," in *Proceedings of the Fifth International Magnesium Symposium, Magnesium in Health and Disease,* ed. Y. Itokawa and J. Durlach (London, England: John Libbey & Company: 1989), 71–78.

Franz, K.B., personal communication, 2002.

Sax, L., "The Institute of Medicine's 'Dietary Reference Intake' for Phosphorus: A Critical Perspective," *Journal of the American College of Nutrition* 20 (2001): 271–278.

Seelig, M.S., "Magnesium Deficiency with Phosphate and Vitamin D Excesses: Role in Pediatric Cardiovascular Disease?" *Cardiovascular Medicine* 3 (1978): 637–650.

Shaoul, R., Wolff, R., Seligmann, H., et al., "Symptoms of Hyperphosphatemia, Hypocalcemia, and Hypomagnesemia in an Adolescent after the Oral Administration of Sodium Phosphate in Preparation for a Colonoscopy," *Gastrointestinal Endoscopy* 53 (2001): 650–652.

Shils, Maurice E., "Magnesium," *Modern Nutrition in Health and Disease,* ed. Maurice E. Shils, James A. Olson, and Moshe Shike (Philadelphia: Lippincott Williams & Wilkins, 1994), 173–175.

Silverberg, S.J., Shane, E., Clemens, T.L., et al., "The Effect of Oral Phosphate Administration on Major Indices of Skeletal Metabolism in Normal Subjects," *Journal of Bone and Mineral Research* 1 (1986): 383–388.

Woodward, J.C., and Jee, W.S., "Effects of Dietary Calcium, Phosphorus, and Magnesium on Intranephronic Calculosis in Rats," *The Journal of Nutrition* 114 (1984): 2331–2338.

VITAMIN D

Seelig, M.S., "Vitamin D—Risk versus Benefit," *Journal of the American College of Nutrition* 2 (1983): 109–110.

Seelig, M.S., "Vitamin D and Cardiovascular, Renal, and Brain Damage in Infancy and Childhood," *Annals of the New York Academy of Sciences* 147 (1969): 539–582.

Shan, J., Resnick, L.M., Lewanczuk, R.Z., et al., "1,25-Dihydroxyvitamin D as a Cardiovascular Hormone. Effects on Calcium Current and Cytosolic Free Calcium in Vascular Smooth Muscle Cells," *American Journal of Hypertension* 6 (1993): 983–988.

Standing Committee on the Scientific Evaluation of Dietary Reference Intakes, Food and Nutrition Board, Institute of Medicine, "Dietary Reference Intakes for Calcium, Phosphorus, Magnesium, Vitamin D, and Fluoride" (Washington, D.C.: National Academy of Sciences, 1997).

Appendix B

COMMON FOODS CLASSIFIED BY MAGNESIUM CONTENT

Pennington, Jean A., *Bowes and Church's Food Values of Portions Commonly Used* (New York: Harper and Row, 1989).

Seelig, M.S., "The Requirement of Magnesium by the Normal Adult," *The American Journal of Clinical Nutrition* 14 (1964): 342–390.

Appendix E

PROBLEMS ASSOCIATED WITH LOW MAGNESIUM LEVELS

Baker, S.M., "Magnesium in Primary Care and Preventive Medicine: Clinical Correlation of Magnesium Loading Studies," *Magnesium and Trace Elements* 10 (1991): 251–262.

Flink, E.B., "Magnesium Deficiency in Human Subjects—A Personal Historical Perspective," *Journal of the American College of Nutrition* 4 (1985): 17–31.

Rude, R.K., and Singer, F.R., "Magnesium Deficiency and Excess," *Annual Review of Medicine* 32 (1981): 245–259.

Shils, Maurice E., "Section B: Magnesium," in *Modern Nutrition in Health and Disease,* ed. Robert Stanley Goodhart and Maurice E. Shils (Philadelphia: Lea & Febiger, 1973), 287–296.

Shils, Maurice E., "Magnesium," in *Mod-*

ern Nutrition in Health and Disease, ed. Maurice E. Shils, James A. Olson, and Moshe Shike (Philadephia: Lippincott Williams & Wilkins, 1994), 173–175.

Appendix F

Guidelines for Magnesium Injections

Burch, G.E., and Giles, T.D., "The Importance of Magnesium Deficiency in Cardiovascular Disease," *American Heart Journal* 94 (1977): 649–657.

Flink, E.B., "Magnesium Deficiency in Human Subjects—A Personal Historical Perspective," *Journal of the American College of Nutrition* 4 (1985): 17–31.

Index